Handbook of Experimental Pharmacology

Volume 188

Giovanna Lombardi • Yanira Riffo-Vasquez
Editors

Dendritic Cells

Contributors

L. Adorini, W. van den Ancker, G. Belz, A. Benlahrech, F. Belardelli, M. Buckland, A.E. Castell-Rodriguez, G. D'Agostino, S.S. Diebold, M. Ferrantini, R. Fischer, K.A. Gelderman, H. Hammad, W. Han, M. Herrera-Enriquez, I. Houtenbos, D. Kahler, A. KleinJan, C. van Kooten, B.N. Lambrecht, A. Lanzavecchia, C. Lapenta, G. Lombardi, A.A. van de Loosdrecht, A. Martín-Fontecha, F. Masson, A.L. Mellor, A. Mount, G.J. Ossenkoppele, T. Papagatsias, S. Patterson, G. Penna, T.R.D.J. Radstake, M.D. Ramirez-Gonzalez, F. Sallusto, S.M. Santini, L. Santodonato, A.S. Stax, T. Taner, A.W. Thomson, H.R. Turnquist, R.E.M. Toes, Y.R. Vasquez, L.G. Villanueva-Rodriguez, M.H. Wenink, T.M. Westers, A.M. Woltman

Springer

Editors
Giovanna Lombardi
Professor of Human Transplant Immunology
MRC Centre in Transplantation
Dep. of Nephrology and Transplantation, DIIID
King's College London
School of Medicine
Guy's Hospital
London, UK
giovanna.lombardi@kcl.ac.uk

Yanira Riffo Vasquez
Research Fellow
The Sackler Institute of Pulmonary Pharmacology
Pharmaceutical Science Division
5th Floor Hodgkin Building
School of Biomedical and Health Sciences
King's College London
London SE1 1UL
United Kingdom
yanira.vasquez@kcl.ac.uk

ISBN 978-3-540-71028-8 e-ISBN 978-3-540-71029-5

Handbook of Experimental Pharmacology ISSN 0171-2004

Library of Congress Control Number: 2008932233

Cover Design: WMXDesign GmbH, Heidelberg

Printed on acid-free paper

springer.com

Preface

The understanding of the role of dendritic cells (DCs) in immune responses has come a long way since Steinmann and colleagues described these cells in 1972. Extensive research during the intervening period has provided a good understanding of the complexity of the DC system and its pivotal role in immunity. It is also now clearer how different subsets of DCs interact and regulate each other and how DC populations affect the function of other cells of the immune system. The improved understanding of their role in immune response has led to the idea that modulation of DC functions by, for example, pharmacological agents could be used as a potential therapeutic approach in some pathological conditions. The actual applicability and therapeutic potential of all these approaches is yet to be fully demonstrated but nonetheless, animal models of human diseases are proving to be very helpful in the evaluation of manipulated DCs as a new treatment in diseases like cancer, autoimmunity or asthma.

DCs are integral to the initiation and regulation of immune response (Banchereau et al. 2000). The outcome of antigen presentation by DCs is determined by their maturation status, which can be induced by their interaction with danger signals. To recognise a wide array of pathogen-associated molecular patterns (PAMP), DCs express a number of pattern recognition receptors (PRR) such as Toll-like receptors (TLRs) and C-type lectin receptors (CLR) that recognise structural components of pathogens and discriminate between self and non-self molecules. The distribution of PRRs by DCs is variable and differs between DC subsets, as reviewed in this issue of Handbook of Experimental Pharmacology. Following an encounter with pathogens, DCs stop sampling the microenviroment and became dedicated antigen presenting cells. These mature DCs migrate to the secondary lymphoid organs and present antigen to lymphocytes. The trafficking of DCs, in particular from skin and blood, has been reviewed in this volume. Mature DCs have a potent capacity to stimulate T cells, while immature DCs fail to fully activate T cells and can induce T cell tolerance through anergy, deletion or induction of Tregs (Bonifaz et al. 2002; Hawiger et al. 2001). More specifically, different DC subsets appear to have distinct effects on T cell behaviour. DCs are in fact a very heterogenous population of cells. In mice there are at least six major subtypes of

DCs (reviewed by Pulendran et al. 2008). In the spleen and lymph nodes, DCs are characterised by the expression of CD11c and MHC class II. In the spleen there are three subsets: (1) $CD11c^{high}CD8\alpha^{+}CD11b^{-}DEC205^{+}$ ($CD8\alpha^{+}$ lymphoid DCs); (2) $CD11c^{high}CD8\alpha^{-}CD11b^{+}DEC205^{-}$ ($CD8\alpha^{-}$ myeloid DCs); (3) $CD11c^{int}CD8\alpha^{+/-}CD11b^{+}B220^{+}Gr\text{-}1^{+-}$ (pDCs). However there is another way in which splenic DCs have been classified, based on the expression of CD4 and CD8 surface markers (Dudziak et al. 2007; Masson et al. 2008). Using these two markers, three populations of DCs can be discerned in the spleen: $CD8\alpha^{+}CD4^{-}$ (CD8α DCs) $CD8\alpha^{-}CD4^{+}$, and $CD8\alpha^{-}CD4^{-}$ (the last two defined as non CD8α DCs). Furthermore, the $CD8\alpha^{+}CD4^{-}$ DCs express the CD205 molecule, while the $CD8\alpha^{-}CD4^{+}$ DCs express a high level of the C-type lectin inhibitory receptor-2 (DCIR2) which can be targeted by the antibody 33D1 (Dudziak et al. 2007). The percentages vary slightly, depending on the mouse strain. More recently, it has been shown that $CD4^{-}CD8\alpha^{+}$ and $CD4^{+}CD8\alpha^{-}$ DC stimulate $CD8^{+}$ and $CD4^{+}$ T cells respectively (Dudziak et al. 2007). These properties are related to differences in the MHC class I and MHC class II antigen presentation pathways (Dudziak et al. 2007). In the lymph nodes there are two additional subsets $CD11c^{high}CD8\alpha^{dull}DEC205^{high}Langerin^{+}$ (Langherans cell-derived DCs-LCDCs) and $CD11c^{high}CD8\alpha^{-}CD11b^{+}DEC205^{+}$ (Dermal DCs). The LCDCs and the Dermal DCs in the lymph nodes are derived from skin (reviewed in this volume). All these subsets of DCs have different locations in the secondary lymphoid organs. The $CD11c^{high}CD8\alpha^{+}$ DCs are localised in the T cell area while the $CD8\alpha^{-}$ DCs are localised in the marginal zones of the spleen and the subcapsular sinuses of the lymph nodes. The $CD8\alpha^{+}$ DC subset secrete IL-12 while the $CD8\alpha^{-}$ produce mostly IL-10. While in vivo data suggests that $CD8\alpha^{+}$ DC stimulation of T cells generally promotes Th1 and $CD8\alpha^{-}$ DCs mainly promote a Th2 response, in vitro stimulation has shown that this division can be overcome (Maldonado-Lopez and Moser 2001). In this issue the role in particular of the anti-viral immune responses of different DCs subsets will be discussed. Apart from the three subsets of DCs present in the skin (LCDCs, Dermal DCs and pDCs) that migrate to the lymph nodes following activation, four different subsets of DCs have been described in three main locations in the intestine (Peyer's patches, lamina propria, and mesenteric LNs). These four subsets are similar to the subsets identified in the spleen with an additional marker, CCR6, to subdivide the $CD11c^{bright}CD8\alpha^{-}CD11b^{+}$ DCs. Very recently an alternative classification of DC subsets has been used, based on the expression of chemokine receptor CX3CR1 and CD103, further confirming the unresolved issue of DC subsets in the mouse.

Plasmacytoid DCs are a specialised DC subset of distinct lineage from $CD11c^{high}$ DCs, and they produce type I IFNs in response to microbial infections. Immature pDCs are poor stimulators of naïve T cell activation, a consequence of their low expression levels of co-stimulatory molecules and intermediate MHC class II expression (Martin et al. 2002), (Asselin-Paturel et al. 2001). As applies to conventional $CD11c^{high}$ DCs, the maturation status of the pDC determines its stimulatory potential, and upon maturation, pDCs acquire the ability to prime T cell responses, albeit less than $CD11c^{high}$ DCs (Salio et al. 2004). Although pDCs have a key role in a number of immune-mediated diseases such as psoriasis and immunity to tumours and pathogens, pDCs have also the ability to down-regulate the immune response (Abe et al. 2005; Moseman et al. 2004; Ochando et al. 2006). Aspects of pDC migration and function are discussed in this book.

In humans there are two major DC subtypes described, classically defined as Myeloid and Lymphoid. Myeloid DCs are divided into steady state DCs, including Langherans cells and Interstitial DCs that continually sample the microenviroment, and inflammatory DCs that are generated in response to inflammation (Shortman and Naik 2007). The other prominent DC subtype in the human is the type-I IFN producing pDCs, that respond to viral infection (14). DCs can be generated in vitro from $CD14^{+}CD11c^{+}$ monocyte with Granulocyte/Macrophage Colony-Stimulating Factor (GM-CSF) and IL-4 (Sallusto and Lanzavecchia 1994). Alternatively it has been shown that the addition of type-I IFN or TGF-β and GM-CSF can result in DCs deficient in the adhesion molecule DC-SIGN that resembles Langherans cells (Relloso et al. 2002). Human Myeloid DCs can also be directly obtained ex vivo from the blood by using an antibody that recognises the Blood Dendritic Cell Antigen-2 ($BDCA\text{-}2^{+}$) marker. Plasmacytoid DCs can also be generated ex vivo from $BDCA\text{-}4^{+}$ precursor and cultured in the presence of IL-3 (Ito et al. 2007).

Altogether the overview of the DC subsets presented here further highlights the complexity of the DC system and raises important questions about the use of DCs in immunotherapy. The growing importance of DCs in the immune system is confirmed by the ever increasing number of published data found in the literature. We felt it timely to commission a contemporary review of the current understanding of DC function in health and disease and their potential manipulation for immunotherapy.

In the first part of this volume, the authors present a very comprehensive review of DCs as pivotal components of the immune system, as already mentioned. In the three initial chapters we will learn what is currently known about activation, migration, and function of DCs as antigen presenting cells and T-cell activators. These chapters lay the foundation for the second part of this volume, which describes the role of DCs in diseases. It is clear that DCs are important in many pathological conditions. However, it would have been very difficult to discuss all of them in one single volume. We have chosen some conditions where significant research has been done in the last few years and where DCs have been shown to be a potential therapeutic target (Rheumatoid Arthritis, Allergic Diseases and Drug Induced Adverse Reaction).

In the last part of the volume we take a closer look at the current status of the specific use of DCs as therapy. The first chapter discusses the intrinsic properties of a subpopulation of pDCs that express IDO following inflammatory conditions and their critical role as regulator of the immune response. The chapter finishes by reviewing the opportunity to manipulate IDO expression in DCs for immunotherapy. This review is followed by four chapters where the authors discuss the manipulation of DCs to induce tolerance in transplantation and autoimmunity, using various drugs (Aspirin, Rapamycin, Dexamethasone and Vitamin D Receptor Antagonists). The last three chapters review the general knowledge on the use of DCs to booster the immune responses in the treatment of viral infections, cancer and in particular, leukaemia. The first chapter focuses on the development of HIV vaccines based on recombinant adenoviruses (rAd). This review discusses the different types of rAd vectors and their effect in stimulating the DCs and the other cells of the immune system. This chapter is followed by a review of our knowledge of the role played by type I IFNs in the differentiation and activation of DCs towards the priming and expansion of protective antitumour responses. The chapter finishes by discussing how the type I IFNs could be exploited to develop strategies for an effective cancer immunotherapy. Finally, the last chapter discusses the use of DC vaccination to overcome the "intrinsic tolerant state" of patients with acute myloid leukaemia. The authors also mention the possibility of using an AML-derived cell line (MUTZ-3), equivalent to $CD34^{+}$DC precursor cells, for vaccination purpose.

Altogether, the genetic or pharmacological manipulations of DCs and their potential use in vaccination have raised expectation and hopes in many areas of research concerning the induction of tolerance in autoimmunity and transplantation and the stimulation of the immune responses in cancer and viral infections such as HIV. A great deal of data derived from animal models of human diseases have been published in the last few years from leading laboratories around the world, suggesting that this type of treatment is a real possibility in the very near future.

We hope that this book will give the reader a better understanding of the biology of DCs and why these cells are such important players in the battle against diseases.

We thank our contributors who, with great professionalism, have shared their knowledge and expertise with us.

London, United Kingdom

Giovanna Lombardi
Yanira Vasquez

References

Abe M, Colvin BL, Thomson AW (2005) Plasmacytoid dendritic cells: in vivo regulators of alloimmune reactivity? Transplant Proc 37: 4119–21

Asselin-Paturel C, Boonstra A, Dalod M, Durand I, Yessaad N, Dezutter-Dambuyant C, Vicari A, O'Garra A, Biron C, Briere F, Trinchieri G (2001) Mouse type I IFN-producing cells are immature APCs with plasmacytoid morphology. Nat Immunol 2: 1144–50

Banchereau J, Briere F, Caux C, Davoust J, Lebecque S, Liu YJ, Pulendran B, Palucka K (2000) Immunobiology of dendritic cells. Annu Rev Immunol 18: 767–811

Bonifaz L, Bonnyay D, Mahnke K, Rivera M, Nussenzweig MC, Steinman RM (2002) Efficient targeting of protein antigen to the dendritic cell receptor DEC-205 in the steady state leads to antigen presentation on major histocompatibility complex class I products and peripheral CD8 + T cell tolerance. J Exp Med 196: 1627–38

Dudziak D, Kamphorst AO, Heidkamp GF, Buchholz VR, Trumpfheller C, Yamazaki S, Cheong C, Liu K, Lee HW, Park CG, Steinman RM, Nussenzweig MC (2007) Differential antigen processing by dendritic cell subsets in vivo. Science 315: 107–11

Hawiger D, Inaba K, Dorsett Y, Guo M, Mahnke K, Rivera M, Ravetch JV, Steinman RM, Nussenzweig MC (2001) Dendritic cells induce peripheral T cell unresponsiveness under steady state conditions in vivo. J Exp Med 194: 769–79

Ito T, Yang M, Wang YH, Lande R, Gregorio J, Perng OA, Qin XF, Liu YJ, Gilliet M (2007) Plasmacytoid dendritic cells prime IL-10-producing T regulatory cells by inducible costimulator ligand. J Exp Med 204: 105–15

Maldonado-Lopez R, Moser M (2001) Dendritic cell subsets and the regulation of Th1/Th2 responses. Semin Immunol 13: 275–82

Martin P, Del Hoyo GM, Anjuere F, Arias CF, Vargas HH, Fernandez LA, Parrillas V, Ardavin C (2002) Characterization of a new subpopulation of mouse CD8alpha + B220 + dendritic cells endowed with type 1 interferon production capacity and tolerogenic potential. Blood 100: 383–90

Masson F, Mount AM, Wilson NS, Belz GT (2008) Dendritic cells: driving the differentiation programme of T cells in viral infections. Immunol Cell Biol 86: 333–42

Moseman EA, Liang X, Dawson AJ, Panoskaltsis-Mortari A, Krieg AM, Liu YJ, Blazar BR, Chen W (2004) Human plasmacytoid dendritic cells activated by CpG oligodeoxynucleotides induce the generation of CD4 + CD25 + regulatory T cells. J Immunol 173: 4433–42

Ochando JC, Homma C, Yang Y, Hidalgo A, Garin A, Tacke F, Angeli V, Li Y, Boros P, Ding Y, Jessberger R, Trinchieri G, Lira SA, Randolph GJ, Bromberg JS (2006) Alloantigen-presenting plasmacytoid dendritic cells mediate tolerance to vascularized grafts. Nat Immunol 7: 652–62

Pulendran B, Tang H, Denning TL (2008) Division of labor, plasticity, and crosstalk between dendritic cell subsets. Curr Opin Immunol 20: 61–7

Relloso M, Puig-Kroger A, Pello OM, Rodriguez-Fernandez JL, de la Rosa G, Longo N, Navarro J, Munoz-Fernandez MA, Sanchez-Mateos P, Corbi AL (2002) DC-SIGN (CD209) expression is IL-4 dependent and is negatively regulated by IFN, TGF-beta, and anti-inflammatory agents. J Immunol 168: 2634–43

Salio M, Palmowski MJ, Atzberger A, Hermans IF, Cerundolo V (2004) CpG-matured murine plasmacytoid dendritic cells are capable of in vivo priming of functional CD8 T cell responses to endogenous but not exogenous antigens. J Exp Med 199: 567–79

Sallusto F, Lanzavecchia A (1994) Efficient presentation of soluble antigen by cultured human dendritic cells is maintained by granulocyte/macrophage colony-stimulating factor plus interleukin 4 and downregulated by tumor necrosis factor alpha. J Exp Med 179: 1109–18

Shortman K, Naik SH (2007) Steady-state and inflammatory dendritic-cell development. Nat Rev Immunol 7: 19–30

Contents

Contributors

Luciano Adorini BioXell, Via Olgettina 58, 20132 Milano, Italy, luciano.adorini@bioxell.com

W. van den Ancker Department of Haematology, VU-Institute of Cancer and Immunology, VU University Medical Center, De Boelelaan 1117, 1081 HV, Amsterdam, The Netherlands

Gabrielle Belz Division of Immunology, The Walter and Eliza Hall Institute of Medical Research, Melbourne, Australia, belz@wehi.edu.au

Adel Benlahrech Department of Immunology, Imperial College, Chelsea and Westminster Hospital, London, UK

Filippo Berlardelli Section of Experimental Immunotherapy, Department of Cell Biology and Neurosciences, Istituto Superiore di Sanità, Viale Regina Elena, 299, 00161 Rome, Italy, belard@iss.it

Matthew Buckland Immunoregulation Laboratory, Department of Nephrology and Transplantation, 5th Floor Thomas Guy House, Guys Hospital Campus, Kings College London School of Medicine, Guys, Kings College and St Thomas Hospitals, London SE1 9RT, UK, matthew.buckland@kcl.ac.uk

Andres Eliu Castell-Rodriguez Department of Pharmacology and Tissue Cells Biology, School of Medicine, National Autonomous University of Mexico, Mexico

Giuseppina D'Agostino Section of Experimental Immunotherapy, Department of Cell Biology and Neurosciences, Istituto Superiore di Sanità, Viale Regina Elena, 299, 00161 Rome, Italy

Sandra S. Diebold Immunobiology Laboratory, Cancer Research UK, London Research Institute, London WC2A 3PX, UK, Sandra.diebold@kcl.ac.uk

Maria Ferrantini Section of Experimental Immunotherapy, Department of Cell Biology and Neurosciences, Istituto Superiore di Sanità, Viale Regina Elena, 299, 00161 Rome, Italy

Ryan Fischer Children's Hospital of Pittsburgh of the University of Pittsburgh Medical Center, Pittsburgh, PA 15213, USA

Kyra A. Gelderman Leiden University Medical Center, Department of Nephrology, C3P, Albinusdreef 2, P.O. Box 9600, NL-2300RC Leiden, The Netherlands

Hamida Hammad Department of Pulmonary Medicine, Erasmus M.C. Dr. Molerwaterplein 50, 3015 GE Rotterdam, The Netherlands

W. Han Department of Rheumatology, Radboud University Nijmegen Medical Centre, Nijmegen, The Netherlands

Miguel Herrera-Enriquez Department of Pharmacology and Tissue Cells Biology, School of Medicine, National Autonomous University of Mexico, Mexico

I. Houtenbos Department of Haematology, VU-Institute of Cancer and Immunology, VU University Medical Center, De Boelelaan 1117, 1081 HV, Amsterdam, The Netherlands

David Kahler Department of Medicine, Program in Molecular Immunology, Institute of Molecular Medicine and Genetics, Medical College of Georgia 1120, 15th Street, Augusta, GA 30912-2600, USA

Alex KleinJan Department of Pulmonary Medicine, Erasmus MC, Room Ee2257b, Dr. Molewaterplein 50, 3015 GE. Rotterdam, The Netherlands, a.kleinjan@erasmusmc.nl

Cees van Kooten Leiden University Medical Center, Department of Nephrology, C3P, Albinusdreef 2, P.O. Box 9600, NL-2300RC Leiden, The Netherlands, C.van_Kooten@lumc.nl

Bart N. Lambrecht Department of Pulmonary Medicine, Erasmus M.C. Dr. Molerwaterplein 50, 3015 GE. Rotterdam, The Netherlands, bart.lambrecht@ugent.be

Antonio Lanzavecchia King's College London and Guy's and St Thomas' Hospital, Department of Nephrology and Transplantation, GKT School of Medicine, King's College London, UK

Caterina Lapenta Section of Experimental Immunotherapy, Department of Cell Biology and Neurosciences, Istituto Superiore di Sanità, Viale Regina Elena, 299, 00161 Rome, Italy

Giovanna Lombardi Immunoregulation Laboratory, Department of Nephrology and Transplantation, GKT School of Medicine, King's College London, 5th Floor Thomas Guy House, London SE1 9RT, UK, giovanna.lombardi@kcl.ac.uk

Alfonso Martín-Fontecha King's College London and Guy's and St Thomas' Hospital, Department of Nephrology and Transplantation, GKT School of Medicine, King's College London, UK, alfonso.martin-fontecha@kcl.ac.uk

Frederick Masson Division of Immunology, The Walter and Eliza Hall Institute of Medical Research, Melbourne, Australia

Andrew L. Mellor Department of Medicine, Program in Molecular Immunology, Institute of Molecular Medicine and Genetics, Medical College of Georgia 1120, 15th Street, Augusta, GA 30912-2600, USA, amellor@mcg.edu

Adele Mount Division of Immunology, The Walter and Eliza Hall Institute of Medical Research, Melbourne, Australia

G.J. Ossenkoppele Department of Haematology, VU-Institute of Cancer and Immunology, VU University Medical Center, De Boelelaan 1117, 1081 HV, Amsterdam, The Netherlands

Timos Papagatsias Department of Immunology, Imperial College London, Chelsea and Westminster Hospital Campus, London, SW10 9NH

Steven Patterson Department of Immunology, Imperial College, Chelsea and Westminster Hospital, London, UK, s.patterson@imperial.ac.uk

Giuseppe Penna BioXell, Via Olgettina 58, 20132 Milano, Italy

T.R.D.J. Radstake Department of Rheumatology, Radboud University Nijmegen Medical Centre, Nijmegen, The Netherlands, t.radstake@reuma.umcn.nl

Maria Dolores Ramirez-Gonzalez Department of Pharmacology and Tissue Cells Biology, School of Medicine, National Autonomous University of Mexico, Mexico, mdrg@servidor.unam.mx

Federica Sallusto King's College London and Guy's and St Thomas' Hospital, Department of Nephrology and Transplantation, GKT School of Medicine, King's College London, UK

Stefano Maria Santini Section of Experimental Immunotherapy, Department of Cell Biology and Neurosciences, Istituto Superiore di Sanità, Viale Regina Elena, 299, 00161 Rome, Italy, stefano.santini@iss.it

Laura Santodonato Section of Experimental Immunotherapy, Department of Cell Biology and Neurosciences, Istituto Superiore di Sanità, Viale Regina Elena, 299, 00161 Rome, Italy

Annelein S. Stax Leiden University Medical Center, Department of Nephrology, C3P, Albinusdreef 2, P.O. Box 9600, NL-2300RC Leiden, The Netherlands

Timuçin Taner Department of Surgery, Mayo Clinic, Rochester, MN 55905, USA

Angus W. Thomson University of Pittsburgh, W1544 Biomedical Science Tower, 200 Lothrop Street, Pittsburgh, PA 15213, USA, thomsonaw@upmc.edu

R.E.M. Toes Department of Rheumatology, Radboud University Nijmegen Medical Centre, Nijmegen, The Netherlands

Heth R. Turnquist Thomas E. Starzl Transplantation Institute, University of Pittsburgh School of Medicine, Pittsburgh, PA 15213, USA

Department of Surgery, University of Pittsburgh School of Medicine, Pittsburgh, PA 15213, USA

A.A. van de Loosdrecht Department of Haematology, VU-Institute of Cancer and Immunology, VU University Medical Center, De Boelelaan 1117, 1081 HV, Amsterdam, The Netherlands, A.vandeloosdrecht@vumc.nl

Yanira Riffo Vasquez The Sackler Institute of Pulmonary Pharmacology, Division of Pharmacology and Therapeutics, GKT School of Biomedical Sciences, King's College London, 5th floor Hodgkin Building, London, SE1 1UL, UK, yanira.vasquez@kcl.ac.uk

Luisa Geraldine Villanueva-Rodriguez Department of Pharmacology and Tissue Cells Biology, School of Medicine, National Autonomous University of Mexico, Mexico

M.H. Wenink Department of Rheumatology, Radboud University Nijmegen Medical Centre, Nijmegen, The Netherlands

T.M. Westers Department of Haematology, VU-Institute of Cancer and Immunology, VU University Medical Center, De Boelelaan 1117, 1081 HV, Amsterdam, The Netherlands

Andrea M. Woltman Leiden University Medical Center, Department of Nephrology, C3P, Albinusdreef 2, P.O. Box 9600, NL-2300RC Leiden, The Netherlands

Part I
Biology of Dendritic Cells

Activation of Dendritic Cells by Toll-Like Receptors and C-Type Lectins

Sandra S. Diebold

Contents

Abstract As sentinels of the immune system, dendritic cells (DC) scan their environment for the presence of pathogens. DC sense pathogens either directly or indirectly via endogenous factors such as cytokines and chemokines, which are produced by other cell types in response to infection. Although indirect signals in form of endogenous factors alert DC, direct activation of DC by pathogen-associated molecular patterns (PAMP) is crucial for the induction of primary T cell responses. Direct recognition of PAMP is mediated by pattern recognition receptors (PRR) such as Toll-like receptors (TLR) and C-type lectin receptors (CLR). The molecular patterns that are recognized by these receptors are indispensable for the life cycle of the pathogens, and their structure or cellular localization is different from that of the host. TLR detect cell-wall components of bacteria, fungi, and protozoa at the cell

S.S. Diebold
Peter Gorer Department of Immunobiology, King's College London, Guy's Hospital, London SE1 9RT, UK
Sandra.diebold@kcl.ac.uk

G. Lombardi, Y. Riffo-Vasquez (eds.), *Dendritic Cells,* Handbook of Experimental Pharmacology 188,

surface or bacterial and viral nucleic acid structures in a specialized endosomal compartment, while CLR that are involved in pattern recognition bind to carbohydrate structures associated with pathogens.

Keywords: Adjuvant · C-type lectins · Dendritic cells · Innate immunity · Pathogen-associated molecular patterns · Pattern recognition receptors · Toll-like receptors

1 Introduction

DC form the link between the innate and the adaptive immune system. Immature DC reside in peripheral tissues where they scan the environment for signs of infection. Upon detection of pathogens, DC become activated and migrate to the draining lymph nodes where they play a crucial role in instructing T cells. The activation of DC is a complex process, which involves a number of different stages. Immediately after the encounter of PAMP in the periphery, DC transiently increase their endocytic activity to allow for the uptake of pathogen-associated exogenous material, and subsequently cease endocytosis (West et al. 2004). As a consequence of activation, DC raise the expression of costimulatory molecules such as CD40 and CD86 and also the levels of major histocompatibility complex (MHC) class II at the cell surface (Lanzavecchia and Sallusto 2001; Mellman and Steinman 2001). While the majority of MHC class II molecules in immature DC is recycled from the cell surface and is present intracellularly, recycling of MHC class II molecules stops after DC activation and the material taken up by DC shortly after activation is processed and presented efficiently on MHC class II at the cell surface (Inaba et al. 2000; Pierre et al. 1997). The activation of DC in the periphery also induces the expression of chemokine receptors such as CCR7 (Sallusto et al. 1999). This enables activated DC to migrate to the draining lymph nodes after having sampled the infected environment in the periphery.

Activation of DC via direct encounter with pathogen-associated material is signified by the induction of cytokines. While up-regulation of maturation markers such as co-stimulatory molecules and MHC class II at the cell surface can be a consequence of indirect DC activation by cytokines such as type I interferon (IFN-I) and tumour necrosis factor alpha (TNFα) that are produced by other cell types in an inflammatory environment, while the induction of cytokines by DC is a marker for direct activation via stimulation of PRR. The functional consequences of direct vs. indirect DC activation are different and only directly activated DC have the capacity to prime naïve T cells and to induce their differentiation into effector T cells (Sporri and Reise Sousa 2005). This has crucial implications for vaccine design i.e., to allow for the priming of naïve T cells, vaccines should employ ligands that trigger direct DC activation via PRR.

Thus, direct activation of DC plays a critical role in the induction of primary T cell responses, and DC express a variety of PRR, which mediate DC activation in response to infection. The presence of PRR on professional antigen-presenting cells (APC) such as DC and the functional consequences of their activation by PAMP were postulated by Charles Janeway (1989). The first PRR that were subsequently identified belonged to the TLR family, which now comprises the best-characterized family of PRR (Uematsu and Akira 2006). TLR are germline-encoded receptors of the innate immune system that recognize general molecular structures shared between entire classes of pathogens, which are indispensable for the life cycle of these pathogens. In addition, the PAMP are either structurally different from the patterns found in the host or their cellular localization is unusual for eukaryotic cells. Pathogens such as bacteria, fungi, and protozoa are largely extracellular and feature characteristic cell wall components in the form of glycolipid and peptidoglycan structures that are fundamentally different from the host and therefore serve as suitable TLR ligands. Viruses, in contrast, are intracellular pathogens that hijack the host metabolism for replication and thus do not create 'foreign' glycolipid and peptidoglycan structures. For detection of virus infections, the immune system has evolved TLR with the ability to sense the genetic material and replication intermediates of viruses in specialized endosomal compartments.

But TLR are not the only PRR that can sense PAMP and lead to direct activation of DC in response to infection. C-type lectin receptors (CLR) are a diverse family of receptors with the ability to bind to carbohydrate moieties (Zelensky and Gready 2005). The physiological functions of CLR vary widely with some family members mediating adhesion between different cell types, while others specific for pathogen-derived carbohydrate structures play a role in pattern recognition. Yet even among the CLR recognizing pathogen-specific carbohydrates, the functional consequences of ligand recognition differ with some receptors serving as scavenger receptors while others act as genuine PRR. The role of CRL in pattern recognition in general and in the activation of DC, in particular, is only now emerging and awaits further investigation.

TLR and CLR both represent PRR families, which are expressed by specialized cell types such as DC playing a crucial role in their function as APC during infections. However, there are other ubiquitously expressed cytoplasmic PRR, which can induce direct activation of DC and may play crucial roles in the induction of immune responses to particular pathogens (Meylan et al. 2006). These cytoplasmic PRR include helicases such as retinoic acid inducible gene I (RIG-I) and melanoma differentiation factor-5 (MDA5) sensing cytoplasmic viral RNA species, and DNA-dependent activator of IFN-regulatory factors (DAI) detecting cytoplasmic viral DNA. In addition to these nucleic acid-sensing PRR, there are a variety of cytoplasmic PRR that recognize bacterial components. However, the role of these cytoplasmic PRR in the activation of DC in response to infection is poorly defined.

The cytoplasmic PRR are expressed ubiquitously, while TLR and CLR are differentially expressed on different DC subsets. These different classes of PRR play distinct roles in the activation of DC. Important aspects of pattern recognition that influence the activation of the immune system in response to particular pathogens are the differential expression patterns of particular PRR, the functional specialization of different DC subsets, and the accessibility of particular pathogen-derived ligands for different PRR.

2 Families of PRR

2.1 Toll-Like Receptors

The TLR family is the best-characterized family of PRR. So far 10 family members have been described in humans and mice (Chuang and Ulevitch 2001; Chuang and Ulevitch 2000; Du et al. 2000; Medzhitov et al. 1997; Rock et al. 1998; Takeuchi et al. 1999b). TLR were named after the Drosophila transmembrane receptor Toll, which is crucial for the establishment of the dorso-ventral organisation in the developing drosophila embryo and also plays a role in innate immunity in the adult fly (Belvin and Anderson 1996; Hashimoto et al. 1988). The endogenous ligand Spätzle binds to Toll upon cleavage by a serine protease, which is activated in response to infection. In this regard, Toll differs from the mammalian TLR, which recognise PAMP directly. Upon binding of cleaved Spätzle, Toll is activated and leads to the expression of the antifungal peptide drosomycin (Levashina et al. 1999). Flies carrying a mutation in the Toll pathway are highly susceptible to fungal and gram-positive bacterial infections confirming that Toll is involved in the induction of innate immune responses in Drosophila (Lemaitre et al. 1996; Rutschmann et al. 2002).

TLR and Toll share a highly conserved cytoplasmic domain, which is crucial for mediating immune activation upon ligand binding (Belvin and Anderson 1996). This so called Toll/interleukin-1 (IL-1) receptor (TIR) domain is also found in the mammalian IL-1/IL-18 receptor. Upon ligand binding, the TIR domain recruits TIR domain-containing adaptor molecules such as myeloid differentiation factor 88 (MyD88), which like the TLR themselves are highly conserved between species (Horng and Medzhitov 2001; Tauszig-Delamasure et al. 2002). The extracellular domain of TLR is characterized by a leucin-rich repeat (LRR) domain, which mediates ligand binding.

Mammalian TLR can be divided into two subfamilies distinguished by their cellular localization and by the type of ligands they recognise. The first subfamily comprises TLR1, TLR2, TLR4–6, TLR10 in humans and TLR11 in mice. These TLR are expressed at the cell surface where they directly encounter their ligands. The other subfamily of TLR, which includes TLR3 and TLR7–9, is localized in a specialized endosomal compartment where they detect the presence of viral and bacterial nucleic acids (Fig. 1).

2.1.1 Detection of Pathogen-Associated Cell Wall Components at the Cell Surface

The TLR that sample the environment at the cell surface are specialized in the recognition of bacterial, fungal, and protozoan PAMP that are directly accessible on the surface of the organisms. TLR4 recognizes bacterial lipopolysaccharide (LPS), a cell wall component of gram-negative bacteria, whereas TLR2 senses the presence

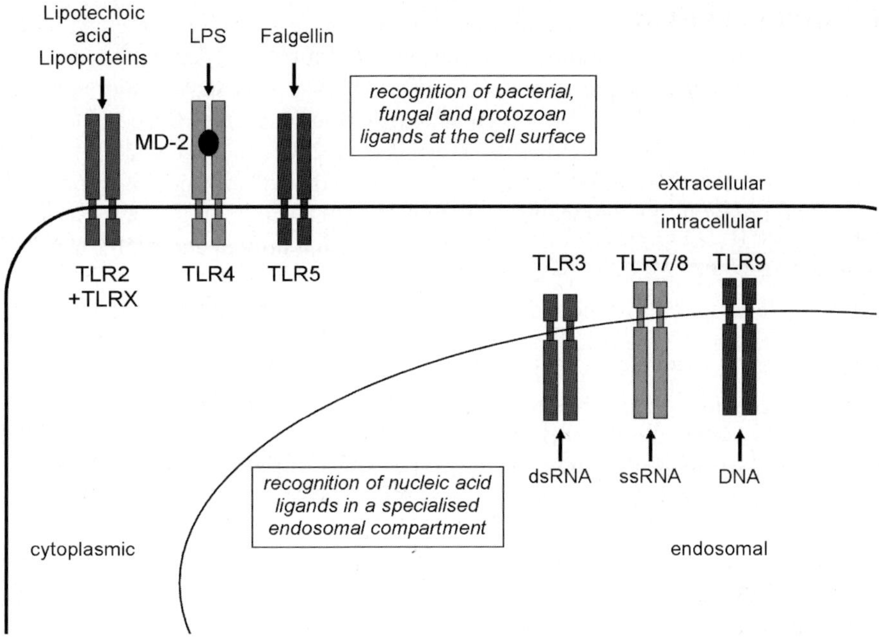

Fig. 1 The Toll-like receptor (TLR) family can be divided into two subfamilies: the TLR at the cell surface primarily detect bacterial, fungal and protozoan cell wall components while the intracellular TLR recognize nucleic acid ligands in a specialized endosomal compartment

of gram-positive and fungal cell wall components such as lipotechoic acid and peptidoglycans (Takeuchi et al. 1999a). TLR2 also forms heterodimers with TLR1 and TLR6, which recognize triacyl and diacyl lipopetides, respectively (Alexopoulou et al. 2002; Takeuchi et al. 2001; Takeuchi et al. 2002). Furthermore, TLR1 and TLR2 were shown to have the ability to heterodimerize with TLR10 (Hasan et al. 2005). Whether heterodimers between TLR10 and other TLRs are formed in vivo and which ligands may be recognized by such heterodimeric TLR is, however, unclear. TLR5 recognizes the bacterial protein flagellin (Hayashi et al. 2001), which is crucial for the motility of certain bacteria, while TLR11 senses uropathogenic bacteria as well as a protozoan profillin-like molecule (Yarovinsky et al. 2005; Zhang et al. 2004). The molecular signatures recognized by these TLR at the cell surface are fundamentally different from the peptidoglycan, glycolipid, and lipoprotein patterns found in the host, and, therefore, allow for discrimination between self and foreign structures by the innate immune system as was originally postulated by the pattern recognition hypothesis (Janeway 1989). The molecular structures of bacteria, fungi, and protozoa that are recognized by TLR are highly conserved and, therefore, enable the innate immune system to use a limited set of PRR for the detection of a wide range of pathogens.

While these TLR are expressed at the cell surface, they, nevertheless, are likely to be recruited to endosomal compartments once pathogens expressing the respective ligands have been taken up by phagocytosis, as was shown for TLR2 and TLR4

(Underhill et al. 1999). Yet, the activation of cells in response to TLR2 and TLR4 ligands is unaffected by inhibitors of endosomal maturation (Ahmad-Nejad et al. 2002; Heil et al. 2003; Lee et al. 2003). For TLR4 it was shown that signaling requires the presence of CD14, which acts as a binding partner for complexes of LPS and LPS-binding protein (da Silva Correia et al. 2001; Jiang et al. 2000). MD-2 is another accessory protein that amplifies TLR4-mediated activation in response to LPS when bound to the extracellular portion of LPS (Akashi et al. 2000; Shimazu et al. 1999). Accessory molecules such as LPS-binding protein and MD-2 have not been identified for any other TLR.

The majority of PAMP recognized by TLR at the cell surface are microbial signatures of bacterial, fungal, and protozoan infections, yet, there are also a few structural proteins of viral origin with the ability to trigger this TLR subfamily. TLR4 recognizes the fusion protein of respiratory syncytial virus and the envelope protein of mouse mammary tumour virus (Kurt-Jones et al. 2000; Rassa et al. 2002).Similarly, TLR2 is involved in the detection of a variety of viruses including herpes simplex virus 1 (HSV-1), measles virus, and human cytomegalovirus (Bieback et al. 2002; Compton et al. 2003; Kurt-Jones et al. 2004). The recognition of these viral structures is rather specific for particular viruses and does not match completely with the concept of PRR, which are supposed to recognize structures conserved among whole classes of pathogens. Therefore, it is unclear, whether the TLR have evolved to recognize these viral structures or whether the viral proteins have evolved to trigger and maybe modulate TLR-mediated immune activation.

2.1.2 Detection of Pathogen-Associated Nucleic Acid Structures in a Specialized Endosomal Compartment

In contrast to the TLR that sense mainly components of extracellular pathogens at the cell surface, the other TLR family members sample the content of a specialized endosomal compartment for the presence of PAMP in form of different classes of viral nucleic acids. TLR3 recognizes double-stranded RNA (dsRNA), while TLR7 and TLR8 are sensors for viral single-stranded RNA (ssRNA), and TLR9 not only detects viral but also bacterial and protozoan DNA (Alexopoulou et al. 2001; Coban et al. 2005; Diebold et al. 2004; Heil et al. 2004; Hemmi et al. 2000; Lund et al. 2003; 2004). The detection of these particular TLR ligands in a specialized endosomal compartment serves two distinct purposes. First, viral nucleic acids are either present inside virus particles or are associated with infected cells. In both cases, the nucleic acids are not directly accessible for recognition by TLR at the cell surface. Uptake of virus particles and material from infected cells is, therefore, a prerequisite for ligand recognition. Partial degradation of the virus particles and the cellular material is necessary to allow for the binding of nucleic acid ligands to the endosomal TLR. Second, restricting ligand recognition to a specialized endosomal compartment allows cells of the innate immune system to detect foreign nucleic acids of pathogens and those associated with infected cells, while averting immune activation in response to endogenous nucleic acids. Self-DNA and

RNA from healthy cells do not gain access to intracellular TLR under physiological conditions and nucleic acids released from necrotic cells are quickly degraded by extracellular nucleases before they can reach the TLR-sensing endosomal compartment (Barton et al. 2006). However, in case of noninfected apoptotic cells, it is less clear how detection of endogenous nucleic acids is prevented.

It is thought that differences in the modification of nucleic acids between eukaryotic cells and microbes such as bacteria and viruses enable the intracellular TLR to discriminate between self and foreign nucleic acid structures. For recognition of bacterial DNA by TLR9, it was argued that the receptor favors the recognition of unmethylated CpG-rich sequences that are abundant in bacterial, but sparse in mammalian DNA (Hemmi et al. 2000; Krieg et al. 1995). Similarly, introduction of methylated nucleosides into synthetic RNA ligands abrogates their TLR7 stimulatory capacity (Kariko et al. 2005). Yet, while those modifications affect ligand recognition, the ability of the intracellular TLR to discriminate between self and foreign nucleic acid ligands is not absolute (Sioud 2006). When introduced into the endosomal compartment in which recognition takes place, mammlian mRNA triggers TLR3 and TLR7-mediated DC activation (Diebold et al. 2006; Kariko et al. 2004). Likewise, mammalian DNA triggers TLR9-mediated immune activation when applied in the form of complexes with cationic lipids that mediate endosomal delivery or in the form of immunocomplexes with nucleic acid-binding antibodies (Boule et al. 2004; Yasuda et al. 2005). Furthermore, the expression of chimeric TLR9 at the cell surface enables recognition of DNA from apoptotic cells (Barton et al. 2006). This indicates that access to the endosomal compartment in which TLR9 recognition takes place is the limiting factor preventing responses to self-DNA rather than the ability of the PRR to discriminate between foreign and self. This is further supported by several studies demonstrating a role for TLR7 and TLR9-mediated immune activation in response to immune complexes containing self nucleic acids in patients with systemic lupus erythematosus (SLE) (Barrat et al. 2005; Boule et al. 2004; Lau et al. 2005; Leadbetter et al. 2002).

2.1.3 Functional Consequences of TLR Stimulation on DC

Upon detection of any of these PAMP via TLR, DC undergo activation, which involves the up-regulation of maturation markers such as the costimulatory molecules CD80, CD86, CD40, and increased presentation of MHC class II molecules at the cell surface. In addition, DC respond with the induction of cytokines. The qualitative and quantitative composition of the cytokine pattern induced in response to TLR stimulation depends on the receptors that are triggered, the ligands that are recognized, and the cell types that are activated (Reise Sousa 2004).

Differences in the TIR-domain-containing adaptors used for downstream signaling by TLR have a crucial influence on the cytokine patterns induced in response to ligand recognition (Fig. 2). All TLR share the adaptor molecule MyD88 except for TLR3, which exclusively signals via the TIR domain-containing adaptor inducing IFNβ (TRIF) (O'Neill and Bowie 2007). While the TIR domain of MyD88 is

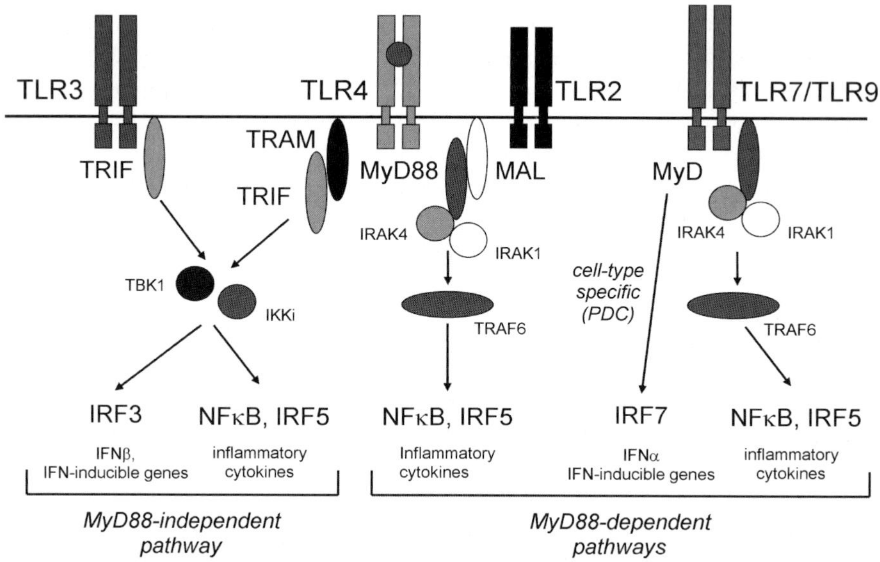

Fig. 2 Signaling pathways mediating Toll-like receptor induced activation

recruited directly to the cytoplasmic TIR domain of most TLR, TLR2 and TLR4 require the MyD88-adaptor-like adaptor (MAL), also called TIR-domain-containing adaptor protein (TIRAP), as a bridge for recruitment of MyD88 (Fitzgerald et al. 2001; Horng et al. 2002; Horng et al. 2001; Kagan and Medzhitov 2006; Yamamoto et al. 2002). In addition to these two TIR-containing adaptor molecules, TLR4 also signals via TRIF and the TRIF-related adaptor molecule (TRAM) (Fitzgerald et al. 2003; Oshiumi et al. 2003; Yamamoto et al. 2003). These differences in adaptor molecule usage between the TLR leads to activation of various transcription factors in the downstream signaling cascade. Triggering of TLR2 homo and heterodimers and TLR5 lead exclusively to NF-κB activation, whereas TLR4 additionally induces interferon regulatory factor 3 (IRF3) in a TRIF/TRAM-dependent manner (Fitzgerald et al. 2003). While IRF3 is crucial for the induction of interferon-β (IFNβ) in response to TLR4, NF-κB-mediated immune activation leads to the rapid induction of pro-inflammatory cytokines such as IL-6 and TNFα. IRF5 was shown to play a crucial role in the induction of proinflammatory cytokines and IFN-I in response to TLR activation in general (Takaoka et al. 2005).

2.2 C-Type Lectin Receptors

In addition to TLR, other PRR have been identified on DC, which belong to the CLR family. CLR, also called C-type lectins, are a diverse family of receptors containing one or more C-type lectin domains. Originally, the C-type lectin domain was identified as a carbohydrate-binding structure, but the structural motif formed by the domain does not mediate interaction with carbohydrates for all CLR. Similarly, some CLR bind carbohydrates in a Ca^{2+}-dependent manner, while for others ligand interaction is Ca^{2+}-independent. CLR are classified into groups according to their domain structure. The different groups vary widely in ligand recognition and function and only a few act as innate PRR mediating the recognition of PAMP by DC (Robinson et al. 2006). A full overview of C-type lectin domain-containing proteins can be found in the review by Zelensky and Gready (Zelensky and Gready 2005).

2.2.1 CLR Involved in Host Defense

The carbohydrate structures of bacteria and fungi are distinct from those generated by mammalian cells. They represent conserved PAMP that can be used by the innate immune system to distinguish foreign from self. Yet not all CLR exclusively recognize pathogen-associated carbohydrate structures. Selectins represent type I transmembrane proteins with a C-type lectin domain that recognizes endogenous carbohydrate structures and mediate adhesion between cells. The transient cellular interactions between selectins on leukocytes and epithelial cells play a role in leukocyte extravasation (Rossiter et al. 1997). Collectins, in contrast, form a group of soluble CLR, which bind to pathogen-associated carbohydrate structures and play a role in innate immunity by activating complement via the lectin pathway (Gupta and Surolia 2007). Despite their role in innate immunity, these CLR are not genuine PRR, as they do not mediate the activation of APC in response to PAMP recognition. Another group of CLR involved in innate immunity comprises NK cell receptors such as NKG2D. NKG2D recognizes endogenous molecules such as MICA and MICB, which are up-regulated in response to cellular stress, and is thus involved in innate immunity but not in pattern recognition (Eagle and Trowsdale 2007). CLR expressed by APC such as DC are dectin-1, DEC-205, and DC-SIGN, which all belong to a separate group of CLR (Zelensky and Gready 2005). Dectin-1 has been shown to act as PRR, whereas DEC-205 and DC-SIGN play a role in uptake, processing, and presentation of antigens from pathogens, but do not induce DC activation.

In mice, DEC-205 is expressed on a subset of DC specialized in cross-priming of cytotoxic T lymphocyte (CTL) responses. Binding of its carbohydrate ligand leads to receptor-mediated internalization into an endosomal compartment that allows for the presentation of antigen by DC (Jiang et al. 1995; Mahnke et al. 2000). The ligand for DEC-205 has not been identified, yet it was shown that DEC-205 participates in the clearance of apoptotic thymocytes by thymic DC suggesting that the receptor recognizes endogenous rather than foreign carbohydrate structures (Small and Kraal 2003). In addition, ligand-receptor interaction does not lead to DC activation further indicating that DEC-205 does not serve as a PRR. Nevertheless, DEC-205 is used as a target receptor for cell type-specific delivery of antigens to DC using antibody–antigen conjugates. Since ligand binding to DEC-205 does not induce immune activation, injection of antigen bound to DEC-205 specific antibody leads to tolerance induction (Bonifaz et al. 2002; Hawiger et al. 2001). For the induction of antigen-specific immune activation, the simultaneous application of an adjuvant in addition to the DEC-205-targeting complex is necessary (Bonifaz et al. 2004; Hawiger et al. 2001). Thus, DEC-205 represents a versatile tool for immunotherapy that can be used to vaccinate against particular antigens, but is equally suitable for the induction of tolerance.

The situation for the DC-specific CLR DC-SIGN is more complicated. DC-SIGN binds to endogenous carbohydrate structures, but also recognizes and interacts with structures on viruses, bacteria, and protozoa (Koppel et al. 2005). Therefore, its role in innate immunity is less clear. DC-SIGN recognizes endogenous ligands such as ICAM-2 and ICAM-3 and serves as an adhesion receptor mediating cellular interactions between DC and T cells and epithelial cells (Geijtenbeek et al. 2000a; Geijtenbeek et al. 2000c). Yet, DC-SIGN also detects a wide range of viruses such as human immunodeficiency virus (HIV), human cytomegalovirus, Ebola virus, Dengue virus, and hepatitis C virus (Alvarez et al. 2002; Geijtenbeek et al. 2000b; Halary et al. 2002; Lozach et al. 2004; Tassaneetrithep et al. 2003). When looking at the functional consequences of viral interaction with DC-SIGN, it appears that the pathogens may have evolved strategies to escape antiviral immune responses by targeting DC-SIGN. HIV-1 for example enters into DEC-205^{+} DC at the mucosal site of entry, stays intact inside a nonlysosomal compartment, and travels with APC to the draining lymph node where the virus then infects CD4 T cells (Geijtenbeek et al. 2000b). Other viruses such as human cytomegalovirus, Ebola, and Dengue virus directly infect DC by interacting with DEC-205 (Alvarez et al. 2002; Halary et al. 2002; Tassaneetrithep et al. 2003). Further evidence of DC-SIGN being used by pathogens to their advantage comes from studies with *Mycobacteria tuberculosis*, which secretes cell wall components that trigger DC-SIGN and induce an inhibitory response leading to the suppression of immune activation via TLR (Geijtenbeek et al. 2003).

Despite its ability to interact with PAMP, DC-SIGN triggering alone is insufficient to induce the induction of cytokines by DC. However, it has been shown that DC-SIGN can modulate signaling by other receptors and increases the induction of IL-10 in response to TLR4 activation, while simultaneously blocking DC maturation (Caparros et al. 2006; Geijtenbeek et al. 2003). Taken together, there is little evidence that DC-SIGN acts as a PRR leading to direct activation of DC. Rather, the receptor seems to be an example of a CLR being exploited by pathogens to gain entry into DC and to alter DC functions for their own means.

2.2.2 CLR Involved in Pattern Recognition

In contrast to DEC-205 and DC-SIGN, dectin-1 has been shown to be involved in pattern recognition resulting in direct DC activation. It recognizes foreign carbohydrate structures in the form of fungal β 1,3-glucans (Brown 2006; Palma et al. 2006). Ligand binding to dectin-1 induces uptake of pathogenic material and triggers DC activation (Rogers et al. 2005). Similarly, the mannose receptor, which mediates uptake of ligands into an endosomal compartment of APC, has the ability to regulate APC function in response to ligand binding (Chieppa et al. 2003; Mahnke et al. 2000).

Upon ligand binding to dectin-1, its cytoplasmic hemITAM motif is phosphorylated by a src family kinase and Syk is recruited (Rogers et al. 2005; Underhill et al. 2005). Downstream of Syk, dectin-1-signaling is transmitted via the adaptor molecule CARD9, which leads to the activation of NFκB (Gross et al. 2006; Rogers et al. 2005; Underhill et al. 2005). Syk recruitment results in the induction of IL-2, IL-10, and IL-23, but little IL-12 (LeibundGut-Landmann et al. 2007; Rogers et al. 2005). When DC activated via dectin-1 interact with CD4 T cells, the functional outcome of this interaction is a T_H-17 response (LeibundGut-Landmann et al. 2007). The role of dectin-1 in antifungal host defense is still somewhat controversial. It is currently unclear whether it acts as a crucial PRR, which is required for controlling fungal infections with *Candida albicans* or whether it only plays a minor role in antifungal defense in comparison to TLR-mediated immune activation (Saijo et al. 2007; Taylor et al. 2007).

Thus some CLR are emerging as a new class of PRR involved in innate immunity. However, their role in innate immunity seems to be qualitatively and quantitatively different from the role of TLR. Although TLR are potent inducers of DC activation and consequently of DC function, the role of CLR in DC function seems less clear. The role of CLR that recognize foreign carbohydrate structure includes the uptake, processing, and presentation of pathogen-associated antigens and may also involve modulation of DC activation. Currently, it seems unlikely that CLR activation can replace TLR activation functionally in the context of host defense.

2.3 Cytoplasmic PRR

TLR and CLR represent PRR expressed on specialized cell types, which are involved in the initiation of an immune response against the invading pathogen. The activation of these receptors on DC, therefore, plays a crucial role in the complex coordination of immune responses and particularly in the initiation of adaptive immune responses. In addition to these PRR whose expression is restricted to a few specialized cells, there are receptors that are expressed ubiquitously and fulfil the characteristics of PRR. These receptors are intracellularly localized, recognize microbial structures, which are indicative of infection and lead to the activation of cells that sense the PAMP. Yet, their role in innate immunity is different from the role of PRR expressed by specialized cell types. The primary role of these receptors is to prevent the spread of the infection locally in the tissue especially in the context of viral infections (Pichlmair and Reise Sousa 2007).

Ubiquitously expressed cytoplasmic PRR can be divided into two groups, the NOD-like receptors (NLR) and the RIG-I-like receptors (RLR), which are specialized in the detection of bacterial and viral PAMP, respectively (Meylan et al. 2006). The NLR senses cytoplasmic microbial products such as specific bacterial peptidoglycans via their LRR domains (Kanneganti et al. 2007). However, the mechanism by which bacterial molecules enter the cytosol for recognition by NLR remains unclear. Furthermore, their exact role in host defence is, to date, poorly defined.

Upon detection of viral PAMP by cytoplasmic PRR specialized in viral recognition, a cellular programme is initiated, which leads to IFN-I production, RNA degradation, and induction of apoptosis (Samuel 2001). The PRR involved in these responses include the protein kinase R (PKR) and 2′–5′-oligoadenylate synthetase (OAS), which are both activated upon binding of viral dsRNA in the cytoplasm of infected cells. Further cytoplasmic PRR were identified more recently, which include the helicases RIG-I and MDA5 and the DNA-sensing molecule DAI (Takaoka et al. 2007; Yoneyama et al. 2005; Yoneyama et al. 2004). As for the nucleic acid-sensing TLR, the cytoplasmic RLR comprise receptors specific for the detection of ssRNA, dsRNA, and DNA. Despite these apparent similarities, the molecular structures mediating recognition are different between the TLR and the cytoplasmic PRR. The structural motif identified by MDA5 has not been characterized in detail, but RIG-I has been shown to recognize the 5′-phosphate group of viral ssRNA (Pichlmair et al. 2006). Mammalian mRNA is capped and therefore not recognized by the receptor. For DAI it is unclear whether the receptor can distinguish between molecular structures of viral or bacterial vs. endogenous dsDNA, but synthetic oligonucleotides with a phosphorothioate backbone as used for TLR9 activation do not trigger the cytoplasmic PRR for DNA (Stetson and Medzhitov 2006).

The functional outcome of stimulation of these cytoplasmic PRR in infected cells is the production of IFNβ, which confers virus resistance to neighbouring uninfected cells, shut-down of protein synthesis, degradation of RNA and induction of apoptosis. All these processes are crucial for limiting virus replication and spread. With regard to the antiviral immune response, factors expressed by infected tissue cells as a consequence of activation via the cytoplasmic PRR may contribute to the induction of the inflammatory response in the infected tissue. However, they have very limited scope to contribute to the induction of an antiviral adaptive immune response.

When DC are infected by viruses such as lymphocytic choriomeningitis virus (LCMV), cytoplasmic recognition of viral nucleic acids leads to their activation (Diebold et al. 2003). However, virus infection of DC renders them into targets for virus-specific CTL and their depletion, as a consequence of CTL killing, can have a detrimental influence on the overall anti-viral immune response as seen for the LCMV strain clone 13 (Borrow et al. 1995).

3 Differential Expression of PRR by Dendritic Cell Subsets

DC are a heterogeneous group of APC with the shared characteristic of being potent stimulators of T cell responses. Activation via PRR is crucial for DC to gain full T cell stimulatory activity during infections (Iwasaki and Medzhitov 2004). As PRR are differentially expressed by different DC subsets, only a selected group of DC is activated in response to PAMP expressed by particular pathogens. Since different DC have specialized functions, this has implications for the overall outcome of the immune response.

DC are divided into two major subsets i.e., plasmacytoid DC (PDC) and the so-called conventional DC. In addition to this classification, there are a variety of different conventional DC subsets. DC subsets are identified by the expression of surface markers, and there remains some debate with regard to the nomenclature of the conventional DC subsets. The lineage to which particular DC belong is one criterion used to divide conventional DC subset into myeloid vs. lymphoid DC. Yet, lineage commitment of different DC subsets still needs further clarification and, therefore, the term lymphoid DC is often avoided (Shortman and Liu 2002). Another way of distinguishing DC is by classifying them according to the tissues in which they reside in the steady state. When using the location of DC as a point of reference, interstitial or tissue-derived DC are discriminated from lymphoid-resident DC, which are also called blood-derived DC. The former are found in peripheral tissue such as skin and mucosal sites where they act as sentinels of the immune system. Upon activation in response to infection, the cells migrate, via lymphatic vessels, to the secondary lymphoid organs to prime T cell response against pathogen-associated antigens. In contrast to this, lymphoid-resident DC are not found in peripheral tissue and enter secondary lymphoid organs such as the spleen and lymph nodes directly from the blood.

3.1 Plasmacytoid Dendritic Cells

PDC correspond to natural interferon producing cells and are specialized in producing high levels of IFNα in response to virus infection (Siegal et al. 1999). Upon activation, they are thought to differentiate into DC with the capacity to prime naïve T cells (Soumelis and Liu 2006). However, their role in antigen-presentation and T cell priming is somewhat controversial, since their T cell stimulatory activity is inferior to that of conventional DC. In addition, it is unclear to what extent PDC take up, process, and present exogenous antigens. In mouse models, it has been shown that they do not present exogenous antigen such as ovalbumin (Krug et al. 2003; Salio et al. 2004). However, there are other reports indicating that PDC are able to present exogenous antigen, but handle antigens differently from conventional DC (Kuwana et al. 2001). Although it is controversial whether or not PDC present exogenous antigen, they clearly present endogenous antigen and are implicated in tolerance induction to self-antigens in the steady state (Kuwana et al. 2001). Furthermore, they have been shown to prime T cell responses against endogenously expressed antigens upon TLR9-mediated activation and virus infection (Dalod et al. 2003; Fonteneau et al. 2003; Salio et al. 2004; Zuniga et al. 2004). Thus PDC could play a crucial role during virus infection not only by producing high levels of IFN-I, but also by priming and/or expanding virus-specific T cells. Their role during bacterial infections or during infections with viruses that do not infect PDC is less clear.

PDC detect viral infections predominantly via TLR7 and TLR9, respectively (Hornung et al. 2002; Kadowaki et al. 2001). Neither human nor mouse PDC express TLR3 (Tables 1 and 2). TLR8 is, in contrast, expressed by mouse but not by

Table 1 Relative differential expression of TLR3, TLR5 and TLR7 on mouse splenic DC subsets as measured on the mRNA level. The mRNA expression levels of TLR1, TLR2, TLR4, TLR6, TLR8 and TLR9 are similar between the different splenic DC subsets [37]

DC subset:	PDC	$CD4^+$ DC	$CD8_\alpha{}^+$DC	DN DC
TLR3	-	+	+++	++
TLR5	+	++	-	+
TLR7	+++	++	-	+

Table 2 Relative differential expression of TLR on human peripheral blood DC subsets as measured on the mRNA level [65, 70, 74]. monoDC: monocyte-derived DC

DC subset:	PDC	myeloid DC	monoDC	monocytes
TLR1	+	-	+	++
TLR2	-	+++	+++	+++
TLR3	-	-	+	-
TLR4	-	+	+++	+++
TLR5	-	+++	+	+
TLR6	+	+	+	+
TLR7	+++	-	-	+
TLR8	-	+	+	+
TLR9	+++	-	-	-
TLR10	+	-	-	-

human PDC. In accordance with this expression pattern, PDC produce high levels of IFNα in response to CpG-rich oligonucleotides triggering TLR9, but also upon stimulation of TLR7 and TLR9 by genomic viral RNA and DNA, respectively (Diebold et al. 2004; Heil et al. 2004; Krug et al. 2001a; Krug et al. 2001b; Lund et al. 2003). Non-fusogenic viruses such as influenza virus enter cells by receptor-mediated uptake mechanism and in PDC, such viruses end up directly in the TLR-sensing compartment where the virus particles are degraded and the genomic ssRNA triggers TLR activation. For viruses that do not infect PDC, uptake is thought to involve FcγR-mediated mechanisms (Guzylack-Piriou et al. 2006; Wang et al. 2007). In contrast for fusogenic viruses such as vesicular stomatitis virus, it has been shown that the viral nucleic acids produced in the cytoplasm of infected PDC are transferred to the TLR expressing endosomal compartment by autophagy (Lee et al. 2007). Thus PDC have multiple strategies to allow for the recognition of viral nucleic acids in their specialized endosomal compartment.

Studies with isolated bacterial DNA have shown that it triggers TLR9, yet the role of TLR9-mediated activation of PDC in host immune responses against bacteria is unclear. The same is true for recognition of bacterial infections via other TLR. Human PDC express TLR1, TLR6, and low levels of TLR10 (Hornung et al. 2002), but whether, and how, PDC respond to the respective ligands is not well understood.

The main function of PDC seems to be the production of IFN-I in response to virus infection. High systemic levels of IFN-I are a hallmark of virus infections and IFN-I acts on a number of cell types including T and B cells. It plays a crucial role in the induction of T_H1 immune responses, in promoting cross-priming of CTL responses and in class switching of B cells (Cousens et al. 1999; Le Bon et al. 2003;

Le Bon et al. 2001; Le Bon et al. 2006). Thus IFN-I is influencing not only the innate immune system, but also the antigen-specific antiviral immune response by acting on the three different effector cell types of the adaptive immune system.

3.2 Conventional Dendritic Cells

In the mouse, conventional DC from spleen comprise three different DC subsets distinguished by their expression of the T cell markers CD4 and CD8 namely $CD4^+$ DC, $CD8\alpha^+$ DC, and double-negative (DN) DC (Vremec et al. 2000). These DC subsets are also present in murine lymph nodes alongside 1–2 additional DC populations, which express moderate and high levels of DEC-205, respectively, and which are thought to represent DC that have recently immigrated from the periphery via lymphatic vessels (Anjuere et al. 1999; Henri et al. 2001). The DC subset with intermediate levels of DEC-205 is found in all lymph nodes, lacks CD4 and CD8α expression, and can be distinguished from the other DN DC subset because they express CD11b. This DC subset is believed to be derived from interstitial DC. In contrast to this, the DC subset with high levels of DEC-205 expresses langerin, which is a marker for epidermal Langerhans cells. These DC are only found in skin-draining lymph nodes and are therefore thought to be derived from Langerhans cells. The TLR expression pattern of murine spleen-resident DC subsets was identified, which revealed differences in expression of TLR3, TLR5, and TLR7 between the different subsets (Table 1) (Edwards et al. 2003).

In humans, blood rather than lymph nodes or spleen are used as a source for primary DC. In human blood, $CD11b^+$ MHC class II-high myeloid DC can be distinguished from PDC phenotypically and functionally. The myeloid DC can be further divided into two separate subsets by their differential expression of CD1c and CD141. However, despite the phenotypic difference between these myeloid DC subsets, differences in their function still have to be elucidated. Another human DC subset that is often studied experimentally is monocyte-derived DC, which are generated in vitro by culturing monocytes in the presence of GM-CSF and IL-4 (Bender et al. 1996; Romani et al. 1996; Sallusto et al. 1994).

The TLR expression of the conventional DC in mice and the human myeloid DC differs widely unlike the TLR expression of mouse and human PDC (Tables 1 and 2) (Jarrossay et al. 2001; Kadowaki et al. 2001). Human myeloid DC express high levels of TLR2 and TLR5, while monocyte-derived DC express high levels of TLR2 and TLR4. In contrast to PDC, human myeloid DC and monocyte-derived DC do not express TLR7 and TLR9. Nevertheless, these non-PDC subsets respond to viral ssRNA via stimulation of TLR8. TLR7 and TLR8 are both activated by viral ssRNA, yet, while PDC respond mainly by producing high levels of IFNα, myeloid DC produce IL-6 and TNFα instead. It was thought that this difference was due to differences in the downstream signaling of the two ssRNA-sensing TLR. However, in mice, TLR8 was thought to be nonfunctional and doesn't seem to be engaged by ssRNA in the presence of TLR7 (Gorden et al. 2006; Jurk et al. 2002). Thus in mouse DC the response to viral ssRNA is mediated via TLR7 for both myeloid DC and PDC. Nevertheless, the two DC subsets show the same cytokine induction pattern that is seen for human DC with PDC primarily producing IFN-I and conventional DC mainly secreting pro-inflammatory cytokines such as IL-6 and TNFα. This difference in cytokine induction is attributed to differences in the signaling pathways downstream of TLR7. PDC recruit the adaptor molecule MyD88 to the early endosomal compartment, which leads to activation of IRF7 and subsequently to induction of IFN-I, while conventional DC recruit MyD88 to a late endosomal compartment, which results in the stimulation of NFκB and the production of IL-6 and TNFα (Guiducci et al. 2006; Hondo et al. 2005). Interestingly, manipulation of endosomal maturation by adding cationic lipids can alter the cytokines that are induced in response to TLR7 ligands in conventional DC and PDC. Thus the functional consequences of TLR activation can be cell-type specific due to differences in the signaling pathways that are engaged in response to ligand recognition.

3.3 Tissue vs. Blood-Derived Dendritic Cells

Interstitial DC interact with pathogens at the site of infection such as skin or mucosal tissue. They encounter PAMP in the periphery and are activated directly. The PRR-mediated activation then induces their migration to the draining lymph node where they instruct the adaptive immune response. For blood-derived DC, which resides in secondary lymphoid tissue such as lymph nodes, it is less clear how they are activated in the absence of direct contact with the pathogen. Under specific circumstances, pathogen-derived factors including antigens and PAMP may drain to lymph nodes via lymphatic vessels or in cases of systemic infections the pathogen itself may reach the secondary lymphoid organs. Under these conditions lymph node-resident DC have direct contact with antigens and PAMP associated with the infection. However, lymph node-resident DC seem to play a role in antigen-presentation even in the absence of systemic infection and direct drainage of antigen. It is thought that tissue-derived DC migrate to the draining lymph node upon activation in the periphery, where they interact with lymph node-resident blood-derived DC and transfer antigen (Carbone et al. 2004). Among the lymph node-resident DC is a DC subset that is specialized in cross-presentation of exogenous antigen on MHC class I. This cell type is thought to be of particular importance for the induction of CTL responses to viral antigens by cross-priming in the absence of direct infection of DC.

3.4 Cross-Priming Dendritic Cells

It has been shown that the lymph node-resident DC specialized in cross-priming present exogenous tissue-derived antigens on MHC class I and II (Belz et al. 2002;

Scheinecker et al. 2002). While the cross-presentation of exogenous antigen by these cells leads to the induction of tolerance in the steady state, they induce anti-viral CTL responses by cross-priming of CD8 T cells upon virus infection (Belz et al. 2002; Belz et al. 2004b; Scheinecker et al. 2002). Their crucial role in inducing anti-viral CTL responses has been shown for a variety of viruses (Belz et al. 2004a).

This cross-priming DC subset was identified in spleen and lymph node of mice expressing CD8$\alpha\alpha$ homodimers and DEC205 (Pooley et al. 2001). These so-called CD8α^+ DC are furthermore specialized in the uptake of cellular material from apoptotic cells and in cross-presentation of antigens associated with the internalized cellular material (Iyoda et al. 2002; Schulz and Reise Sousa 2002). CD8α^+ DC express TLR1–4, TLR6, TLR8, TLR9, and TLR11 and are, therefore, responsive to a wide array of different PAMP. Upon TLR activation with stimuli such as CpG or extracts from *Toxoplasma gondii*, these cells produce high levels of IL-12 p70 (Schulz et al. 2000). As a result of the high production of IL-12 in response to activation, CD8α^+ DC bias CD4 T cell priming toward a T_H1 response (Maldonado-Lopez et al. 1999). Furthermore, it has been shown that activation of CD8α^+ DC via TLR3 and TLR9 promotes cross-priming (Heit et al. 2003; Schulz et al. 2005). These two TLR are involved in the detection of viral PAMP and TLR3 has been shown to allow the CD8α^+ DC subset to discriminate between noninfected and infected apoptotic cells by sensing viral dsRNA associated with the cellular material of the latter (Schulz et al. 2005). It is of interest to note that CD8α^+ DC do not express TLR7. Since the nucleic acid sensing TLR are unable to clearly discriminate between foreign and self nucleic acids, one can speculate that TLR7 expression by this subset could potentially lead to the initiation of autoimmune responses upon detection of endogenous RNA associated with apoptotic cells. Thus, the inability of the cross-priming DC subset to sense viral ssRNA may have evolved as a safety mechanism to prevent the induction of autoimmunity.

The human equivalent of the murine CD8α^+ DC subset has not been identified so far due to the lack of expression of CD8$\alpha\alpha$ homodimers on human DC. However, there is immense interest in the identification of this subset in humans, since these cross-priming DC are an ideal target for immunotherapeutic approaches. The lack of immunization strategies that mediate strong cellular immunity to exogenous antigens has hampered the development of better vaccines against a variety of pathogens such as HIV. Delivering antigens to CD8α^+ DC in mice by antibody-mediated methods that target the CLR DEC-205 has been shown to be a promising strategy to achieve tolerance induction or immunity against exogenous antigens (Bonifaz et al. 2002; Bonifaz et al. 2004; Hawiger et al. 2001). Since DEC-205 mediated uptake does not induce DC activation, the presence of an adjuvant such as a suitable TLR ligand is crucial for the induction of cellular immunity rather than tolerance. This underlines again the importance of TLR-mediated DC activation for the outcome of DC–T cell interactions.

4 Endogenous Ligands for PRR

While there is overwhelming evidence that TLR recognize primarily PAMP, endogenous ligands for particular TLR have been described. It has been shown that heat shock proteins (Hsp) can trigger TLR activation, with mammalian Hsp70 and Hsp60 being recognized by TLR4 and TLR2, respectively (Asea et al. 2002; Vabulas et al. 2001; Vabulas et al. 2002). Similarly, breakdown products of hyaluronan bind to TLR4 as does high mobility group box 1 (HMGB1) protein (Apetoh et al. 2007; Taylor et al. 2004; Termeer et al. 2002). According to the danger model, this is the evidence that the immune system does not discriminate between foreign and self, but rather responds to exogenous and endogenous danger signals (Matzinger 2002). Such danger signals may collectively expose hydrophobic structures, which can bind to the LRR domains of TLR (Seong and Matzinger 2004). While endogenous danger signals clearly alert the immune system during infections, they do not seem to compare favorably with the immunostimulatory activity of PAMP and it is unclear whether immune activation triggered by endogenous ligands alone is sufficient for the induction of immune responses capable of eliminating pathogens.

In contrast to the endogenous ligands that trigger TLR2 and TLR4 at the cell surface, there is a body of evidence that self nucleic acids trigger activation of intracellular TLR. Mammalian DNA activates TLR9 and mammalian mRNA induces stimulation of TLR3 and TLR7 (Sioud 2006). According to the danger model, nucleic acids released from necrotic cells serve as endogenous danger signals, which alert the immune system to tissue damage in a similar way to the detection of Hsp and hyaluronan breakdown products (Matzinger 2002). However, there is little evidence that release of nucleic acids from dying cells leads to the activation of intracellular nucleic acid sensing TLR under physiological conditions. It is thought that extracellular nucleases eliminate such responses against self nucleic acids (Barton et al. 2006). Furthermore, detection of self-RNA and DNA only became evident in the context of autoimmune responses such as SLE. In SLE patients, anti-RNA and DNA autoantibodies are present, which lead to the internalization of antibody–nucleic acid immune complexes by PDC and B cells via Fcγ receptor-mediated uptake mechanisms. The immune activation by endogenous nucleic acids and the humoral autoimmune response against self-RNA and DNA are central for the progress of the autoimmune disease. Thus, in SLE the endogenous RNA and DNA serve as adjuvant and antigen, simultaneously. In contrast to the evidence indicating a detrimental role for recognition of self nucleic acids by TLR in the context of autoimmunity, there is no direct evidence supporting a beneficial role for detection of endogenous RNA and DNA as a danger signal during infections.

5 Conclusions

Just as T cells require activation to turn into effector cells, DC must be activated to gain their full T cell stimulatory activity and to induce T cell priming. While T cells become activated when interacting with activated DC, DC activation is initiated by the encounter of PAMP via PRR. The PRR that have been shown to induce potent DC activation and to play a crucial role in T cell priming all belong to the TLR family. Some other PRR belonging to the CLR family can induce DC activation, yet their role in linking the innate with the adaptive immune response is still only partially understood. Understanding what turns DC into potent T cell stimulatory cells is crucial for the development of better vaccines aimed at inducing humoral but especially cellular immunity.

Acknowledgements S.D. is funded by a Cancer Research UK Career Development Award. I thank Amy Lewis for her critical reading of the manuscript.

References

Ahmad-Nejad P, Hacker H, Rutz M, Bauer S, Vabulas RM, Wagner H (2002) Bacterial CpG-DNA and lipopolysaccharides activate Toll-like receptors at distinct cellular compartments. Eur J Immunol 32:1958–1968

Akashi S, Shimazu R, Ogata H, Nagai Y, Takeda K, Kimoto M, Miyake K (2000) Cutting edge: cell surface expression and lipopolysaccharide signaling via the toll-like receptor 4-MD-2 complex on mouse peritoneal macrophages. J Immunol 164:3471–3475

Alexopoulou L, Holt AC, Medzhitov R, Flavell RA (2001) Recognition of double-stranded RNA and activation of NF-kappaB by Toll-like receptor 3. Nature 413:732–738

Alexopoulou L, Thomas V, Schnare M, Lobet Y, Anguita J, Schoen RT, Medzhitov R, Fikrig E, Flavell RA (2002) Hyporesponsiveness to vaccination with Borrelia burgdorferi OspA in humans and in TLR1- and TLR2-deficient mice. Nat Med 8:878–884

Alvarez CP, Lasala F, Carrillo J, Muniz O, Corbi AL, Delgado R (2002) C-type lectins DC-SIGN and L-SIGN mediate cellular entry by Ebola virus in cis and in trans. J Virol 76:6841–6844

Anjuere F, Martin P, Ferrero I, Fraga ML, del Hoyo GM, Wright N, Ardavin C (1999) Definition of dendritic cell subpopulations present in the spleen, Peyer's patches, lymph nodes, and skin of the mouse. Blood 93:590–598

Apetoh L, Ghiringhelli F, Tesniere A, Obeid M, Ortiz C, Criollo A, Mignot G, Maiuri MC, Ullrich E, Saulnier P, Yang H, Amigorena S, Ryffel B, Barrat FJ, Saftig P, Levi F, Lidereau R, Nogues C, Mira JP, Chompret A, Joulin V, Clavel-Chapelon F, Bourhis J, Andre F, Delaloge S, Tursz T, Kroemer G, Zitvogel L (2007) Toll-like receptor 4-dependent contribution of the immune system to anticancer chemotherapy and radiotherapy. Nat Med 13:1050–1059

Asea A, Rehli M, Kabingu E, Boch JA, Bare O, Auron PE, Stevenson MA, Calderwood SK (2002) Novel signal transduction pathway utilized by extracellular HSP70: role of toll-like receptor (TLR) 2 and TLR4. J Biol Chem 277:15028–15034

Barrat FJ, Meeker T, Gregorio J, Chan JH, Uematsu S, Akira S, Chang B, Duramad O, Coffman RL (2005) Nucleic acids of mammalian origin can act as endogenous ligands for Toll-like receptors and may promote systemic lupus erythematosus. J Exp Med 202:1131–1139

Barton GM, Kagan JC, Medzhitov R (2006) Intracellular localization of Toll-like receptor 9 prevents recognition of self DNA but facilitates access to viral DNA. Nat Immunol 7:49–56

Belvin MP, Anderson KV (1996) A conserved signaling pathway: the Drosophila toll-dorsal pathway. Annu Rev Cell Dev Biol 12:393–416

Belz GT, Behrens GM, Smith CM, Miller JF, Jones C, Lejon K, Fathman CG, Mueller SN, Shortman K, Carbone FR, Heath WR (2002) The CD8alpha(+) dendritic cell is responsible for inducing peripheral self-tolerance to tissue-associated antigens. J Exp Med 196: 1099–1104

Belz GT, Smith CM, Eichner D, Shortman K, Karupiah G, Carbone FR, Heath WR (2004a) Cutting edge: conventional CD8 alpha+ dendritic cells are generally involved in priming CTL immunity to viruses. J Immunol 172:1996–2000

Belz GT, Smith CM, Kleinert L, Reading P, Brooks A, Shortman K, Carbone FR, Heath WR (2004b) Distinct migrating and nonmigrating dendritic cell populations are involved in MHC class I-restricted antigen presentation after lung infection with virus. Proc Natl Acad Sci USA 101:8670–8675

Bender A, Sapp M, Schuler G, Steinman RM, Bhardwaj N (1996) Improved methods for the generation of dendritic cells from nonproliferating progenitors in human blood. J Immunol Methods 196:121-135

Bieback K, Lien E, Klagge IM, Avota E, Schneider-Schaulies J, Duprex WP, Wagner H, Kirschning CJ, Ter Meulen V, Schneider-Schaulies S (2002) Hemagglutinin protein of wild-type measles virus activates toll-like receptor 2 signaling. J Virol 76:8729-8736

Bonifaz L, Bonnyay D, Mahnke K, Rivera M, Nussenzweig MC, Steinman RM (2002) Efficient targeting of protein antigen to the dendritic cell receptor DEC-205 in the steady state leads to antigen presentation on major histocompatibility complex class I products and peripheral CD8+ T cell tolerance. J Exp Med 196:1627–1638

Bonifaz LC, Bonnyay DP, Charalambous A, Darguste DI, Fujii S, Soares H, Brimnes MK, Moltedo B, Moran TM, Steinman RM (2004) In vivo targeting of antigens to maturing dendritic cells via the DEC-205 receptor improves T cell vaccination. J Exp Med 199:815–824

Borrow P, Evans CF, Oldstone MB (1995) Virus-induced immunosuppression: immune system-mediated destruction of virus-infected dendritic cells results in generalized immune suppression. J Virol 69:1059–1070

Boule MW, Broughton C, Mackay F, Akira S, Marshak-Rothstein A, Rifkin IR (2004) Toll-like receptor 9-dependent and -independent dendritic cell activation by chromatin-immunoglobulin G complexes. J Exp Med 199:1631–1640

Brown GD (2006) Dectin-1: a signalling non-TLR pattern-recognition receptor. Nat Rev Immunol 6:33–43

Caparros E, Munoz P, Sierra-Filardi E, Serrano-Gomez D, Puig-Kroger A, Rodriguez-Fernandez JL, Mellado M, Sancho J, Zubiaur M, Corbi AL (2006) DC-SIGN ligation on dendritic cells results in ERK and PI3K activation and modulates cytokine production. Blood 107:3950–3958

Carbone FR, Belz GT, Heath WR (2004) Transfer of antigen between migrating and lymph node-resident DCs in peripheral T-cell tolerance and immunity. Trends Immunol 25:655–658

Chieppa M, Bianchi G, Doni A, Del Prete A, Sironi M, Laskarin G, Monti P, Piemonti L, Biondi A, Mantovani A, Introna M, Allavena P (2003) Cross-linking of the mannose receptor on monocyte-derived dendritic cells activates an anti-inflammatory immunosuppressive program. J Immunol 171:4552–4560

Chuang T, Ulevitch RJ (2001) Identification of hTLR10: a novel human Toll-like receptor preferentially expressed in immune cells. Biochim Biophys Acta 1518:157–161

Chuang TH, Ulevitch RJ (2000) Cloning and characterization of a sub-family of human toll-like receptors: hTLR7, hTLR8 and hTLR9. Eur Cytokine Netw 11:372–378

Coban C, Ishii KJ, Kawai T, Hemmi H, Sato S, Uematsu S, Yamamoto M, Takeuchi O, Itagaki S, Kumar N, Horii T, Akira S (2005) Toll-like receptor 9 mediates innate immune activation by the malaria pigment hemozoin. J Exp Med 201:19–25

Compton T, Kurt-Jones EA, Boehme KW, Belko J, Latz E, Golenbock DT, Finberg RW (2003) Human cytomegalovirus activates inflammatory cytokine responses via CD14 and Toll-like receptor 2. J Virol 77:4588–4596

Cousens LP, Peterson R, Hsu S, Dorner A, Altman JD, Ahmed R, Biron CA (1999) Two roads diverged: interferon alpha/beta- and interleukin 12-mediated pathways in promoting T cell interferon gamma responses during viral infection. J Exp Med 189:1315–1328

da Silva Correia J, Soldau K, Christen U, Tobias PS, Ulevitch RJ (2001) Lipopolysaccharide is in close proximity to each of the proteins in its membrane receptor complex. transfer from CD14 to TLR4 and MD-2. J Biol Chem 276:21129–21135

Dalod M, Hamilton T, Salomon R, Salazar-Mather TP, Henry SC, Hamilton JD, Biron CA (2003) Dendritic cell responses to early murine cytomegalovirus infection: subset functional specialization and differential regulation by interferon alpha/beta. J Exp Med 197:885–898

Diebold SS, Kaisho T, Hemmi H, Akira S, Reise Sousa C (2004) Innate antiviral responses by means of TLR7-mediated recognition of single-stranded RNA. Science 303:1529–1531

Diebold SS, Massacrier C, Akira S, Paturel C, Morel Y, Reise Sousa C (2006) Nucleic acid agonists for Toll-like receptor 7 are defined by the presence of uridine ribonucleotides. Eur J Immunol 36:3256–3267

Diebold SS, Montoya M, Unger H, Alexopoulou L, Roy P, Haswell LE, Al-Shamkhani A, Flavell R, Borrow P, Reise Sousa C (2003) Viral infection switches non-plasmacytoid dendritic cells into high interferon producers. Nature 424:324–328

Du X, Poltorak A, Wei Y, Beutler B (2000) Three novel mammalian toll-like receptors: gene structure, expression, and evolution. Eur Cytokine Netw 11:362–371

Eagle RA, Trowsdale J (2007) Promiscuity and the single receptor: NKG2D. Nat Rev Immunol 7:737–44

Edwards AD, Diebold SS, Slack EM, Tomizawa H, Hemmi H, Kaisho T, Akira S, Reis e Sousa C (2003) Toll-like receptor expression in murine DC subsets: lack of TLR7 expression by CD8 alpha+ DC correlates with unresponsiveness to imidazoquinolines. Eur J Immunol 33:827–833

Fiebiger E, Meraner P, Weber E, Fang IF, Stingl G, Ploegh H, Maurer D (2001) Cytokines regulate proteolysis in major histocompatibility complex class II-dependent antigen presentation by dendritic cells. J Exp Med 193:881–892

Fitzgerald KA, Palsson-McDermott EM, Bowie AG, Jefferies CA, Mansell AS, Brady G, Brint E, Dunne A, Gray P, Harte MT, McMurray D, Smith DE, Sims JE, Bird TA, O'Neill LA (2001) Mal (MyD88-adapter-like) is required for Toll-like receptor-4 signal transduction. Nature 413:78–83

Fitzgerald KA, Rowe DC, Barnes BJ, Caffrey DR, Visintin A, Latz E, Monks B, Pitha PM, Golenbock DT (2003) LPS-TLR4 signaling to IRF-3/7 and NF-kappaB involves the toll adapters TRAM and TRIF. J Exp Med 198:1043–1055

Fonteneau JF, Gilliet M, Larsson M, Dasilva I, Munz C, Liu YJ, Bhardwaj N (2003) Activation of influenza virus-specific CD4+ and CD8+ T cells: a new role for plasmacytoid dendritic cells in adaptive immunity. Blood 101:3520–3526

Geijtenbeek TB, Krooshoop DJ, Bleijs DA, van Vliet SJ, van Duijnhoven GC, Grabovsky V, Alon R, Figdor CG, van Kooyk Y (2000a) DC-SIGN-ICAM-2 interaction mediates dendritic cell trafficking. Nat Immunol 1:353–357

Geijtenbeek TB, Kwon DS, Torensma R, van Vliet SJ, van Duijnhoven GC, Middel J, Cornelissen IL, Nottet HS, KewalRamani VN, Littman DR, Figdor CG, van Kooyk Y (2000b) DC-SIGN, a dendritic cell-specific HIV-1-binding protein that enhances trans-infection of T cells. Cell 100:587–597

Geijtenbeek TB, Torensma R, van Vliet SJ, van Duijnhoven GC, Adema GJ, van Kooyk Y, Figdor CG (2000c) Identification of DC-SIGN, a novel dendritic cell-specific ICAM-3 receptor that supports primary immune responses. Cell 100:575–585

Geijtenbeek TB, Van Vliet SJ, Koppel EA, Sanchez-Hernandez M, Vandenbroucke-Grauls CM, Appelmelk B, Van Kooyk Y (2003) Mycobacteria target DC-SIGN to suppress dendritic cell function. J Exp Med 197:7–17

Gorden KK, Qiu XX, Binsfeld CC, Vasilakos JP, Alkan SS (2006) Cutting edge: activation of murine TLR8 by a combination of imidazoquinoline immune response modifiers and polyT oligodeoxynucleotides. J Immunol 177:6584–6587

Gross O, Gewies A, Finger K, Schafer M, Sparwasser T, Peschel C, Forster I, Ruland J (2006) Card9 controls a non-TLR signalling pathway for innate anti-fungal immunity. Nature 442:651–656

Guiducci C, Ott G, Chan JH, Damon E, Calacsan C, Matray T, Lee KD, Coffman RL, Barrat FJ (2006) Properties regulating the nature of the plasmacytoid dendritic cell response to Toll-like receptor 9 activation. J Exp Med 203:1999–2008

Gupta G, Surolia A (2007) Collectins: sentinels of innate immunity. Bioessays 29:452–464

Guzylack-Piriou L, Bergamin F, Gerber M, McCullough KC, Summerfield A (2006) Plasmacytoid dendritic cell activation by foot-and-mouth disease virus requires immune complexes. Eur J Immunol 36:1674–1683

Halary F, Amara A, Lortat-Jacob H, Messerle M, Delaunay T, Houles C, Fieschi F, Arenzana-Seisdedos F, Moreau JF, Dechanet-Merville J (2002) Human cytomegalovirus binding to DC-SIGN is required for dendritic cell infection and target cell trans-infection. Immunity 17: 653–664

Hasan U, Chaffois C, Gaillard C, Saulnier V, Merck E, Tancredi S, Guiet C, Briere F, Vlach J, Lebecque S, Trinchieri G, Bates EE (2005) Human TLR10 is a functional receptor, expressed by B cells and plasmacytoid dendritic cells, which activates gene transcription through MyD88. J Immunol 174:2942–2950

Hashimoto C, Hudson KL, Anderson KV (1988) The Toll gene of Drosophila, required for dorsal-ventral embryonic polarity, appears to encode a transmembrane protein. Cell 52:269–279

Hawiger D, Inaba K, Dorsett Y, Guo M, Mahnke K, Rivera M, Ravetch JV, Steinman RM, Nussenzweig MC (2001) Dendritic cells induce peripheral T cell unresponsiveness under steady state conditions in vivo. J Exp Med 194:769–779

Hayashi F, Smith KD, Ozinsky A, Hawn TR, Yi EC, Goodlett DR, Eng JK, Akira S, Underhill DM, Aderem A (2001) The innate immune response to bacterial flagellin is mediated by Toll-like receptor 5. Nature 410:1099–1103

Heil F, Ahmad-Nejad P, Hemmi H, Hochrein H, Ampenberger F, Gellert T, Dietrich H, Lipford G, Takeda K, Akira S, Wagner H, Bauer S (2003) The Toll-like receptor 7 (TLR7)-specific stimulus loxoribine uncovers a strong relationship within the TLR7, 8 and 9 subfamily. Eur J Immunol 33:2987–2997

Heil F, Hemmi H, Hochrein H, Ampenberger F, Kirschning C, Akira S, Lipford G, Wagner H, Bauer S (2004) Species-specific recognition of single-stranded RNA via toll-like receptor 7 and 8. Science 303:1526–1529

Heit A, Maurer T, Hochrein H, Bauer S, Huster KM, Busch DH, Wagner H (2003) Cutting edge: Toll-like receptor 9 expression is not required for CpG DNA-aided cross-presentation of DNA-conjugated antigens but essential for cross-priming of CD8 T cells. J Immunol 170:2802–2805

Hemmi H, Takeuchi O, Kawai T, Kaisho T, Sato S, Sanjo H, Matsumoto M, Hoshino K, Wagner H, Takeda K, Akira S (2000) A Toll-like receptor recognizes bacterial DNA. Nature 408:740–745

Henri S, Vremec D, Kamath A, Waithman J, Williams S, Benoist C, Burnham K, Saeland S, Handman E, Shortman K (2001) The dendritic cell populations of mouse lymph nodes. J Immunol 167:741–748

Honda K, Ohba Y, Yanai H, Negishi H, Mizutani T, Takaoka A, Taya C, Taniguchi T (2005) Spatiotemporal regulation of MyD88-IRF-7 signalling for robust type-I interferon induction. Nature 434: 1035–1040

Horng T, Barton GM, Flavell RA, Medzhitov R (2002) The adaptor molecule TIRAP provides signalling specificity for Toll-like receptors. Nature 420:329–333

Horng T, Barton GM, Medzhitov R (2001) TIRAP: an adapter molecule in the Toll signaling pathway. Nat Immunol 2:835–841

Horng T, Medzhitov R (2001) Drosophila MyD88 is an adapter in the Toll signaling pathway. Proc Natl Acad Sci USA 98:12654–12658

Hornung V, Rothenfusser S, Britsch S, Krug A, Jahrsdorfer B, Giese T, Endres S, Hartmann G (2002) Quantitative expression of toll-like receptor 1–10 mRNA in cellular subsets of human peripheral blood mononuclear cells and sensitivity to CpG oligodeoxynucleotides. J Immunol 168:4531–4537

Inaba K, Turley S, Iyoda T, Yamaide F, Shimoyama S, Reise Sousa C, Germain RN, Mellman I, Steinman RM (2000) The formation of immunogenic major histocompatibility complex class II-peptide ligands in lysosomal compartments of dendritic cells is regulated by inflammatory stimuli. J Exp Med 191:927–936

Iwasaki A, Medzhitov R (2004) Toll-like receptor control of the adaptive immune responses. Nat Immunol 5:987–995

Iyoda T, Shimoyama S, Liu K, Omatsu Y, Akiyama Y, Maeda Y, Takahara K, Steinman RM, Inaba K (2002) The CD8+ dendritic cell subset selectively endocytoses dying cells in culture and in vivo. J Exp Med 195:1289–1302

Janeway CA, Jr. (1989) Approaching the asymptote? Evolution and revolution in immunology. Cold Spring Harb Symp Quant Biol 54 Pt 1:1–13

Jarrossay D, Napolitani G, Colonna M, Sallusto F, Lanzavecchia A (2001) Specialization and complementarity in microbial molecule recognition by human myeloid and plasmacytoid dendritic cells. Eur J Immunol 31:3388–3393

Jiang Q, Akashi S, Miyake K, Petty HR (2000) Lipopolysaccharide induces physical proximity between CD14 and toll-like receptor 4 (TLR4) prior to nuclear translocation of NF-kappa B. J Immunol 165:3541–3544

Jiang W, Swiggard WJ, Heufler C, Peng M, Mirza A, Steinman RM, Nussenzweig MC (1995) The receptor DEC-205 expressed by dendritic cells and thymic epithelial cells is involved in antigen processing. Nature 375:151–155

Jurk M, Heil F, Vollmer J, Schetter C, Krieg AM, Wagner H, Lipford G, Bauer S (2002) Human TLR7 or TLR8 independently confer responsiveness to the antiviral compound R-848. Nat Immunol 3: 499

Kadowaki N, Ho S, Antonenko S, Malefyt RW, Kastelein RA, Bazan F, Liu YJ (2001) Subsets of human dendritic cell precursors express different toll-like receptors and respond to different microbial antigens. J Exp Med 194:863–869

Kagan JC, Medzhitov R (2006) Phosphoinositide-mediated adaptor recruitment controls Toll-like receptor signaling. Cell 125:943–955

Kanneganti TD, Lamkanfi M, Nunez G (2007) Intracellular NOD-like receptors in host defense and disease. Immunity 27:549–559

Kariko K, Buckstein M, Ni H, Weissman D (2005) Suppression of RNA recognition by Toll-like receptors: the impact of nucleoside modification and the evolutionary origin of RNA. Immunity 23:165–175

Kariko K, Ni H, Capodici J, Lamphier M, Weissman D (2004) mRNA is an endogenous ligand for Toll-like receptor 3. J Biol Chem 279:12542–12550

Koppel EA, van Gisbergen KP, Geijtenbeek TB, van Kooyk Y (2005) Distinct functions of DC-SIGN and its homologues L-SIGN (DC-SIGNR) and mSIGNR1 in pathogen recognition and immune regulation. Cell Microbiol 7:157–165

Krieg AM, Yi AK, Matson S, Waldschmidt TJ, Bishop GA, Teasdale R, Koretzky GA, Klinman DM (1995) CpG motifs in bacterial DNA trigger direct B-cell activation. Nature 374:546–549

Krug A, Rothenfusser S, Hornung V, Jahrsdorfer B, Blackwell S, Ballas ZK, Endres S, Krieg AM, Hartmann G (2001a) Identification of CpG oligonucleotide sequences with high induction of IFN-alpha/beta in plasmacytoid dendritic cells. Eur J Immunol 31:2154–2163

Krug A, Towarowski A, Britsch S, Rothenfusser S, Hornung V, Bals R, Giese T, Engelmann H, Endres S, Krieg AM, Hartmann G (2001b) Toll-like receptor expression reveals CpG DNA as a unique microbial stimulus for plasmacytoid dendritic cells which synergizes with CD40 ligand to induce high amounts of IL-12. Eur J Immunol 31:3026–3037

Krug A, Veeraswamy R, Pekosz A, Kanagawa O, Unanue ER, Colonna M, Cella M (2003) Interferon-producing cells fail to induce proliferation of naive T cells but can promote expansion and T helper 1 differentiation of antigen-experienced unpolarized T cells. J Exp Med 197:899–906

Kurt-Jones EA, Chan M, Zhou S, Wang J, Reed G, Bronson R, Arnold MM, Knipe DM, Finberg RW (2004) Herpes simplex virus 1 interaction with Toll-like receptor 2 contributes to lethal encephalitis. Proc Natl Acad Sci U S A 101: 1315–1320

Kurt-Jones EA, Popova L, Kwinn L, Haynes LM, Jones LP, Tripp RA, Walsh EE, Freeman MW, Golenbock DT, Anderson LJ, Finberg RW (2000) Pattern recognition receptors TLR4 and CD14 mediate response to respiratory syncytial virus. Nat Immunol 1: 398–401

Kuwana M, Kaburaki J, Wright TM, Kawakami Y, Ikeda Y (2001) Induction of antigen-specific human CD4(+) T cell anergy by peripheral blood DC2 precursors. Eur J Immunol 31: 2547–2557

Lanzavecchia A, Sallusto F (2001) Regulation of T cell immunity by dendritic cells. Cell 106: 263–6

Lau CM, Broughton C, Tabor AS, Akira S, Flavell RA, Mamula MJ, Christensen SR, Shlomchik MJ, Viglianti GA, Rifkin IR, Marshak-Rothstein A (2005) RNA-associated autoantigens activate B cells by combined B cell antigen receptor/Toll-like receptor 7 engagement. J Exp Med 202:1171–1177

Le Bon A, Etchart N, Rossmann C, Ashton M, Hou S, Gewert D, Borrow P, Tough DF (2003) Cross-priming of CD8+ T cells stimulated by virus-induced type I interferon. Nat Immunol 4:1009–1015

Le Bon A, Schiavoni G, D'Agostino G, Gresser I, Belardelli F, Tough DF (2001) Type i interferons potently enhance humoral immunity and can promote isotype switching by stimulating dendritic cells in vivo. Immunity 14:461–470

Le Bon A, Thompson C, Kamphuis E, Durand V, Rossmann C, Kalinke U, Tough DF (2006) Cutting edge: enhancement of antibody responses through direct stimulation of B and T cells by type I IFN. J Immunol 176:2074–2078

Leadbetter EA, Rifkin IR, Hohlbaum AM, Beaudette BC, Shlomchik MJ, Marshak-Rothstein A (2002) Chromatin-IgG complexes activate B cells by dual engagement of IgM and Toll-like receptors. Nature 416:603–607

Lee HK, Lund JM, Ramanathan B, Mizushima N, Iwasaki A (2007) Autophagy-dependent viral recognition by plasmacytoid dendritic cells. Science 315:1398–1401

Lee J, Chuang TH, Redecke V, She L, Pitha PM, Carson DA, Raz E, Cottam HB (2003) Molecular basis for the immunostimulatory activity of guanine nucleoside analogs: activation of Toll-like receptor 7. Proc Natl Acad Sci USA 100:6646–6651

LeibundGut-Landmann S, Gross O, Robinson MJ, Osorio F, Slack EC, Tsoni SV, Schweighoffer E, Tybulewicz V, Brown GD, Ruland J, Reise Sousa C (2007) Syk- and CARD9-dependent coupling of innate immunity to the induction of T helper cells that produce interleukin 17. Nat Immunol 8:630–638

Lemaitre B, Nicolas E, Michaut L, Reichhart JM, Hoffmann JA (1996) The dorsoventral regulatory gene cassette spatzle/Toll/cactus controls the potent antifungal response in Drosophila adults. Cell 86:973–983

Levashina EA, Langley E, Green C, Gubb D, Ashburner M, Hoffmann JA, Reichhart JM (1999) Constitutive activation of toll-mediated antifungal defense in serpin-deficient Drosophila. Science 285:1917–1919

Lozach PY, Amara A, Bartosch B, Virelizier JL, Arenzana-Seisdedos F, Cosset FL, Altmeyer R (2004) C-type lectins L-SIGN and DC-SIGN capture and transmit infectious hepatitis C virus pseudotype particles. J Biol Chem 279:32035–32045

Lund J, Sato A, Akira S, Medzhitov R, Iwasaki A (2003) Toll-like receptor 9-mediated recognition of Herpes simplex virus-2 by plasmacytoid dendritic cells. J Exp Med 198:513–520

Lund JM, Alexopoulou L, Sato A, Karow M, Adams NC, Gale NW, Iwasaki A, Flavell RA (2004) Recognition of single-stranded RNA viruses by Toll-like receptor 7. Proc Natl Acad Sci U S A 101: 5598–5603

Mahnke K, Guo M, Lee S, Sepulveda H, Swain SL, Nussenzweig M, Steinman RM (2000) The dendritic cell receptor for endocytosis, DEC-205, can recycle and enhance antigen presentation via major histocompatibility complex class II-positive lysosomal compartments. J Cell Biol 151:673–684

Maldonado-Lopez R, De Smedt T, Michel P, Godfroid J, Pajak B, Heirman C, Thielemans K, Leo O, Urbain J, Moser M (1999) CD8alpha+ and CD8alpha− subclasses of dendritic cells direct the development of distinct T helper cells in vivo. J Exp Med 189:587–592

Matzinger P (2002) The danger model: a renewed sense of self. Science 296:301–305

Medzhitov R, Preston-Hurlburt P, Janeway CA, Jr. (1997) A human homologue of the Drosophila Toll protein signals activation of adaptive immunity. Nature 388:394–397

Mellman I, Steinman RM (2001) Dendritic cells: specialized and regulated antigen processing machines. Cell 106:255–258

Meylan E, Tschopp J, Karin M (2006) Intracellular pattern recognition receptors in the host response. Nature 442:39–44
O'Neill LA, Bowie AG (2007) The family of five: TIR-domain-containing adaptors in Toll-like receptor signalling. Nat Rev Immunol 7:353–364
Oshiumi H, Sasai M, Shida K, Fujita T, Matsumoto M, Seya T (2003) TIR-containing adapter molecule (TICAM)-2, a bridging adapter recruiting to toll-like receptor 4 TICAM-1 that induces interferon-beta. J Biol Chem 278:49751–49762
Palma AS, Feizi T, Zhang Y, Stoll MS, Lawson AM, Diaz-Rodriguez E, Campanero-Rhodes MA, Costa J, Gordon S, Brown GD, Chai W (2006) Ligands for the beta-glucan receptor, Dectin-1, assigned using "designer" microarrays of oligosaccharide probes (neoglycolipids) generated from glucan polysaccharides. J Biol Chem 281:5771–5779
Pichlmair A, Reise Sousa C (2007) Innate recognition of viruses. Immunity 27:370–383
Pichlmair A, Schulz O, Tan CP, Naslund TI, Liljestrom P, Weber F, Reise Sousa C (2006) RIG-I-mediated antiviral responses to single-stranded RNA bearing 5′-phosphates. Science 314: 997–1001
Pierre P, Turley SJ, Gatti E, Hull M, Meltzer J, Mirza A, Inaba K, Steinman RM, Mellman I (1997) Developmental regulation of MHC class II transport in mouse dendritic cells. Nature 388:787–792
Pooley JL, Heath WR, Shortman K (2001) Cutting edge: intravenous soluble antigen is presented to CD4 T cells by CD8− dendritic cells, but cross-presented to CD8 T cells by CD8+ dendritic cells. J Immunol 166:5327–5330
Rassa JC, Meyers JL, Zhang Y, Kudaravalli R, Ross SR (2002) Murine retroviruses activate B cells via interaction with toll-like receptor 4. Proc Natl Acad Sci U S A 99: 2281–2286
Reise Sousa C (2004) Toll-like receptors and dendritic cells: for whom the bug tolls. Semin Immunol 16:27–34
Robinson MJ, Sancho D, Slack EC, LeibundGut-Landmann S, Reise Sousa C (2006) Myeloid C-type lectins in innate immunity. Nat Immunol 7:1258–1265
Rock FL, Hardiman G, Timans JC, Kastelein RA, Bazan JF (1998) A family of human receptors structurally related to Drosophila Toll. Proc Natl Acad Sci USA 95:588–593
Rogers NC, Slack EC, Edwards AD, Nolte MA, Schulz O, Schweighoffer E, Williams DL, Gordon S, Tybulewicz VL, Brown GD, Reise Sousa C (2005) Syk-dependent cytokine induction by Dectin-1 reveals a novel pattern recognition pathway for C type lectins. Immunity 22:507–517
Romani N, Reider D, Heuer M, Ebner S, Kampgen E, Eibl B, Niederwieser D, Schuler G (1996) Generation of mature dendritic cells from human blood. An improved method with special regard to clinical applicability. J Immunol Methods 196: 137–151
Rossiter H, Alon R, Kupper TS (1997) Selectins, T-cell rolling and inflammation. Mol Med Today 3:214–222
Rutschmann S, Kilinc A, Ferrandon D (2002) Cutting edge: the toll pathway is required for resistance to gram-positive bacterial infections in Drosophila. J Immunol 168:1542–1546
Saijo S, Fujikado N, Furuta T, Chung SH, Kotaki H, Seki K, Sudo K, Akira S, Adachi Y, Ohno N, Kinjo T, Nakamura K, Kawakami K, Iwakura Y (2007) Dectin-1 is required for host defense against Pneumocystis carinii but not against Candida albicans. Nat Immunol 8:39–46
Salio M, Palmowski MJ, Atzberger A, Hermans IF, Cerundolo V (2004) CpG-matured murine plasmacytoid dendritic cells are capable of in vivo priming of functional CD8 T cell responses to endogenous but not exogenous antigens. J Exp Med 199:567–579
Sallusto F, Lanzavecchia A (1994) Efficient presentation of soluble antigen by cultured human dendritic cells is maintained by granulocyte/macrophage colony-stimulating factor plus interleukin 4 and downregulated by tumor necrosis factor alpha. J Exp Med 179: 1109–1118
Sallusto F, Palermo B, Lenig D, Miettinen M, Matikainen S, Julkunen I, Forster R, Burgstahler R, Lipp M, Lanzavecchia A (1999) Distinct patterns and kinetics of chemokine production regulate dendritic cell function. Eur J Immunol 29:1617–1625
Samuel CE (2001) Antiviral actions of interferons. Clin Microbiol Rev 14:778–809, table of contents

Scheinecker C, McHugh R, Shevach EM, Germain RN (2002) Constitutive presentation of a natural tissue autoantigen exclusively by dendritic cells in the draining lymph node. J Exp Med 196:1079–1090
Schulz O, Diebold SS, Chen M, Naslund TI, Nolte MA, Alexopoulou L, Azuma YT, Flavell RA, Liljestrom P, Reise Sousa C (2005) Toll-like receptor 3 promotes cross-priming to virus-infected cells. Nature 433:887–892
Schulz O, Edwards AD, Schito M, Aliberti J, Manickasingham S, Sher A, Reise Sousa C (2000) CD40 triggering of heterodimeric IL-12 p70 production by dendritic cells in vivo requires a microbial priming signal. Immunity 13:453–462
Schulz O, Reise Sousa C (2002) Cross-presentation of cell-associated antigens by CD8alpha+ dendritic cells is attributable to their ability to internalize dead cells. Immunology 107: 183–189
Schwandner R, Dziarski R, Wesche H, Rothe M, Kirschning CJ (1999) Peptidoglycan- and lipoteichoic acid-induced cell activation is mediated by toll-like receptor 2. J Biol Chem 274: 17406–17409
Seong SY, Matzinger P (2004) Hydrophobicity: an ancient damage-associated molecular pattern that initiates innate immune responses. Nat Rev Immunol 4:469–478
Shimazu R, Akashi S, Ogata H, Nagai Y, Fukudome K, Miyake K, Kimoto M (1999) MD-2, a molecule that confers lipopolysaccharide responsiveness on Toll-like receptor 4. J Exp Med 189:1777–1782
Shortman K, Liu YJ (2002) Mouse and human dendritic cell subtypes. Nat Rev Immunol 2: 151–161
Siegal FP, Kadowaki N, Shodell M, Fitzgerald-Bocarsly PA, Shah K, Ho S, Antonenko S, Liu YJ (1999) The nature of the principal type 1 interferon-producing cells in human blood. Science 284:1835–1837
Sioud M (2006) Innate sensing of self and non-self RNAs by Toll-like receptors. Trends Mol Med 12:167–176
Small M, Kraal G (2003) In vitro evidence for participation of DEC-205 expressed by thymic cortical epithelial cells in clearance of apoptotic thymocytes. Int Immunol 15:197–203
Soumelis V, Liu YJ (2006) From plasmacytoid to dendritic cell: morphological and functional switches during plasmacytoid pre-dendritic cell differentiation. Eur J Immunol 36: 2286–2292
Sporri R, Reise Sousa C (2005) Inflammatory mediators are insufficient for full dendritic cell activation and promote expansion of CD4+ T cell populations lacking helper function. Nat Immunol 6:163–170
Stetson DB, Medzhitov R (2006) Recognition of cytosolic DNA activates an IRF3-dependent innate immune response. Immunity 24:93–103
Takaoka A, Wang Z, Choi MK, Yanai H, Negishi H, Ban T, Lu Y, Miyagishi M, Kodama T, Honda K, Ohba Y, Taniguchi T (2007) DAI (DLM-1/ZBP1) is a cytosolic DNA sensor and an activator of innate immune response. Nature 448:501–505
Takaoka A, Yanai H, Kondo S, Duncan G, Negishi H, Mizutani T, Kano S, Honda K, Ohba Y, Mak TW, Taniguchi T (2005) Integral role of IRF-5 in the gene induction programme activated by Toll-like receptors. Nature 434:243–249
Takeuchi O, Hoshino K, Kawai T, Sanjo H, Takada H, Ogawa T, Takeda K, Akira S (1999a) Differential roles of TLR2 and TLR4 in recognition of gram-negative and gram-positive bacterial cell wall components. Immunity 11:443–451
Takeuchi O, Kawai T, Muhlradt PF, Morr M, Radolf JD, Zychlinsky A, Takeda K, Akira S (2001) Discrimination of bacterial lipoproteins by Toll-like receptor 6. Int Immunol 13:933–940
Takeuchi O, Kawai T, Sanjo H, Copeland NG, Gilbert DJ, Jenkins NA, Takeda K, Akira S (1999b) TLR6: A novel member of an expanding toll-like receptor family. Gene 231:59–65
Takeuchi O, Sato S, Horiuchi T, Hoshino K, Takeda K, Dong Z, Modlin RL, Akira S (2002) Cutting edge: role of Toll-like receptor 1 in mediating immune response to microbial lipoproteins. J Immunol 169:10–14

Tassaneetrithep B, Burgess TH, Granelli-Piperno A, Trumpfheller C, Finke J, Sun W, Eller MA, Pattanapanyasat K, Sarasombath S, Birx DL, Steinman RM, Schlesinger S, Marovich MA (2003) DC-SIGN (CD209) mediates dengue virus infection of human dendritic cells. J Exp Med 197:823–829

Tauszig-Delamasure S, Bilak H, Capovilla M, Hoffmann JA, Imler JL (2002) Drosophila MyD88 is required for the response to fungal and Gram-positive bacterial infections. Nat Immunol 3:91–97

Taylor KR, Trowbridge JM, Rudisill JA, Termeer CC, Simon JC, Gallo RL (2004) Hyaluronan fragments stimulate endothelial recognition of injury through TLR4. J Biol Chem 279: 17079–17084

Taylor PR, Tsoni SV, Willment JA, Dennehy KM, Rosas M, Findon H, Haynes K, Steele C, Botto M, Gordon S, Brown GD (2007) Dectin-1 is required for beta-glucan recognition and control of fungal infection. Nat Immunol 8:31–38

Termeer C, Benedix F, Sleeman J, Fieber C, Voith U, Ahrens T, Miyake K, Freudenberg M, Galanos C, Simon JC (2002) Oligosaccharides of Hyaluronan activate dendritic cells via toll-like receptor 4. J Exp Med 195:99–111

Uematsu S, Akira S (2006) Toll-like receptors and innate immunity. J Mol Med 84:712–725

Underhill DM, Ozinsky A, Hajjar AM, Stevens A, Wilson CB, Bassetti M, Aderem A (1999) The Toll-like receptor 2 is recruited to macrophage phagosomes and discriminates between pathogens. Nature 401:811–815

Underhill DM, Rossnagle E, Lowell CA, Simmons RM (2005) Dectin-1 activates Syk tyrosine kinase in a dynamic subset of macrophages for reactive oxygen production. Blood 106: 2543–2550

Vabulas RM, Ahmad-Nejad P, da Costa C, Miethke T, Kirschning CJ, Hacker H, Wagner H (2001) Endocytosed HSP60s use toll-like receptor 2 (TLR2) and TLR4 to activate the toll/interleukin-1 receptor signaling pathway in innate immune cells. J Biol Chem 276:31332–31339

Vabulas RM, Ahmad-Nejad P, Ghose S, Kirschning CJ, Issels RD, Wagner H (2002) HSP70 as endogenous stimulus of the Toll/interleukin-1 receptor signal pathway. J Biol Chem 277:15107–15112

Vremec D, Pooley J, Hochrein H, Wu L, Shortman K (2000) CD4 and CD8 expression by dendritic cell subtypes in mouse thymus and spleen. J Immunol 164: 2978–2986

Wang JP, Asher DR, Chan M, Kurt-Jones EA, Finberg RW (2007) Cutting Edge: Antibody-mediated TLR7-dependent recognition of viral RNA. J Immunol 178:3363–3367

West MA, Wallin RP, Matthews SP, Svensson HG, Zaru R, Ljunggren HG, Prescott AR, Watts C (2004) Enhanced dendritic cell antigen capture via toll-like receptor-induced actin remodeling. Science 305:1153–1157

Yamamoto M, Sato S, Hemmi H, Sanjo H, Uematsu S, Kaisho T, Hoshino K, Takeuchi O, Kobayashi M, Fujita T, Takeda K, Akira S (2002) Essential role for TIRAP in activation of the signalling cascade shared by TLR2 and TLR4. Nature 420:324–329

Yamamoto M, Sato S, Hemmi H, Uematsu S, Hoshino K, Kaisho T, Takeuchi O, Takeda K, Akira S (2003) TRAM is specifically involved in the Toll-like receptor 4-mediated MyD88-independent signaling pathway. Nat Immunol 4:1144–1150

Yarovinsky F, Zhang D, Andersen JF, Bannenberg GL, Serhan CN, Hayden MS, Hieny S, Sutterwala FS, Flavell RA, Ghosh S, Sher A (2005) TLR11 activation of dendritic cells by a protozoan profilin-like protein. Science 308:1626–1629

Yasuda K, Yu P, Kirschning CJ, Schlatter B, Schmitz F, Heit A, Bauer S, Hochrein H, Wagner H (2005) Endosomal translocation of vertebrate DNA activates dendritic cells via TLR9-dependent and -independent pathways. J Immunol 174:6129–6136

Yoneyama M, Kikuchi M, Matsumoto K, Imaizumi T, Miyagishi M, Taira K, Foy E, Loo YM, Gale M, Jr., Akira S, Yonehara S, Kato A, Fujita T (2005) Shared and unique functions of the DExD/H-box helicases RIG-I, MDA5, and LGP2 in antiviral innate immunity. J Immunol 175:2851–2858

Yoneyama M, Kikuchi M, Natsukawa T, Shinobu N, Imaizumi T, Miyagishi M, Taira K, Akira S, Fujita T (2004) The RNA helicase RIG-I has an essential function in double-stranded RNA-induced innate antiviral responses. Nat Immunol 5:730–737

Yoshimura A, Lien E, Ingalls RR, Tuomanen E, Dziarski R, Golenbock D (1999) Cutting edge: recognition of Gram-positive bacterial cell wall components by the innate immune system occurs via Toll-like receptor 2. J Immunol 163: 1–5

Zelensky AN, Gready JE (2005) The C-type lectin-like domain superfamily. Febs J 272:6179–217

Zhang D, Zhang G, Hayden MS, Greenblatt MB, Bussey C, Flavell RA, Ghosh S (2004) A toll-like receptor that prevents infection by uropathogenic bacteria. Science 303:1522–1526

Zuniga EI, McGavern DB, Pruneda-Paz JL, Teng C, Oldstone MB (2004) Bone marrow plasmacytoid dendritic cells can differentiate into myeloid dendritic cells upon virus infection. Nat Immunol 5:1227–1234

Dendritic Cell Migration to Peripheral Lymph Nodes

Alfonso Martín-Fontecha, Antonio Lanzavecchia, and Federica Sallusto

Contents

Abstract Dendritic cells are potent antigen-presenting cells endowed with the unique ability to prime T-cell responses. To present foreign antigens to naïve T cells, dendritic cells must migrate from inflamed or injured peripheral tissues to the closest draining lymph nodes through afferent lymphatic vessels. In addition, conventional dendritic cells, plasmacytoid dendritic cells and monocytes enter lymph nodes from blood crossing high endothelial venules. The selective migration of dendritic cells and their residence in non lymphoid as well as in lymphoid organs are tightly regulated events, whose molecular control is being unraveled rapidly. In this chapter, we review key aspects of what is known about dendritic cell traffic to peripheral nodes from tissues, in particular skin, and from blood. A better understanding of the regulation of dendritic cell migration for optimal priming of T-cell responses is essential for future advances in manipulating dendritic cell traffic as a means to improve immune responses in clinical settings.

A. Martín-Fontecha (✉)
King's College London and Guy's and St Thomas' Hospital, Department of Nephrology and Transplantation, School of Medicine, King's College London, UK
alfonso.martin-fontecha@kcl.ac.uk

G. Lombardi, Y. Riffo-Vasquez (eds.), *Dendritic Cells,* Handbook of Experimental Pharmacology 188,

1 Introduction

Dendritic cells (DCs) are unique antigen presenting cells owing to their capacity to acquire and process antigens, and their potential to express high levels of co-stimulatory molecules that trigger naïve T-cell activation (Banchereau and Steinman 1998). In addition, DCs induce immune responses by driving T-cell memory differentiation and polarization. Indeed, DCs transmit a distinct set of information to T cells, based on their state of differentiation or maturation, and these instructions determine different outcomes that range from Th1, Th2, Th17 effectors to memory and regulatory T-cell responses (Lanzavecchia and Sallusto 2001).

A crucial attribute of DCs at various differentiation stages is their mobility, which allows them to be present in the right place at the right time for regulation of immunity (Austyn et al. 1988). DC precursors migrate from bone marrow to all bodily tissues where they reside in an immature state to exert a sentinel function for incoming antigens, and they readily relocate to secondary lymphoid organs, particularly lymph nodes (LNs), to ensure an efficient encounter with naïve and with central memory T cells (T_{CM}) (Banchereau et al. 2000; Steinman et al. 2003). Chemokines are mediators of cell migration during steady state immune surveillance and inflammation. Chemokines bind to G protein–coupled receptors that trigger intracellular signaling pathways involved in cell movement and activation (Moser et al. 2004). Chemokines and chemokine receptors play a determinant role in the trafficking of DCs to LNs through afferent lymphatic vessels (Gunn et al. 1999; Martín-Fontecha et al. 2003; Ohl et al. 2004) and from blood (Diacovo et al. 2005; Yoneyama et al. 2004) and, thus, have become relevant targets for immune intervention (Proudfoot 2002).

The current model describes a linear route between antigen uptake in the periphery and T-cell priming in the LNs. This model is based primarily on observations of the migration of Langerhans cells (LCs) following administration of skin-sensitizing agents (Macatonia et al. 1987), carcinogens, or upon infection (Dandie et al. 1994; Merad et al. 2000). By applying sensitizers admixed with haptens and fluorescent molecules in the skin, it was possible to detect antigen-carrying DCs in draining LNs, where they initiate adaptive immune response (Ruedl et al. 2001; Stoitzner et al. 2003). Models of *Leishmania major* infection have shown that LCs take up *L. major* upon subcutaneous or intradermal infection and subsequently migrate to LNs to induce T-cell priming (Moll et al. 1993). Infection with other pathogens also induce a strong migration of DCs and their precursors from the blood stream, increasing antigen presentation capabilities in LNs. Thus, monocytes (Palframan et al. 2001), conventional DCs (Martin et al. 2002) and plasmacytoid DCs (PDCs) (Diacovo et al. 2005; Yoneyama et al. 2004) can gain access to peripheral LNs via high endothelial venules (HEVs) with subsequent impact on T cell-mediated responses.

Here, we will review what is known about the mechanisms that govern DC migration to subcutaneous LNs and the main regulation check points in the context of triggering T cell-mediated immune responses. A comprehensive view on how mucosal DCs integrate signals from the epithelial cells and other stromal cells, and migrate to mucosa-draining LNs to mount regulatory and stimulatory immune responses can be found in a recent review (Iwasaki 2007).

2 From Skin to Draining Lymph Nodes

The skin is the body's largest exposed interface with the environment and has evolved as a barrier to shield external pathogens from entering the body. DCs are strategically present near superficial surfaces like the skin to initiate immune defense responses when pathogens succeed in breaching peripheral barriers. Well-known examples of skin resident DCs are LCs, a subset of immature DCs settled in the epidermis, and dermal DCs (dDCs) in the dermis (Caux et al. 2000). On their way from the epidermis, LCs must cross the basement membrane and move through connective tissue until they reach a lymph vessel, which they enter to travel further to the draining LNs. The pathway through the collagenous connective tissue is the same for dDCs. Proteinases are, therefore, important for DC migration, particularly when these cells must pass relatively solid tissues such as basement membranes. Matrix metalloproteinases (MMPs) constitute a family of proteinases (including collagenases) that participate in cell migration (Salmi and Jalkanen 2005). MMPs may be expressed on the surface of cells, thus allowing for precise, localized proteolysis that creates a path for migrating cells (Murphy and Gavrilovic 1999). MMP-9 is expressed by epidermal LCs, up-regulated by inflammatory cytokines (TNF-α, IL-1β) (Saren et al. 1996) and it has been shown to be released following topical application of skin sensitizers (Kobayashi 1997). Further confirmation on the role of MMPs comes from experiments, where the migration of both LCs and dDCs was prevented by broad spectrum MMP inhibitors (BB-3103), by antibodies to MMP-9 and MMP-2, and by the natural tissue inhibitors of metalloproteinases (TIMP), TIMP-1 and TIMP-2 (Ratzinger et al. 2002). In vivo evidence of the importance of extracellular matrix-DC interaction for migration stems from mice deficient for the secreted protein, acidic and rich in cysteine (SPARC). SPARC is a calcium-binding matricellular glycoprotein that binds a range of extracellular matrix components (Bradshaw et al. 2002). LCs and dDCs in SPARC-deficient and SPARC-sufficient mice show striking differences in terms of mobility to draining LNs (Sangaletti et al. 2005). Although similar numbers of LCs populate the ear skin of SPARC$^{-/-}$ and SPARC$^{+/+}$ mice, more LCs are found in the LNs draining antigen-sensitized ears of SPARC$^{-/-}$ mice and significantly more LCs migrate from null-mice-derived ear skin explants. Importantly, the increased DC migration had a profound influence on contact-induced, delayed type-hypersensitivity and naïve T-cell priming.

Enzymatic digestion of surrounding tissues is thus a critical step in the initiation of the complex process of DC relocation to LNs. However, DCs may be situated far away (millimeters) from the closest skin lymphatic vessel and targeting into lymph flow may be facilitated by additional guidance provided by chemokines. Based on the chemokine receptor expression profile of DCs, as well as on chemokines found to be expressed in the inflamed skin, it has been proposed that CCL22 (Campbell et al. 1999), CCL17 (Katou et al. 2001), CCL20 (Dieu-Nosjean et al. 2000), CXCL9, CXCL10, and CXCL11 (Flier et al. 2001) play an important role in recruiting bone marrow-derived immature DCs to these sites. Most of the receptors recognizing these chemokines are expressed on immature DCs, while mature DCs express chemokine receptors CCR7 and CXCR4, (Sallusto et al. 1998) indicating a role for CCL19, CCL21 and possibly CXCL12 in driving DC exit from sites of inflammation and migration to T-cell zones of draining LNs.

Most in vivo studies of DC migration are based either on models that induce some degree of inflammation of the skin (Thomas et al. 1980) or in settings in which bone marrow-derived DCs (BMDCs) are activated in vitro with inflammatory stimuli before in vivo transfer (Martín-Fontecha et al. 2003). These experimental conditions are known to trigger the maturation of skin LCs, dDCs and BMDCs. Nevertheless, tissue-derived DCs are also found in the draining LNs in the absence of an inflammatory event, suggesting a continuous migration of DCs, a process described as steady-state migration (Merad et al. 2002). A recent report has provided strong evidence that CCR7 is involved in the steady-state migration of skin DCs (Ohl et al. 2004), indicating that maturation and migration can be independently regulated events. In support of this idea, Geissman and colleagues found that LCs present in T-cell areas of skin-draining LNs of dermatopathic lymphadenitis patients were largely immature (Geissmann et al. 2002). Furthermore, in vitro–generated LCs maintained their immature phenotype when cultured in the presence of TGF-β1 and TNF-α, in spite of acquisition of CCR7 expression and responsiveness to LN homing chemokines.

Adoptive transfer experiments of in vitro generated CCR7-deficient BMDCs to normal CCR7-sufficient hosts (Martín-Fontecha et al. 2003) it have shown that upon inflammation, DCs need to express CCR7 to migrate efficiently to LNs. Transfer of CCR7-deficient BMDCs resulted in the recovery of less than one-tenth the number of DCs from draining LNs compared with transfer of CCR7$^+$ DCs. Further, FITC-bearing skin-derived, CD11c$^+$ MHCII^{high} cells are absent in the draining LN after skin sensitization of CCR7-deficient mice (Ohl et al. 2004). Together, these data provide strong evidence to suggest that CCR7 is involved in recruiting LCs as well as other skin-derived DC into skin-draining LN under inflammatory conditions.

The genes encoding the CCR7 ligands CCL19 and CCL21 have been duplicated and modified during evolution such that there is now more than one gene encoding for each chemokine. In mice, there are two known functional genes that encode CCL21: CCL21Leu protein is expressed in the periphery by lymphatic vessels, while CCL21Ser is expressed in LNs, including lymphatic vessels in subcapsular sinus. It is not clear, however, which of these CCL21 gene products is expressed in skin lymphatic vessels. In contrast, functional CCL19 expression is restricted to mature DCs and to stromal cells in LNs. In a naturally occurring mouse mutant, the *plt/plt* (paucity of lymph-node T cells) mouse, some of the genes that encode CCL19 and the CCL21Ser variant are absent (Luther et al. 2000; Vassileva et al. 1999), while CCL21Leu is preserved. Consistent with a role for CCR7 ligands in DC trafficking, a number of laboratories have reported impaired DC migration to LNs in *plt/plt* mice after FITC painting (Gunn et al. 1999), lipopolysaccharide administration (Yoshino et al. 2003) or injection of microsphers (Qu et al. 2004). Although appealing, the hypothesis that lymphatic-vessel expression of CCR7 ligands guides DCs towards these vessels for subsequent entry has not yet been formally proven. When DCs become activated for maturation and migration, they begin to secrete CCL19 (Sallusto et al. 1999). Hence, it is possible that DCs, in addition to following chemokine gradients to move, might use autocrine CCR7-dependent mechanisms to migrate towards lymphatics and LNs. A recent study proposed that CCR8 and its cognate ligand CCL1 are also involved in the emigration of mouse monocyte-derived DC from the skin. Considering the anatomical expression of CCL1 in the subcapsule of LNs, it is possible that, in addition to CCR7/CCL21Leu interactions, the CCL1/CCR8 pair may function downstream the entry of DCs into the lymphatic vessel by regulating the exit from the afferent terminals towards the subcapsular sinus of LNs.

The relevance of intracytoplasmic events, including chemotactic receptor signaling, on DC migration has been clearly documented in mice, lacking the gamma isoform of phosphoinositide-3 kinase (PI3Kγ). PI3Kγ is located downstream of seven trans-membrane chemotatic receptors, and plays a non redundant role in cell responses to chemotatic agonists. DCs from PI3Kγ deficient mice show a profound migration defect both in vivo and in vitro settings in response to chemokines, and this defect is associated with a defective ability to mount antigen specific T-cell responses (Del Prete et al. 2004). Cytoskeletal rearrangements in LCs are also critical for determining LC ability to dislodge and transmigrate. For example, epidermal LCs deficient in the Wiskott–Aldrich syndrome protein (WASp) show impaired migration to LNs following contact sensitization (de Noronha et al. 2005). Importantly, the observed impaired migration of in vitro generated WASp deficient DCs when transferred into wild type C57BL/6 mice was associated with a reduced capacity to prime CD4 and CD8 T cells in vivo (Bouma et al. 2007).

Consistent with a requirement for molecular interactions between DCs and the skin lymphatic endothelium, some data point to a role for intercellular adhesion molecule 1 (ICAM-1) expressed by a peripheral cell type, namely lymphatic endothelial cells, in mediating the migration of DCs to LNs (Ma et al. 1994; Xu et al. 2001). Also JAM-1 (junctional adhesion molecule 1), an adhesion molecule expressed by DCs and by the lymphatic endothelium, affects DC mobility since the absence of JAM-1 expression in DCs facilitates their migration to LNs (Cera et al. 2004).

3 From Blood to Lymph Nodes

It has become widely accepted that the trafficking of naïve T and B cells from blood stream into peripheral LNs is controlled by a sequence of at least three distinct adhesion and signaling events (Butcher and Picker 1996; Springer 1994; von Andrian and Mackay 2000). A slow rolling step along the vessel follows an initial tethering that allows leukocytes to bind to endothelial cells. Chemotactic stimuli from the endothelium engage and trigger specific chemokine receptors on the surface of the rolling lymphocyte, a step that, in turn, induces intracellular signals leading to conformational changes on endothelium integrins. This results in firm adhesion, which enables cells to emigrate through the vessel wall (von Andrian and Mempel 2003).

Intravital microscopy (IVM) has been instrumental in defining the molecular mechanisms behind adhesion cascades that mediate T-cell homing to LNs (Stein et al. 2000; Warnock et al. 1998). Tethering and rolling are mediated by L-selectin (CD62L); the endothelial L-selectin ligand is PNAd, an O-linked carbohydrate moiety, the main components of which are recognized by the monoclonal antibody MECA-79 (Streeter et al. 1988). Stick of naive and central memory T cells to HEVs is mediated by the CCL21 chemokine which is constitutively expressed by HEVs and binds to CCR7 (Gunn et al. 1999). The second CCR7 agonist, CCL19, is expressed by the lymphatic endothelium and interstitial cells in LNs, but not by HEVs. Nonetheless, perivascular CCL19 can be transported to the luminal surface of HEVs and induce integrin activation on rolling T cells (Baekkevold et al. 2001). The relative contribution of CCL19 versus CCL21 in T-cell homing has remained elusive, but some clues will likely be provided in the near future as a result of the recent development of CCL19 deficient but CCL21 sufficient mice (Link et al. 2007). Firm arrest of sticking T cells is mediated by the integrin leukocyte function-associated antigen 1 (LFA-1), which interacts with ICAM-1 and ICAM-2 on HEVs (Hamann et al. 1988).

Currently available data support the concept that the extravasation of DCs into peripheral LNs follows the same rules as those described for naïve T and B cells, with a major role for selectins, chemokine receptors and integrins. The mechanisms for conventional DC precursor recruitment during inflammatory responses was addressed by Ardavín and colleagues (Martin et al. 2002) in a model of infection with the mouse mammary tumor virus MMTV. The authors reported a strong increase of blood-borne CD8 DCs in peripheral LNs following subcutaneous administration of MMTV. This dramatic increase was prevented in mice that were injected with anti-L-selectin antibodies, suggesting that DC precursor recruitment occur via HEVs. Furthermore, conventional, blood borne-DCs have also been found in resting LNs (Ruedl et al. 2000), indicating that, in the steady state a continuous migration of circulating DC precursors may occur, although the molecular requirements for entry in these conditions remain to be established.

PDC represent a rare subset of DCs present in blood and in secondary lymphoid organs (Colonna et al. 2004), that have the extraordinary capacity to produce high amounts of type I interferons following viral infections (Cella et al. 1999). PDCs express several adhesion molecules and chemokine receptors on their surface that could promote interactions with HEVs and support their migration from the blood into peripheral LNs. Indeed, L-selectin is constitutively expressed on these cells, and may play a role in PDC migration to secondary lymphoid organs, as the number of PDCs in non inflamed LNs of L-selectin-deficient mice is reduced compared to controls (Nakano et al. 2001). However, in vivo experiments have shown that blockade of L-selectin inhibits mobilization of PDC precursors in the circulation, but not their migration across HEVs (Yoneyama et al. 2004). Concerning the role of particular chemokine receptors in this process, it was initially proposed to be solely dependent on CXCR3 (Yoneyama et al. 2004). However, other chemokine receptors, such as CCR5, known to regulate PDC trafficking into sites of inflammation (Penna et al. 2001) may also regulate PDC migration to inflamed LNs. Diacovo and colleagues used IVM to study the behavior of murine PDCs in the microvasculature of subiliac LNs in the absence or presence of an inflammatory stimulus. The results of this study provided the first direct evidence that PDCs can emigrate from the blood into peripheral LNs by interacting with HEVs through a coordinated multistep process. The authors showed that PDCs rolled on HEVs of resting LNs but little transmigration was observed. They also demonstrated that entry into activated LNs was dependent upon the expression of E-selectin on LNs and, in contrast to previous studies (Yoneyama et al. 2004), of CCR5 on PDCs. Discrepancies may relate to the use of different adjuvants that may deliver different signals to draining LNs and the expression of a different set of chemokines on HEVs.

4 Dendritic Cell Localization Within Lymph Nodes

The visualization of DC behavior within LNs through the use of two photon microscopy has advanced our understanding of DC function in the context of triggering T-cell responses (Celli et al. 2007). Nonetheless, this powerful technique has not allowed the identification of the precise route followed by DCs to migrate from the subcapsular sinus to the T-cell zone of the LN cortex. Although mouse LNs are thought to be simple with regard to lymphatic-vessel entry, a great complexity of interstitial lymphatic-vessel structure in mouse LNs has been appreciated and gained much interest in recent years (Gretz et al. 1997; Sixt et al. 2005). Whether migrating DCs use such structures connecting the subcapsular sinus to perivenular spaces around HEVs in order to relocate into deeper areas of the LNs is presently unknown.

Initial studies indicated that DCs migrating from nearby tissues primarily relocate to areas next to HEVs for efficient encounter with naïve T cells. The immune system may have developed this strategy to optimize encounter of rare antigen-specific T cells and DCs presenting the relevant antigen. Indeed, by using confocal microscopy, Bajenoff and colleagues (Bajenoff et al. 2003) showed, that DCs that have picked up antigens within the skin are preferentially located in the vicinity of HEVs, and that most antigen-specific T cells passing the HEVs are selectively trapped by the relevant DCs (Bajenoff et al. 2003). A more detailed picture in the interstitial localization of different subsets of tissue-derived DCs within LNs comes from recent work by B. Malissen's group (Kissenpfennig et al. 2005). In order to track and discriminate LCs from dermal DCs in vivo, this group developed knockin mice expressing enhanced green fluorescent protein (EGFP) under the control of the langerin (CD207) gene. The study showed that most EGFP$^+$ LCs were sessile under steady-state conditions, whereas skin inflammation induced LC motility and emigration to LNs. After epicutaneous painting, dDCs and LCs were not evenly intermingled in the paracortex of draining LNs. They occupied distinct, contiguous areas within this T cell-rich zone suggesting the existence of a previously unrecognized microanatomy of the paracortex of LNs. Whether these distinct locations confer LC-derived DCs and dDCs the ability to encounter distinct T-cell subsets remains to be established.

Refined studies using two-photon microscopy have also revealed that DC micromotility within LNs is a critical step for efficient T-cell priming (Bousso and Robey 2003; Celli et al. 2007). By using transgenic mice in which all DCs expressed enhanced yellow fluorescent protein (EYFP) controlled by the CD11c promoter, Lindquist and colleagues studied the behavior of endogenous and adoptively transferred DCs (Lindquist et al. 2004). Most endogenous DCs in the network were involved in continuous probing movements toward T cells, but did not change position and thus seem to be sessile. The dynamics of DC migration into the LNs from peripheral tissue were studied by intradermal injection of DCs marked with green fluorescent protein. It was shown that injected DCs moved faster than resident DCs, and were found mainly at the boundary between the T and B cell zone. Subsequently, these cells became progressively dispersed into the resident network and lost motility by 2–3 days after transfer. The authors proposed a model whereby the initial motility of DCs mainly serves the function of dispersing the cells in the network rather than in promoting encounters with T cells.

A recent study by Bajenoff et al. (2006) has provided evidence that the fibroblastic reticular cell network essentially defines and supports the apparent random walk movement of naive T cells within the LN paracortex. Importantly, CCR7 ligands immobilized on fibroblastic reticular cells or extracellular matrix surfaces, rather than soluble chemokines, mediate the observed CCR7-dependent induction of intranodal T-cell motility (Worbs et al. 2007). Whether similar mechanisms are used by DCs, and whether the contribution of CCL21 and CCL19 on guiding DCs in T-cell areas is redundant, is not clear at present.

5 Regulation of Dendritic Cell Migration to Lymph Nodes

DC migration in vivo is a tightly regulated process controlled at different levels. Primarily, much attention has been paid to the production of chemokines and the expression of relevant chemokine receptors, yet modulation of certain selectins on HEVs and structural changes on stimulated LNs may also affect DC migration. A dramatic change in the repertoire of chemokine receptors is promoted by Toll-like receptor (TLR)-mediated stimulation of DCs (Sallusto et al. 1998), including the upregulation of CCR7. Exogenous administration of the TLR-4 agonist LPS promotes in vivo mobilization of DCs from the periphery within a few hours (De Smedt et al. 1996; Ruedl et al. 2000), and mice treated with neutralizing antibodies to IL-1 or TNF show an impaired migration of DCs (De Smedt et al. 1996). Activation of DCs is also associated with down-regulation of inflammatory chemokine receptors to facilitate unidirectional migration towards draining LNs and release from the inflammatory site.

Although the expression of CCR7 is necessary for the migration of tissue resident DC to draining LNs, it is not sufficient, as this chemokine receptor can be expressed in a biologically inactive state resulting in failure to undergo chemotaxis towards CCR7 ligands (Scandella et al. 2002) or requiring a high concentration of CCR7 ligands (Robbiani et al. 2000). Signals found at sites of inflammation, including the lipid mediators leukotrienes and prostaglandin E2 (Robbiani et al. 2000; Scandella et al. 2002), and the ADP-ribosyl cyclase CD38 (Partida-Sanchez et al. 2004), sensitize CCR7 to CCL19 and CCL21 (Scandella et al. 2004).

P- and E-selectins are transiently expressed in non lymphoid tissues following stimulation with a variety of inflammatory stimuli (Ley 2003). P- and E-selectin ligands are fucosylated oligosaccharides expressed by several proteins such as P-selectin glycoprotein ligand-1 (PSGL-1) that enable a rapid traffic of effector T cells to injured tissues to control pathogen spread (Agace 2006). Adoptive transfer of fluorescently-labeled wild type PDCs into E-selectin-sufficient or into E-selectin-deficient mice showed that transmigration of PDCs to LNs was E-selectin-dependent (Diacovo et al. 2005), suggesting that acutely stimulated LNs undergo changes in HEVs that result in recruitment of PDCs.

DC migration can also be regulated indirectly. For instance, lymphatic vessel structure within LNs is not static, and lymphatic vessel expansion directly correlates with alterations in the magnitude of DC accumulation in LNs (Angeli et al. 2006). Indeed, Angeli and colleagues reported that B cell-derived signals produced in activated draining LNs, i.e. VGEF-A, increased the migration of skin DCs. Thus, mobilization of DCs to LNs can be regulated by signals initiated within LNs themselves. In line with the idea of an indirect check point control we found that inflammatory stimuli present in the skin influence DC migration not only by modulating the expression of CCR7 by DCs, but also through up-regulation of CCL21 which is induced by TNF and IL-1β (Fig. 1) (Martín-Fontecha et al. 2003).

One alternative recruitment pathway for increased migration of monocytes to peripheral LNs via HEVs involves the transport of inflammatory chemokines from skin to draining LNs. Palframan and colleagues showed that inhibition of monocyte chemoattractant protein-1 (MCP-1, CCL2) blocked this inflammation-induced monocyte homing to LNs (Palframan et al. 2001). They reported that CCL2 mRNA in inflamed skin was over 100-fold upregulated and paralleled by CCL2 protein levels, whereas in draining LNs CCL2 mRNA induction was much weaker and occurred only after a pronounced rise in CCL2 protein expression, suggesting that CCL2 in draining LNs was primarily derived from inflamed skin. In CCL2-deficient mice, intracutaneously injected CCL2 accumulated rapidly in the draining LNs, where it enhanced monocyte recruitment. IVM showed that skin-derived CCL2 was transported via the lymph to the luminal surface of HEVs, where it triggered integrin-dependent arrest of rolling monocytes. These findings demonstrate that inflamed peripheral tissues project their local chemokine profile to HEVs in draining LNs, and thereby exerting *remote control* over the composition of leukocyte populations that home to these organs from the blood.

Pathogens, in their quest for survival, have evolved several ways to escape immunity eventually by subverting DC function, especially through the manipulation

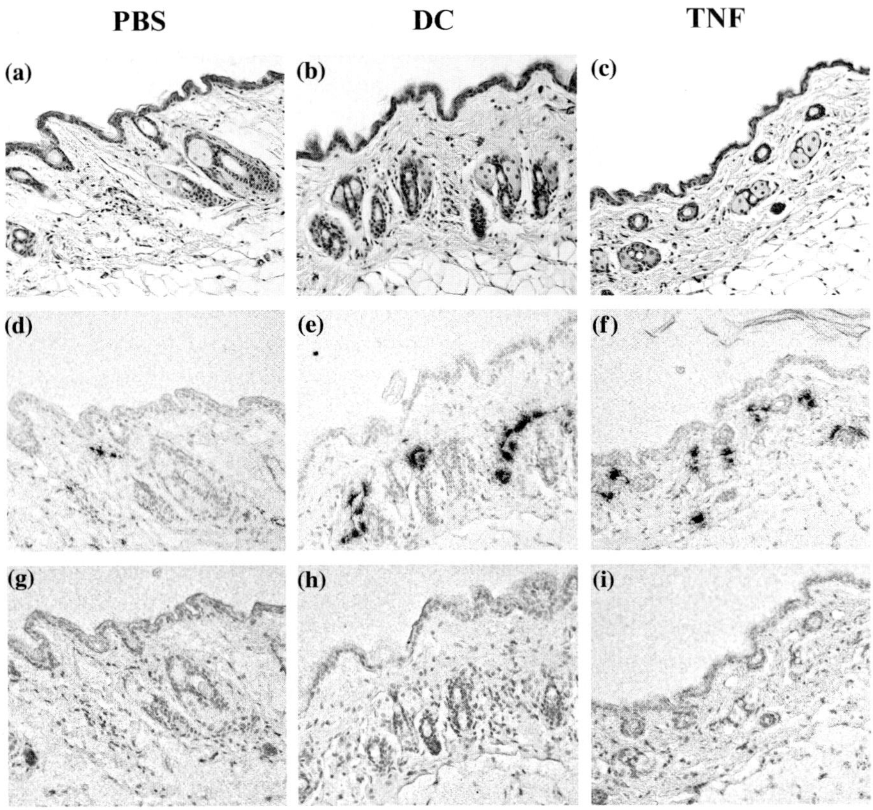

Fig. 1 CCL21 is up-regulated on lymphatic endothelial cells after injection of mature DCS or TNF. Mice were injected intradermally with PBS, 10^5 syngeneic dcs, or 10 ng TNF. 8 h later, skin samples were collected and embedded in paraffin. Serial sections were stained with hematoxylin and eosin **(a)**–**(c)**, or hybridized with antisense **(d)**–**(f)** or sense (inset) ^{35}S-labeled CCL21 riboprobe or stained with a polyclonal antibody to mouse CCL21 **(g)**–**(i)**. X20. This figure is reproduced with the kind permission of the *Journal of Experimental Medicine*. (Martín-Fontecha et al. 2003, Copyright 2003. Rockefeller University Press)

of pathogen-recognition receptors (PRRs), and also by modulating DC migration. A number of studies have indeed appreciated that many viruses, including MMTV (Martin et al. 2002), Rauscher leukaemia virus (RLV) (Gabrilovich et al. 1994), simian immunodeficiency virus (SIV) (Barratt-Boyes et al. 2002), human cytomegalovirus (HCMV) (Moutaftsi et al. 2004) and herpes simplex virus (Prechtel et al. 2005) have found ways to inhibit DC migration to draining LNs. Although the mechanisms for such control is not clear, adhesion molecules like ICAM-1 and CD44 (Gabrilovich et al. 1994) and chemokines (Moutaftsi et al. 2004; Prechtel et al. 2005) may be targets for viral control of DC mobilization.

6 Dendritic Cells-Based Vaccines Against Cancer

Recent advances have been made in understanding DC biology, in the context of prevention and therapy of immune disorders (Steinman and Banchereau 2007). In particular, ex vivo generated cancer vaccines based on DCs are currently applied in the clinic (Banchereau and Palucka 2005). DC migration must be taken into consideration in order to improve strategies to deliver such immunological tools into sites of T-cell priming for induction of an antitumour immune response (Tacken et al. 2007). Indeed, mouse studies show that DC migration directly correlates with the extent of T-cell proliferation and effector cell differentiation (Martín-Fontecha et al. 2003). Therefore, efforts to enhance the delivery of ex vivo generated DCs into LNs of cancer patients might prove to be beneficial. Several clinical trials have been carried out or are in progress to determine the efficacy of therapeutic vaccines that use ex vivo-matured DCs as the main component.

The discovery that DCs can be generated from monocytes in the presence of granulocyte-macrophage colony-stimulating factor and interleukin-4 boosted the clinical application of monocyte-derived DCs (moDCs) (Sallusto and Lanzavecchia 1994). Recently completed patient trials, applying 111-indium labeled moDC as cancer vaccines, revealed that although immature moDCs migrate much less than mature moDCs in vivo, in general less than 5% of intradermally administered mature moDCs reach the draining LNs (De Vries et al. 2003). Data from mouse models employing ex vivo generated BMDCs labeled with either 111-indium or carboxyfluorescein diacetate succinimidyl ester (CFSE) and BMDCs endogenously expressing green fluorescent protein revealed, that DC migration from the intradermal injection site is in the same efficiency range (Eggert et al. 2003; Martín-Fontecha et al. 2003).

In addition to the intradermal injection of DCs, alternative routes of administration have been explored in both mice and humans. In mice, intravenous injection of DCs resulted in the accumulation of DCs in the spleen, as expected (Eggert et al. 1999). Nevertheless, a few but detectable DCs can be found in peripheral LNs in mice following i.v. injection (Cavanagh et al. 2005). Also, we have observed that following i.v. injection of high numbers of OVA-loaded LPS-matured DCs, antigen-specific DO11.10 CD4 T cells were primed in peripheral LNs (Fig. 2; AMF, unpublished observation). To exclude that CD4 T cells were primed in spleen and emigrated to peripheral LNs, we also analyzed the activation of CD4 T cells in mice that were splenectomized (spleen-X) before transfer of DCs i.v. Figure 3 (AMF, unpublished observation) shows a similar CFSE profile in CD4 T cells in LNs whether antigen-loaded DCs were transferred in spleen-X mice or control mice, suggesting that CD4 T cells were primed in LNs. Although we cannot formally rule out that mature DCs injected i.v. migrated to LNs from afferent lymphatics, the fact that the CFSE profile is essentially the same in the LNs of spleen-X mice and control mice suggest that, under certain circumstances, DCs may gain access to peripheral LNs across HEVs and prime T cells. As CD62L is not expressed by ex vivo generated DCs (Robert et al. 2003), the molecular requirements governing DC extravasation from blood remain unknown. In human trials, DC migration following intravenous injection has so far not been monitored. Alternative strategies that are currently

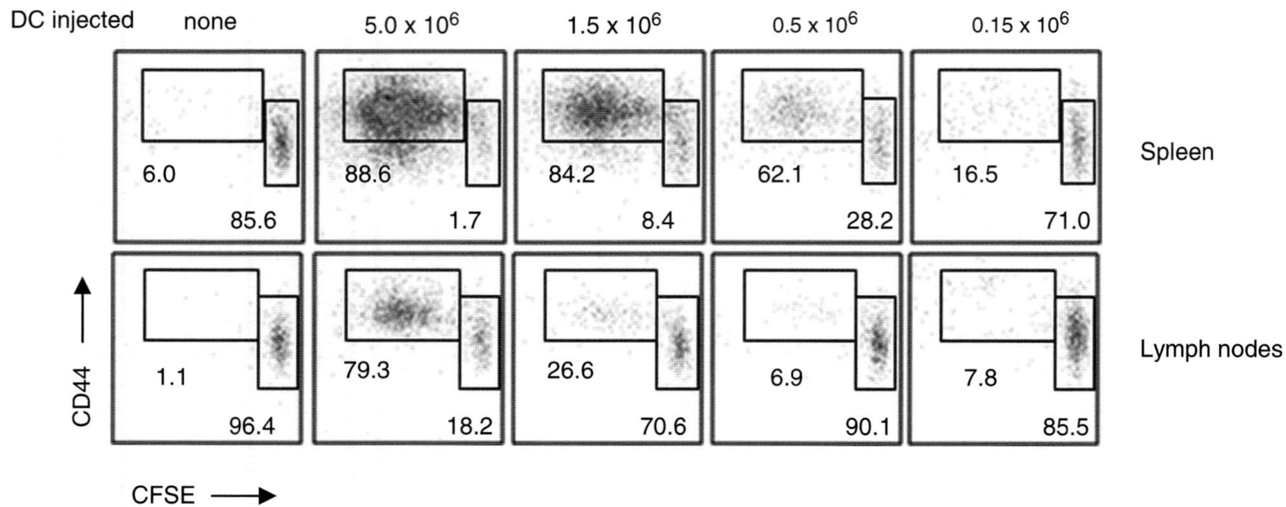

Fig. 2 Antigen carrying DC injected i.v. prime CD4 T cells in subcutaneous lymph nodes. 3×10^6 naïve rag2 −/− DO11.10 CD4 T cells were labeled with CFSE and adoptively transferred into syngeneic BALB/c mice. Mice were primed by increasing numbers of $OVA_{323-339}$-pulsed LPS-matured DCS injected i.v. Shown are the expression of CD44 and the CFSE profiles of $CD4^+/KJ1.26^+$ cells in spleen and subcutaneous lymph nodes three days after priming. Numbers represent the percentage within the indicated gates

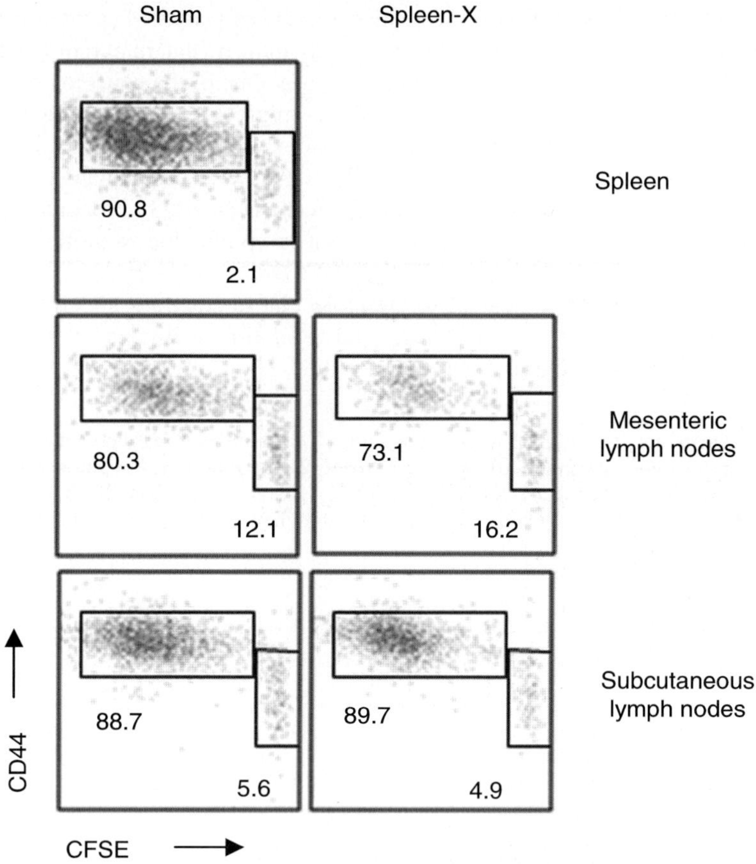

Fig. 3 CD4 T cells are primed in subcutaneous lymph nodes in splenectomized mice. 3×10^6 naïve rag2 −/− DO11.10 CD4 T cells were labeled with CFSE and adoptively transferred into syngeneic BALB/c mice. Mice were splenectomized (Spleen-X) or sham operated and primed by an i.v. injection of 5×10^6 $OVA_{323-339}$-pulsed LPS-matured DCS. Shown are the expression of CD44 and the CFSE profiles of $CD4^+/KJ1.26^+$ cells in spleen and subcutaneous lymph nodes three days after priming. Numbers represent the percentage within the indicated gates

employed to facilitate DC migration following intradermal injection include pretreatment of the vaccine injection site with inflammatory cytokines such as TNF-α (Martín-Fontecha et al. 2003). Similarly, pretreatment with TLR ligands is used to induce an inflammatory environment to improve DC migration (Nair et al. 2003).

An alternative approach that circumvents the skin migration problem involves the direct injection of DCs into the LNs (Jonuleit et al. 2001; Nestle et al. 1998). Although intranodal injection may destroy the architecture of the injected node, migration to subsequent nodes has been observed and follows the physiological path through lymph vessels. Therefore, intranodal versus intradermal administration of peptide-loaded DC vaccines remains to be explored in much more detail, including the quality of the induced T-cell response.

Several studies in which DC vaccination of cancer patients has been explored demonstrate that DC vaccines are safe, and clearly indicate that maturation of DCs is mandatory to induce an effective immune response. One of the concerns relating to ex vivo generated DCs is, how to ensure effective migration to the T-cell areas in the LN. In this context, enhancement of migration of ex vivo generated DC vaccines by pre-*conditioning* peripheral tissue like the skin with either inflammatory cytokines or TLR agonists is worth pursuing (Martín-Fontecha et al. 2003). Preclinical studies also suggest that multiple routes of vaccination are preferable to induce systemic immunity.

In summary a deeper knowledge of the molecular interactions underpinning DC migration may enable us to better understand regulation of immune responses and to better use DCs in the clinical setting.

Acknowledgements The original work in the authors' laboratories was supported by the Swiss National Science Foundation (31-101962 and 31-109832), the European Commission FP6 'Network of Excellence' initiative (N. LSHG-CT-2003-502935 MAIN, LSHB-CT-2004-512074 DC-THERA and LSHG-CT-2005-005203 MUGEN), and the Helmut Horten Foundation (for the Institute for Research in Biomedicine).

References

Agace WW (2006) Tissue-tropic effector T cells: generation and targeting opportunities. Nat Rev 6:682–692

Angeli V, Ginhoux F, Llodra J, Quemeneur L, Frenette PS, Skobe M, Jessberger R, Merad M, Randolph GJ (2006) B cell-driven lymphangiogenesis in inflamed lymph nodes enhances dendritic cell mobilization. Immunity 24:203–215

Austyn JM, Kupiec-Weglinski JW, Hankins DF, Morris PJ (1988) Migration patterns of dendritic cells in the mouse. Homing to T cell-dependent areas of spleen, and binding within marginal zone. J Exp Med 167:646–651

Baekkevold ES, Yamanaka T, Palframan RT, Carlsen HS, Reinholt FP, von Andrian UH, Brandtzaeg P, Haraldsen G (2001) The CCR7 ligand elc (CCL19) is transcytosed in high endothelial venules and mediates T cell recruitment. J Exp Med 193:1105–1112

Bajenoff M, Granjeaud S, Guerder S (2003) The strategy of T cell antigen-presenting cell encounter in antigen-draining lymph nodes revealed by imaging of initial T cell activation. J Exp Med 198:715–724

Bajenoff M, Egen JG, Koo LY, Laugier JP, Brau F, Glaichenhaus N, Germain RN (2006) Stromal cell networks regulate lymphocyte entry, migration, and territoriality in lymph nodes. Immunity 25:989–1001

Banchereau J, Palucka AK (2005) Dendritic cells as therapeutic vaccines against cancer. Nat Rev 5:296–306

Banchereau J, Steinman RM (1998) Dendritic cells and the control of immunity. Nature 392: 245–252

Banchereau J, Briere F, Caux C, Davoust J, Lebecque S, Liu YJ, Pulendran B, Palucka K (2000) Immunobiology of dendritic cells. Annu Rev Immunol 18:767–811

Barratt-Boyes SM, Zimmer MI, Harshyne L (2002) Changes in dendritic cell migration and activation during SIV infection suggest a role in initial viral spread and eventual immunosuppression. J Med Primatol 31:186–193

Bouma G, Burns S, Thrasher AJ (2007) Impaired T cell priming in vivo resulting from dysfunction of WASp-deficient dendritic cells. Blood 110:4278–4284

Bousso P, Robey E (2003) Dynamics of CD8 + T cell priming by dendritic cells in intact lymph nodes. Nat Immunol 4:579–585

Bradshaw AD, Reed MJ, Sage EH (2002) SPARC-null mice exhibit accelerated cutaneous wound closure. J Histochem Cytochem 50:1–10

Butcher EC, Picker LJ (1996) Lymphocyte homing and homeostasis. Science (New York, N.Y) 272:60–66

Campbell JJ, Haraldsen G, Pan J, Rottman J, Qin S, Ponath P, Andrew DP, Warnke R, Ruffing N, Kassam N, et al (1999) The chemokine receptor CCR4 in vascular recognition by cutaneous but not intestinal memory T cells. Nature 400:776–780

Caux C, Ait-Yahia S, Chemin K, de Bouteiller O, Dieu-Nosjean MC, Homey B, Massacrier C, Vanbervliet B, Zlotnik A, Vicari A (2000) Dendritic cell biology and regulation of dendritic cell trafficking by chemokines. Springer Semin Immunopathol 22:345–369

Cavanagh LL, Bonasio R, Mazo IB, Halin C, Cheng G, van der Velden AW, Cariappa A, Chase C, Russell P, Starnbach MN, et al (2005) Activation of bone marrow-resident memory T cells by circulating, antigen-bearing dendritic cells. Nat Immunol 6:1029–1037

Cella M, Jarrossay D, Facchetti F, Alebardi O, Nakajima H, Lanzavecchia A, Colonna M (1999) Plasmacytoid monocytes migrate to inflamed lymph nodes and produce large amounts of type I interferon. Nat Med 5:919–923

Celli S, Lemaitre F, Bousso P (2007) Real-Time Manipulation of T Cell-Dendritic Cell Interactions In Vivo Reveals the Importance of Prolonged Contacts for CD4(+) T Cell Activation. Immunity 27:625–634

Cera MR, Del Prete A, Vecchi A, Corada M, Martin-Padura I, Motoike T, Tonetti P, Bazzoni G, Vermi W, Gentili F, et al (2004) Increased DC trafficking to lymph nodes and contact hypersensitivity in junctional adhesion molecule-A-deficient mice. J Clin Investig 114:729–738

Colonna M, Trinchieri G, Liu YJ (2004) Plasmacytoid dendritic cells in immunity. Nat Immunol 5:1219–1226

Dandie GW, Watkins FY, Ragg SJ, Holloway PE, Muller HK (1994) The migration of Langerhans' cells into and out of lymph nodes draining normal, carcinogen and antigen-treated sheep skin. Immunol Cell Biol 72:79–86

de Noronha S, Hardy S, Sinclair J, Blundell MP, Strid J, Schulz O, Zwirner J, Jones GE, Katz DR, Kinnon C, Thrasher AJ (2005) Impaired dendritic-cell homing in vivo in the absence of Wiskott-Aldrich syndrome protein. Blood 105:1590–1597

De Smedt T, Pajak B, Muraille E, Lespagnard L, Heinen E, De Baetselier P, Urbain J, Leo O, Moser M (1996) Regulation of dendritic cell numbers and maturation by lipopolysaccharide in vivo. J Exp Med 184:1413–1424

De Vries IJ, Krooshoop DJ, Scharenborg NM, Lesterhuis WJ, Diepstra JH, Van Muijen GN, Strijk SP, Ruers TJ, Boerman OC, Oyen WJ, et al (2003) Effective migration of antigen-pulsed dendritic cells to lymph nodes in melanoma patients is determined by their maturation state. Cancer Res 63:12–17

Del Prete A, Vermi W, Dander E, Otero K, Barberis L, Luini W, Bernasconi S, Sironi M, Santoro A, Garlanda C, et al (2004) Defective dendritic cell migration and activation of adaptive immunity in PI3Kgamma-deficient mice. The EMBO J 23:3505–3515

Diacovo TG, Blasius AL, Mak TW, Cella M, Colonna M (2005) Adhesive mechanisms governing interferon-producing cell recruitment into lymph nodes. J Exp Med 202:687–69

Dieu-Nosjean MC, Massacrier C, Homey B, Vanbervliet B, Pin JJ, Vicari A, Lebecque S, Dezutter-Dambuyant C, Schmitt D, Zlotnik A, Caux C (2000) Macrophage inflammatory protein 3alpha is expressed at inflamed epithelial surfaces and is the most potent chemokine known in attracting Langerhans cell precursors. J Exp Med 192:705–718

Eggert AA, Schreurs MW, Boerman OC, Oyen WJ, de Boer AJ, Punt CJ, Figdor CG, Adema GJ (1999) Biodistribution and vaccine efficiency of murine dendritic cells are dependent on the route of administration. Cancer Res 59:3340–3345

Eggert AA, van der Voort R, Torensma R, Moulin V, Boerman OC, Oyen WJ, Punt CJ, Diepstra H, de Boer AJ, Figdor CG, Adema GJ (2003) Analysis of dendritic cell trafficking using EGFP-transgenic mice. Immunol Lett 89:17–24

Flier J, Boorsma DM, van Beek PJ, Nieboer C, Stoof TJ, Willemze R, Tensen CP (2001) Differential expression of CXCR3 targeting chemokines CXCL10, CXCL9, and CXCL11 in different types of skin inflammation. J Pathol 194:398–405

Gabrilovich DI, Woods GM, Patterson S, Harvey JJ, Knight SC (1994) Retrovirus-induced immunosuppression via blocking of dendritic cell migration and down-regulation of adhesion molecules. Immunology 82:82–87

Geissmann F, Dieu-Nosjean MC, Dezutter C, Valladeau J, Kayal S, Leborgne M, Brousse N, Saeland S, Davoust J (2002) Accumulation of immature Langerhans cells in human lymph nodes draining chronically inflamed skin. J Exp Med 196:417–430

Gretz JE, Anderson AO, Shaw S (1997) Cords, channels, corridors and conduits: critical architectural elements facilitating cell interactions in the lymph node cortex. Immunol Rev 156:11–24

Gunn MD, Kyuwa S, Tam C, Kakiuchi T, Matsuzawa A, Williams LT, Nakano H (1999) Mice lacking expression of secondary lymphoid organ chemokine have defects in lymphocyte homing and dendritic cell localization. J Exp Med 189:451–460

Hamann A, Jablonski-Westrich D, Duijvestijn A, Butcher EC, Baisch H, Harder R, Thiele HG (1988) Evidence for an accessory role of LFA-1 in lymphocyte-high endothelium interaction during homing. J Immunol 140:693–699

Iwasaki A (2007) Mucosal dendritic cells. Annu Rev Immunol 25:381–418

Jonuleit H, Giesecke-Tuettenberg A, Tuting T, Thurner-Schuler B, Stuge TB, Paragnik L, Kandemir A, Lee PP, Schuler G, Knop J, Enk AH (2001) A comparison of two types of dendritic cell as adjuvants for the induction of melanoma-specific T-cell responses in humans following intranodal injection. Int J Cancer 93:243–251

Katou F, Ohtani H, Nakayama T, Ono K, Matsushima K, Saaristo A, Nagura H, Yoshie O, Motegi K (2001) Macrophage-derived chemokine (MDC/CCL22) and CCR4 are involved in the formation of T lymphocyte-dendritic cell clusters in human inflamed skin and secondary lymphoid tissue. Am J Pathol 158:1263–1270

Kissenpfennig A, Ait-Yahia S, Clair-Moninot V, Stossel H, Badell E, Bordat Y, Pooley JL, Lang T, Prina E, Coste I, et al (2005) Disruption of the langerin/CD207 gene abolishes Birbeck granules without a marked loss of Langerhans cell function. Mol Cell Biol 25: 88–99

Kobayashi Y (1997) Langerhans' cells produce type IV collagenase (MMP-9) following epicutaneous stimulation with haptens. Immunology 90:496–501

Lanzavecchia A, Sallusto F (2001) The instructive role of dendritic cells on T cell responses: lineages, plasticity and kinetics. Curr opin Immunol 13:291–298

Ley K (2003) The role of selectins in inflammation and disease. Trends Mol Med 9:263–268

Lindquist RL, Shakhar G, Dudziak D, Wardemann H, Eisenreich T, Dustin ML, Nussenzweig MC (2004) Visualizing dendritic cell networks in vivo. Nat Immunol 5:1243–1250

Link A, Vogt TK, Favre S, Britschgi MR, Acha-Orbea H, Hinz B, Cyster JG, Luther SA (2007) Fibroblastic reticular cells in lymph nodes regulate the homeostasis of naive T cells. Nature immunology 8:1225–1265

Luther SA, Tang HL, Hyman PL, Farr AG, Cyster JG (2000) Coexpression of the chemokines ELC and SLC by T zone stromal cells and deletion of the ELC gene in the plt/plt mouse. Proc. Natl. Acad. Sci. USA 97:12694–12699

Ma J, Wang JH, Guo YJ, Sy MS, Bigby M (1994) In vivo treatment with anti-ICAM-1 and anti-LFA-1 antibodies inhibits contact sensitization-induced migration of epidermal Langerhans cells to regional lymph nodes. Cell Immunol 158:389–399

Macatonia SE, Knight SC, Edwards AJ, Griffiths S, Fryer P (1987) Localization of antigen on lymph node dendritic cells after exposure to the contact sensitizer fluorescein isothiocyanate. Functional and morphological studies. J Exp Med 166:1654–1667

Martín-Fontecha A, Sebastiani S, Hopken UE, Uguccioni M, Lipp M, Lanzavecchia A, Sallusto F (2003) Regulation of dendritic cell migration to the draining lymph node: impact on T lymphocyte traffic and priming. J Exp Med 198:615–621

Martin P, Ruiz SR, del Hoyo GM, Anjuere F, Vargas HH, Lopez-Bravo M, Ardavin C (2002) Dramatic increase in lymph node dendritic cell number during infection by the mouse mammary tumor virus occurs by a CD62L-dependent blood-borne DC recruitment. Blood 99:1282–1288
Merad M, Fong L, Bogenberger J, Engleman EG (2000) Differentiation of myeloid dendritic cells into CD8alpha-positive dendritic cells in vivo. Blood 96:1865–1872
Merad M, Manz MG, Karsunky H, Wagers A, Peters W, Charo I, Weissman IL, Cyster JG, Engleman EG (2002) Langerhans cells renew in the skin throughout life under steady-state conditions. Nature Immunol 3:1135–1141
Moll H, Fuchs H, Blank C, Rollinghoff M (1993) Langerhans cells transport Leishmania major from the infected skin to the draining lymph node for presentation to antigen-specific T cells. European J Immunol 23:1595–1601
Moser B, Wolf M, Walz A, Loetscher P (2004) Chemokines: multiple levels of leukocyte migration control. Trends Immunol 25:75–84
Moutaftsi M, Brennan P, Spector SA, Tabi Z (2004) Impaired lymphoid chemokine-mediated migration due to a block on the chemokine receptor switch in human cytomegalovirus-infected dendritic cells. Journal Virol 78:3046–3054
Murphy G, Gavrilovic J (1999) Proteolysis and cell migration: creating a path? Curr Opin Cell Biol 11:614–621
Nair S, McLaughlin C, Weizer A, Su Z, Boczkowski D, Dannull J, Vieweg J, Gilboa E (2003) Injection of immature dendritic cells into adjuvant-treated skin obviates the need for ex vivo maturation. J Immunol 171:6275–6282
Nakano H, Yanagita M, Gunn MD (2001) CD11c(+)B220(+)Gr-1(+) cells in mouse lymph nodes and spleen display characteristics of plasmacytoid dendritic cells. J Exp Med 194:1171–1178
Nestle FO, Alijagic S, Gilliet M, Sun Y, Grabbe S, Dummer R, Burg G, Schadendorf D (1998) Vaccination of melanoma patients with peptide- or tumor lysate-pulsed dendritic cells. Nat Med 4:328–332
Ohl L, Mohaupt M, Czeloth N, Hintzen G, Kiafard Z, Zwirner J, Blankenstein T, Henning G, Forster R (2004) CCR7 governs skin dendritic cell migration under inflammatory and steady-state conditions. Immunity 21:279–288
Palframan RT, Jung S, Cheng G, Weninger W, Luo Y, Dorf M, Littman DR, Rollins BJ, Zweerink H, Rot A, von Andrian UH (2001) Inflammatory chemokine transport and presentation in HEV: a remote control mechanism for monocyte recruitment to lymph nodes in inflamed tissues. J Exp Med 194:1361–1373
Partida-Sanchez S, Goodrich S, Kusser K, Oppenheimer N, Randall TD, Lund FE (2004) Regulation of dendritic cell trafficking by the ADP-ribosyl cyclase CD38: impact on the development of humoral immunity. Immunity 20:279–291
Penna G, Sozzani S, Adorini L (2001) Cutting edge: selective usage of chemokine receptors by plasmacytoid dendritic cells. J Immunol 167:1862–1866
Prechtel AT, Turza NM, Kobelt DJ, Eisemann JI, Coffin RS, McGrath Y, Hacker C, Ju X, Zenke M, Steinkasserer A (2005) Infection of mature dendritic cells with herpes simplex virus type 1 dramatically reduces lymphoid chemokine-mediated migration. J Gen Virol 86:1645–1657
Proudfoot AE (2002) Chemokine receptors: multifaceted therapeutic targets. Nat Rev 2:106–115
Qu C, Edwards EW, Tacke F, Angeli V, Llodra J, Sanchez-Schmitz G, Garin A, Haque NS, Peters W, van Rooijen N, et al (2004) Role of CCR8 and other chemokine pathways in the migration of monocyte-derived dendritic cells to lymph nodes. J Exp Med 200:1231–1241
Ratzinger G, Stoitzner P, Ebner S, Lutz MB, Layton GT, Rainer C, Senior RM, Shipley JM, Fritsch P, Schuler G, Romani N (2002) Matrix metalloproteinases 9 and 2 are necessary for the migration of Langerhans cells and dermal dendritic cells from human and murine skin. J Immunol 168:4361–4371
Robbiani DF, Finch RA, Jager D, Muller WA, Sartorelli AC, Randolph GJ (2000) The leukotriene C(4) transporter MRP1 regulates CCL19 (MIP-3beta, ELC)-dependent mobilization of dendritic cells to lymph nodes. Cell 103:757–768
Robert C, Klein C, Cheng G, Kogan A, Mulligan RC, von Andrian UH, Kupper TS (2003) Gene therapy to target dendritic cells from blood to lymph nodes. Gene Therap 10:1479–1486

Ruedl C, Koebel P, Bachmann M, Hess M, Karjalainen K (2000) Anatomical origin of dendritic cells determines their life span in peripheral lymph nodes. J Immunol 165:4910–4916

Ruedl C, Koebel P, Karjalainen K (2001) In vivo-matured Langerhans cells continue to take up and process native proteins unlike in vitro-matured counterparts. J Immunol 166:7178–7182

Sallusto F, Lanzavecchia A (1994) Efficient presentation of soluble antigen by cultured human dendritic cells is maintained by granulocyte/macrophage colony-stimulating factor plus interleukin 4 and downregulated by tumor necrosis factor alpha. J Exp Med 179:1109–1118

Sallusto F, Schaerli P, Loetscher P, Schaniel C, Lenig D, Mackay CR, Qin S, Lanzavecchia A (1998) Rapid and coordinated switch in chemokine receptor expression during dendritic cell maturation. Eur J Immunol 28:2760–2769

Sallusto F, Palermo B, Lenig D, Miettinen M, Matikainen S, Julkunen I, Forster R, Burgstahler R, Lipp M, Lanzavecchia A (1999) Distinct patterns and kinetics of chemokine production regulate dendritic cell function. Eur J Immunol 29:1617–1625

Salmi M, Jalkanen S (2005) Cell-surface enzymes in control of leukocyte trafficking. Nature Rev 5:760–771

Sangaletti S, Gioiosa L, Guiducci C, Rotta G, Rescigno M, Stoppacciaro A, Chiodoni C, Colombo MP (2005) Accelerated dendritic-cell migration and T-cell priming in SPARC-deficient mice. J Cell Sci 118:3685–3694

Saren P, Welgus HG, Kovanen PT (1996) TNF-alpha and IL-1beta selectively induce expression of 92-kDa gelatinase by human macrophages. J Immunol 157:4159–4165

Scandella E, Men Y, Gillessen S, Forster R, Groettrup M (2002) Prostaglandin E2 is a key factor for CCR7 surface expression and migration of monocyte-derived dendritic cells. Blood 100:1354–1361

Scandella E, Men Y, Legler DF, Gillessen S, Prikler L, Ludewig B, Groettrup M (2004) CCL19/CCL21-triggered signal transduction and migration of dendritic cells requires prostaglandin E2. Blood 103:1595–1601

Sixt M, Kanazawa N, Selg M, Samson T, Roos G, Reinhardt DP, Pabst R, Lutz MB, Sorokin L (2005) The conduit system transports soluble antigens from the afferent lymph to resident dendritic cells in the T cell area of the lymph node. Immunity 22:19–29

Springer TA (1994) Traffic signals for lymphocyte recirculation and leukocyte emigration: the multistep paradigm. Cell 76:301–314

Stein JV, Rot A, Luo Y, Narasimhaswamy M, Nakano H, Gunn MD, Matsuzawa A, Quackenbush EJ, Dorf ME, von Andrian UH (2000) The CC chemokine thymus-derived chemotactic agent 4 (TCA-4, secondary lymphoid tissue chemokine, 6Ckine, exodus-2) triggers lymphocyte function-associated antigen 1-mediated arrest of rolling T lymphocytes in peripheral lymph node high endothelial venules. J Exp Med 191:61–76

Steinman RM, Banchereau J (2007) Taking dendritic cells into medicine. Nature 449:419–426

Steinman RM, Hawiger D, Nussenzweig MC (2003) Tolerogenic dendritic cells. Annu Rev Immunol 21:685–711

Stoitzner P, Holzmann S, McLellan AD, Ivarsson L, Stossel H, Kapp M, Kammerer U, Douillard P, Kampgen E, Koch F, et al (2003) Visualization and characterization of migratory Langerhans cells in murine skin and lymph nodes by antibodies against Langerin/CD207. J Investig Dermatol 120:266–274

Streeter PR, Rouse BT, Butcher EC (1988) Immunohistologic and functional characterization of a vascular addressin involved in lymphocyte homing into peripheral lymph nodes. J Cell Biol 107:1853–1862

Tacken PJ, de Vries IJ, Torensma R, Figdor CG (2007) Dendritic-cell immunotherapy: from ex vivo loading to in vivo targeting. Nature Rev 7:790–802

Thomas WR, Edwards AJ, Watkins MC, Asherson GL (1980) Distribution of immunogenic cells after painting with the contact sensitizers fluorescein isothiocyanate and oxazolone. Different sensitizers form immunogenic complexes with different cell populations. Immunology 39: 21–27

Vassileva G, Soto H, Zlotnik A, Nakano H, Kakiuchi T, Hedrick JA, Lira SA (1999) The reduced expression of 6Ckine in the plt mouse results from the deletion of one of two 6Ckine genes. J Exp Med 190:1183–1188

von Andrian UH, Mackay CR (2000) T-cell function and migration. Two sides of the same coin. The New England J Med 343:1020–1034

von Andrian UH, Mempel TR (2003) Homing and cellular traffic in lymph nodes. Nat Rev 3: 867–878

Warnock RA, Askari S, Butcher EC, von Andrian UH (1998) Molecular mechanisms of lymphocyte homing to peripheral lymph nodes. J Exp Med 187:205–216

Worbs T, Mempel TR, Bolter J, von Andrian UH, Forster R (2007) CCR7 ligands stimulate the intranodal motility of T lymphocytes in vivo. J Exp Med 204:489–495

Xu H, Guan H, Zu G, Bullard D, Hanson J, Slater M, Elmets CA (2001) The role of ICAM-1 molecule in the migration of Langerhans cells in the skin and regional lymph node. Eur J Immunol 31:3085–3093

Yoneyama H, Matsuno K, Zhang Y, Nishiwaki T, Kitabatake M, Ueha S, Narumi S, Morikawa S, Ezaki T, Lu B, et al (2004) Evidence for recruitment of plasmacytoid dendritic cell precursors to inflamed lymph nodes through high endothelial venules. Int Immunol 16:915–928

Yoshino M, Yamazaki H, Nakano H, Kakiuchi T, Ryoke K, Kunisada T, Hayashi S (2003) Distinct antigen trafficking from skin in the steady and active states. Int Immunol 15:773–779

Dendritic Cells in Viral Infections

Gabrielle Belz, Adele Mount, and Frederick Masson

Contents

Abstract Antigen presenting cells (APCs) are recognized as key initiators of adaptive immunity, particularly to pathogens, by eliciting a rapid and potent immune attack on infected cells. Amongst APCs, dendritic cells (DCs) are specially equipped to initiate and regulate immune responses in a manner that depends on signals they receive from microbes and their cellular environment. To achieve this, they are equipped with highly efficient mechanisms that allow them to detect pathogens,

G. Belz (✉)
Division of Immunology, The Walter and Eliza Hall Institute of Medical Research, Melbourne, Australia
belz@wehi.edu.au

G. Lombardi, Y. Riffo-Vasquez (eds.), *Dendritic Cells,* Handbook of Experimental Pharmacology 188,

to capture, process and present antigens, and to activate and guide the differentiation of T cells into effector and memory cells. DCs can no longer be considered as a homogeneous cell type performing a single function, but are heterogeneous both in phenotype, function and dependence on inflammatory stimuli for their formation and responsiveness. Recent studies of DC subtypes have highlighted the contrasting roles of different professional APCs in activating divergent arms of the immune response towards pathogens. In this review, we discuss the progress that has been made in dissecting the attributes of different DC subsets that migrate into, or reside permanently, within lymphoid tissues and their putative roles in the induction of the anti-viral immune response.

Abbreviations

APC	Antigen presenting cell(s)
DC	Dendritic cell
cDC	Conventional DC
pDC	plasmacytoid DC
HEL	Hen egg lysosome
HSV	Herpes simplex virus
IFN	Interferon
LC	Langerhans cell(s)
L. major	*Leishmania major*
MCMV	Murine cytomegalovirus
MHC	Major histocompatibility complex
PRR	Pattern recognition receptors
TLR	Toll-like receptor

1 Background

1.1 Introduction

The body is constantly exposed to a diverse array of infectious agents. The body surface is protected from such organisms by the barrier provided by the epithelial lining. Stationed beneath the body surface is a specialized surveillance system, formed by professional antigen-presenting cells (APCs), such as macrophages and dendritic cells (DCs) that guard the body against overt infection. Over the last decade, it is our increased ability to isolate and characterise the phenotypic and functional qualities of these heterogeneous populations of cells that has illuminated their very potent and distinct roles in driving the generation of immune tolerance to self-antigens, or the generation of immunity against invading pathogens resulting in protective immunity. In addition, the pathogens themselves, have evolved novel ways to capitalize on the body's essential dependence on APCs to initiate immune responses to ensure their own survival in the face of immunity.

Table 1 Specialization of different professional antigen presenting cells

	Dendritic cells	Macrophages	B cells
Antigen uptake	Phagocytosis, macropinocytosis, receptor-mediated endocytosis	Phagocytosis, receptor-mediated endocytosis	Receptor-mediated endocytosis via immunoglobulin
Major histocompatibility class II expression	Constitutive high level expression, inducible	Low level expression, inducible	Constitutive expression, inducible
Antigen presenting function	Activation of naïve T cells	Recruitment of helper $CD4^{+}$ T cells activation of naïve B cells	Recruitment of helper T cells for antibody production

1.2 Antigen Presenting Cells

The term professional APC describes the restricted expression of major histocompatibility complex (MHC) class II to cells such as macrophages, DCs and B cells that have the capacity to endocytose antigens and communicate with T cells. Although all professional APCs share the same essential machinery to enable antigen presentation, each cell type differs markedly in their capacity to perform these functions (Table 1). It is these functional specializations that partly determine the individual contributions of each cell type to the immune response.

1.3 DCs: Critical Initiators of the Immune Response

DCs are a rare population of cells comprising only about 1% of lymphoid cells. They possess several properties which make them ideally suited to capture and present antigens for T cell 'priming'. First, they form an extensive interweaving network under epithelial surfaces that are the key sites of pathogen entry to the body. In addition they are armed with an array of pathogen recognition receptors (PRR) which serve the important role of detecting molecular patterns present in microorganisms and initiating the alert to the immune system that a pathogen has breached the body's protective barriers. Second, although several cell types express the MHC class I and II molecules necessary for antigen presentation, DCs appear to be the only cell type which can efficiently activate, or prime, naive T cells (Banchereau et al. 2000; Belz et al. 2006; Jung et al. 2002; Zammit et al. 2005). Third, DCs have the capacity to take up antigens, in addition to specialized machinery to efficiently process and present antigens, and they possess high levels of T cell costimulatory molecules. In addition, they express chemokine receptors, such as CCR7, that allow them to migrate from sites of infection in peripheral tissues to the secondary lymphoid organs (Guermonprez et al. 2002). During this migration, DCs undergo a process of 'maturation' that results in further upregulation of costimulatory molecules and translocation of MHC class II molecules to the cell surface. Within the secondary lymphoid tissues, DCs can present both self and pathogen-derived antigens to T cells and induce the activation and differentiation of these cells.

1.4 An Historical Perspective

Historically, the lifecycle of the DCs was drawn from studying the behaviour of the prototypical DC, the Langerhans cell (LC). LCs are the prominent DCs found in the epidermis of the skin and when freshly isolated were found to capture antigens, but express relatively low levels of MHC class II and the costimulatory molecules required for efficient antigen presentation and T cell stimulation. However, after a period of in vitro culture, LCs underwent a process of 'maturation' which significantly enhanced their ability to efficiently present antigens they captured earlier in their development (Romani et al. 1989). In parallel, their capacity to effectively activate T cells improved significantly. Other studies investigated the capacity of LCs to migrate from peripheral tissues to local lymph nodes using fluorescent trackers applied to the skin. This work identified that LCs clearly migrated to the regional lymph nodes and pointed to an important function of LCs in acting as a link between the skin and lymph nodes for T cell activation (Macatonia et al. 1987). Steinman and Cohn (Steinman and Cohn 1973) recognized that splenic DCs also possessed strong T cell stimulatory properties leading to the view of DCs as an important immunosurveillance network composed of different populations of DCs (Steinman 1991). Over the last two and a half decades since the first discovery of this cell type, careful dissection of location, lifecycle and intrinsic abilities of different DC populations and their distinct contributions to the immune response highlight the implications and importance of the seminal findings of Steinman and Cohn (Steinman and Cohn 1973).

2 Heterogeneity of the DC Network

DCs are heterogenous population of cells that are phenotypically delineated based on an extensive array of surface markers (see Table 2). The first major division of DCs can be made between conventional DCs (cDCs) and plasmacytoid DCs (pDCs).

2.1 Conventional DCs

Conventional DCs can be divided into three major groups of DCs, all of which are important in viral infections (Fig. 1). These are (a) the *migratory DCs* which originate in the peripheral tissues, such as the skin and mucosal tissues, and (b) the

Table 2 The different types of dendritic cells in murine lymphoid organs

DC type	Subset	CD11c	MHC II	CD8αα	CD11b	CD4	CD205	Sirpα	Langerin
Migratory (tissue-derived) DC	LC	+	+++	Low	+	−	++	+	++
	Dermal	++	+++	−	+++	−	++	+	−
Lymphoid organ DC	$CD8\alpha^+$	++	++	++	−	−	+	−	+
	$CD8\alpha^-CD4^+$	++	++	−	++	−	−	+	−
	$CD8\alpha^-CD4^-$	++	++	−	++	++	−	+	−
	pDC	+	+	+/−	−	−	−		−
Monocyte-derived DC	Inflammatory	+		−	+++	−	−		−

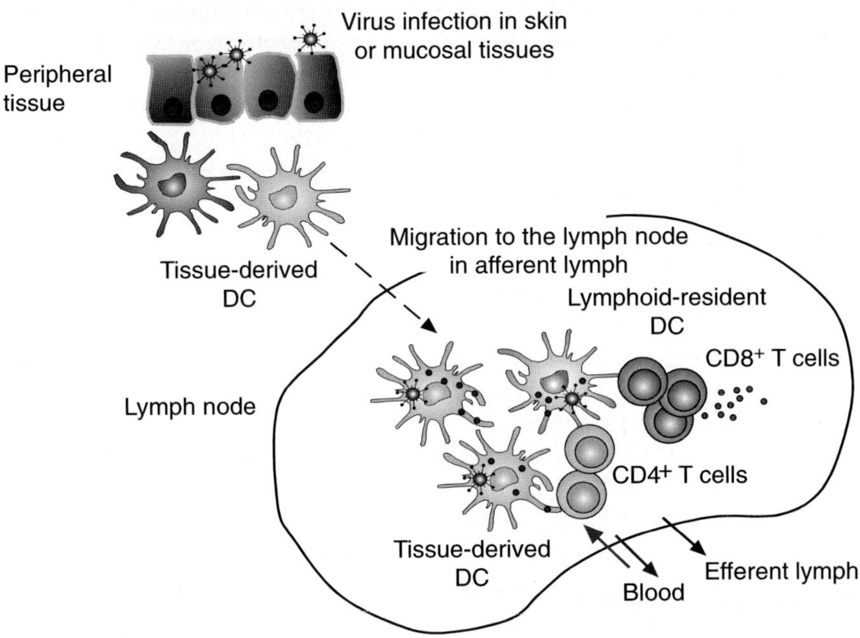

Fig. 1 In the peripheral tissues, migratory DCs have an immature phenotype and form a surveillance network underlying the epithelium. These cells are ideally positioned to continuously sample antigenic material from the environment and endocytose extracellular material. They constitutively migrate to the draining lymph node and in the lymph node acquire a mature phenotype. The lymph nodes also contain lymphoid-resident DCs that develop *in situ* in the lymphoid tissues themselves. They spend their entire lifespan as immature cells unless they encounter pathogen products which initiates an inflammatory cascade and the process of 'maturation'. In the absence of such stimulation at steady-state, most of the lymphoid-resident DCs have an immature phenotype while the migratory DCs are mature. Almost all DCs in the spleen are lymphoid-resident DCs (as they do not contain tissue-derived migratory DCs) and about one half of DCs in the lymph node are resident DCs

lymphoid tissue-resident DCs that appear not to migrate from outside the lymphoid organs but develop *in situ* and live their entire life within the lymphoid tissues, and (c) *monocyte-derived* or *inflammatory DCs* which appear to differentiate into DCs in response to inflammation.

2.1.1 Migratory DCs

The migratory DCs are derived from precursor cells that develop in the tissues themselves, or traffic from the bone marrow. LCs are the specialized prototypical DC subtype found in the squamous epithelium of the skin, while DCs migrating from the subcutaneous tissue (dermis/submucosa/lamina propria and interstitial layers underlying the epithelium) are collectively known as interstitial DCs (Bell et al. 1999; Schuler and Steinman 1985). Migratory DCs constitutively migrate to lymph nodes via the afferent lymphatics, potentially providing a mechanism by which the immune system can continuously receive information about the tissue environment, even in the absence of infection.

2.1.2 Lymphoid-Resident DCs

Resident DCs comprise approximately half the DCs found in lymph nodes, and are the only DC types found in the spleen and thymus since, these lymphoid tissues lack connections with the lymphatic system. Lymphoid-resident DCs are discriminated by differential expression of the T cell co-receptors CD4 and CD8 (Henri et al. 2001; Vremec et al. 2000; Vremec and Shortman 1997; Vremec et al. 1992). These surface molecules divide these DCs into three smaller populations, namely, $CD8\alpha^{+}$ $CD4^{-}$ (CD8 DCs), $CD8\alpha^{-}$ $CD4^{+}$ (CD4 DCs) and $CD8\alpha^{-}CD4^{-}$ (or double-negative) DCs. These DC populations appear to be derived from precursors seeded from the blood and develop into their different lineages in situ (Naik et al. 2006). Of the conventional DCs, the functions of the CD8α DCs in viral infections have been most clearly elucidated (Belz et al. 2002; Heath et al. 2004). For example, CD8α DCs possess specialized machinery for cross-presentation of antigens and play an indispensable role in the initial activation of protective T cells in viral infection (Allan et al. 2003; Belz et al. 2005; den Haan et al. 2000; Schnorrer et al. 2006).

2.1.3 Monocyte-Derived or Inflammatory DCs

Monocytes circulate in the blood and are best known for their capacity to give rise to macrophages in tissues. However, under inflammatory conditions, these monocytes can also differentiate into DCs (Geissmann et al. 2003; Naik et al. 2006). This $Ly6C^{+}$ DC forms major infiltrates in murine skin infected with *Leishmania major* (*L. major*) and a similar type of DC accumulates in a form of leprosy (Krutzik et al. 2005). The importance of inflammatory DCs has only recently become apparent but their role in viral infections has yet to be investigated. It has been suggested that the influx of monocyte-derived DCs represent precursors of migratory DCs; however, the direct lineage development of this DC type remains controversial (Shortman and Naik 2007). Initiation of the immune response to cutaneous *L. major* is mediated largely by interstitial/dermal DCs (Filippi et al. 2003; Lemos et al. 2004) with inflammatory DCs entering the site of infection later, potentially providing a rapid blood-derived source of DCs (sometimes referred to as ‘emergency DCs’) (Leon et al. 2007).

2.2 Plasmacytoid DCs

Plasmacytoid DCs (pDC) were originally described as interferon(IFN)-producing cells for their ability to rapidly release IFN-α during pathogen infections (Asselin-Paturel et al. 2001; Barchet et al. 2005; Liu 2005; O’Keeffe et al. 2002). Phenotypically, pDCs appear to be relatively immature, expressing virtually no co-stimulatory molecules and only low levels of MHC class II molecules. In general, pDCs are considered to be poor stimulators of T cells compared with conventional DCs during viral infection, their main role being to enter lymphoid tissues from blood during infection and produce large amounts of type I IFN to suppress viral invasion (Asselin-Paturel et al. 2001; Cella et al. 1999; Zuniga et al. 2004).

2.3 The DC-Maturation Paradigm and Immunity

Within the tissues of the body, DCs are found as both ‘immature’ and ‘mature’ cells. Immature DCs are highly phagocytic and express low levels of MHC class I and II molecules and co-stimulatory molecules such as CD40, CD80 and CD86 (Inaba et al. 2000; Mellman and Steinman 2001; Pierre et al. 1997; Turley et al. 2000; Wilson et al. 2003). On stimulation with pathogen products or activatory signals, immature DCs transiently increase their phagocytic capacity (West et al. 2004) and rapidly undergo a phenotypic switch. This switch is characterised by an increase in the expression of MHC molecules, co-stimulatory molecules (Caux et al. 1994; Reise Sousa 2006; Sharpe and Freeman 2002), and subsequently down-regulation in their ability to take up antigens and migrate to T cell areas of lymphoid tissues for T cell priming (Guermonprez et al. 2002; Wilson et al. 2003). These changes in DCs appeared to endow them with superior T cell stimulatory capacity giving rise to the idea that, ‘immunogenicity’ is intrinsically linked to ‘maturation’ (Banchereau and Steinman 1998). This classical model, known as the DC-maturation paradigm, suggests that immature DCs induce tolerance while mature DCs induce immunity. This view of DC development was an attractive proposition as it has long been appreciated that TCR stimulation alone is not in itself sufficient to generate productive T cell responses.

Historically, this model has provided an important framework for investigating the function of DCs, but increasingly the limitations of this model are evident (Reise Sousa 2006). Deviations from the classical model includes (a) poor correlation between the in vivo activation status of DCs (migratory DCs appear constitutively mature, even in the absence of infection or other stimulatory factors, while DCs that develop within lymphoid tissues are relatively immature); (b) poor correlation between maturation state and induction of immunity (ie. T cell proliferation is the common pathway DC-T cell engagement that precedes the induction of both T cell tolerization or immunity); (c) differences in DC origin or activation status are capable of polarizing T cell development and influencing imprinting of the homing capacity. Thus, DCs do not exist in simply an 'on' or 'off' functional state but immature DCs undergo progressive differentiation in response to endogenous (e.g. cytokines, hormones or dying cells) or exogenous (e.g. microbial or viral pathogens) stimuli that evoke effector qualities in DCs (e.g. cytokine production) that guide the ultimate effector outcome for T cells.

2.4 DC Heterogeneity and the Complexity of the DC Lifecycle

As we gain an increased understanding of the complexity of DC subsets both phenotypically and functionally, it is important to understand how DCs derived from different tissues, and at different degrees of maturation conform to the schema outlined in the LC paradigm (Pulendran et al. 1997; Shortman and Naik 2007). Anatomically, different DC subsets are localized in different tissues. This means that DCs in lymph nodes draining tissues exposed to the environment (skin and mucosal LN) are likely to receive activatory signals from the periphery via the afferent lymph or blood. In contrast, the spleen lacks afferent lymphatics and receives its major supply of antigens from the blood. The origin of all DCs (except a population of Langerin-expressing DCs (Merad 2002) is from the bone marrow (Akashi et al. 2000; D'Amico and Wu 2003; Ginhoux et al. 2006; Karsunky et al. 2003; Kondo et al. 1997). Precursor DCs from the bone marrow seed the secondary lymphoid tissues from the blood. Within the spleen the major subtypes of DCs must be derived from the blood while those in lymph nodes are composed of three populations of migratory DCs in addition to the blood-derived DCs. Analysis of features of tissue-derived and blood-derived DCs in lymph nodes, including lifespan and migratory ability, suggest that these migratory cells develop within the peripheral tissues themselves and migrate to the regional lymph nodes constitutively, acquiring features of the 'mature' DCs phenotype (Belz et al. 2004b; Henri et al. 2001; Legge and Braciale 2003; Macatonia et al. 1987; Salomon et al. 1998; Stoitzner et al. 2003; Vermaelen et al. 2001; Wilson et al. 2008). In contrast, splenic DCs express very low levels of CD40, CD80, CD86, retain their MHC class II within endosomal compartments and have a high capacity to endocytose antigens (Henri et al. 2001; Inaba et al. 1992; Salomon et al. 1998; Wilson et al. 2003; Wilson and Villadangos 2004). These cells therefore show the classical hallmarks of immature

DCs elucidated from examining freshly isolated LC (Pierre et al. 1997; Witmer-Pack et al. 1993) or bone marrow-derived DCs (Pierre et al. 1997; Winzler et al. 1997). The contrast in maturation profiles between migratory tissue-derived DCs found in the lymph node is closely paralleled by strong stimulatory capacity of migratory DCs and relatively weak capacity for splenic DCs to activate T cells. What then is the role of splenic DCs? Perhaps it is to provide a mechanism to sample continuously self-antigens and antigens derived from blood-borne pathogens (e.g. malaria) that enter the circulation and would flow through this secondary lymphoid tissue.

3 Antigen Presentation in Pathogen Infections

All DC subsets are able to present peptide antigens on their MHC class I and II molecules but presentation of viral antigens are differentially restricted within subsets of DCs (Table 3). This reflects the capacity of these different populations of DCs to generate peptides derived from particular pathogen proteins and incorporate them into peptide-MHC complexes that can be efficiently loaded into the antigen processing pathway of the cell. Antigens can be classified as endogenous (that is, synthesised within the cell itself) or exogenous (that is, taken up from outside the cell) (Ackerman and Cresswell 2004; Yewdell and Haeryfar 2005; Yewdell et al. 1999). At steady state, endogenous peptides are derived from the normal components of the cellular machinery including endocytic proteins, membrane proteins and cytosolic proteins. Therefore, DCs constitutively present peptides on MHC class I and II molecules that are derived from their own components.

When cells become infected with virus, the synthesis of the cells own proteins is down modulated, the dominant cytosolic protein species generated are derived from the virus. This allows preferential incorporation of viral peptides into the antigen-processing pathways and MHC-peptide complexes. Concurrently, when DCs are infected with virus they rapidly upregulate MHC class I and II molecules together with co-stimulatory molecules and very efficiently present viral peptides leading to potent T cell stimulatory activity. Some viruses, such as influenza virus, do not directly interfere with antigen presentation but are cytopathic and can rapidly induce apoptosis (Albert et al. 1998a, b; Bhardwaj et al. 1994), while persistent viruses often express molecules that interfere with DC death and with antigen-processing pathways (Lilley and Ploegh 2005; Loureiro and Ploegh 2006; Ploegh 1998; Yewdell and Hill 2002). Both strategies would potentially cripple the ability of DCs to initiate the early anti-viral response if DCs become infected. Despite the potential of viruses to significantly disable DCs, the consequences are not so simplistic – in most viral infections, a highly efficient virus-specific T cell response is initiated indicating that the level of DC infection is likely to be tightly regulated so as to balance direct pathogen invasion of DCs with the capacity to generate an immune response. Features such as anatomical location of DC populations and cell-type specific expression of viral ‘evasins’ (e.g. targeting of non-classical MHC 1b molecules by murine K3 (from murine γ-herpes 68) is substantially limited to B cells, the major

Table 3 Dendritic cell populations associated with pathogen infections

Infection	DC subset	Naïve T cell activated	Origin/Function	Reference
HSV-1 (cutaneous, subcutaneous)	$CD8\alpha^+$	$CD8^+$ T cell[a]	Blood-derived, Ag presentation	(Belz et al. 2004b); (Allan et al. 2003); (Smith et al. 2003)
HSV-2 (vaginal)	$CD11b^+$	$CD4^+$ T cell[b]	Tissue-derived, Ag presentation	(Zhao et al. 2003)
Influenza A, HSV-1 (intranasal)	$CD8\alpha^+$	$CD8^+$ T cell	Blood-derived Ag presentation	(Belz et al. 2004b) and unpublished (GTB)
	$CD11b^-$	$CD8^+$ T cell	Tissue-derived Ag presentation	
LCMV, vaccinia virus (intravenous, intraperitoneal)	$CD8\alpha^+$	$CD8^+$ T cell[a]	Blood-derived Ag presentation	(Belz et al. 2004a, 2005)
Reovirus	$CD8\alpha^+$	$CD4^+$ T cell	Blood-derived Ag presentation	(Fleeton et al. 2004)
	$CD11b^{low}$	$CD4^+$ T cell	Tissue-derived Ag presentation	
Listeria monocytogenes	$CD8\alpha^+$	$CD8^+$ T cell[a]	blood-derived Ag presentation	(Belz et al. 2005)
	TipDC	[c]	iNOS Antigen presentation	(Serbina et al. 2003a, b)
Leishmania major	$CD11b^+$ (dermal DC)	$CD4^+$ T cell[b]	Tissue-derived Ag presentation	(Lemos et al. 2004)
	$CD8\alpha^+$ inflammatory DC		Blood derived	

[a] Presentation to $CD4^+$ T cells has not been examined
[b] Presentation to $CD8^+$ T cells has not been examined
[c] T cell subset has not been determined

viral reservoir of persistent virus (Boname et al. 2004)) are likely to be important in determining to what extent DCs are directly infected with virus.

The presentation of exogenous antigens via MHC class I, the phenomena of cross-presentation, is less well understood (Ackerman and Cresswell 2004; Heath et al. 2004; Yewdell et al. 1999). *In vitro*, DCs readily capture antigens from live and dying cells (Harshyne et al. 2001). However, in vivo, only the CD8α DC subset is able to efficiently cross-present cell-associated or soluble antigens (den Haan et al. 2000; Pooley et al. 2001; Schnorrer et al. 2006). Whether such apparent specialization is attributable to this subset expressing specialized molecular machinery for cross-presentation, or depends on the unique ability to selectively endocytose antigens is controversial (Ackerman and Cresswell 2004; den Haan et al. 2000; Iyoda et al. 2002; Pooley et al. 2001; Schnorrer et al. 2006; Schulz and Reise Sousa 2002). Despite this, it is interesting to speculate that the dominant role of CD8α DCs in presenting viral antigens is integral to effecting cross-presentation during infection (see Sect. 3.3) (Bevan 1976; Norbury et al. 2001; Sigal et al. 1999; Yewdell and Haeryfar 2005).

3.1 DC Subsets in Acute Viral Infections

3.1.1 DC Subsets and $CD8^+$ T Cell Activation

Activation of naïve and memory T cells responding to a viral infection is thought to be almost exclusively restricted to DCs (Belz et al. 2007; Belz et al. 2006; Zammit et al. 2005). They present viral antigens generated during intracellular replication following direct infection of the cell, or alternately, antigens may be acquired by uptake of viral components from other infected cells by the process of cross-presentation (Basta and Alatery 2007; Belz et al. 2002; Heath et al. 2004; Yewdell and Haeryfar 2005). This may be true for infections such as HSV-1 and 2, and influenza virus, where viral replication is largely restricted to the skin and lung (Allan et al. 2003; Belz et al. 2004b; Smith et al. 2003; Zhao et al. 2003). In some cases, such as systemic infection with vaccinia virus (VV), vesicular stomatitis virus (VSV), and lymphocytic choriomeningitis virus (LCMV) which infect a wide variety of cell types, antigen presentation by nonhaemopoietic-derived cells has been found to drive modest expansion of effector $CD8^+$ T cells. This appears to follow the initial activation events by DCs, but raises the possibility that other cell types can be involved in determining the overall quality and quantity of T cells generated during the anti-viral response (Thomas et al. 2007).

Studies on the presentation of antigens in pathogen infections have focussed on understanding the complex interplay of different DC populations – this encompasses cDCs, pDCs and novel subsets of DCs, such as the Tip DCs (Borrow et al. 1995; Odermatt et al. 1991; Serbina et al. 2003b). In the case of LCMV infection, the influx of IFN-α producing pDCs is crucial to limit viral replication (Asselin-Paturel et al. 2001), while Tip DCs ($CD11c^+$ $CD11b^+$ DCs), a type of inflammatory DCs, characteristically produce tumor necrosis factor-α (TNF-α) and inducible nitric oxide synthase (iNOS) have been described in bacterial infections (Serbina et al. 2003b). Both pDCs and Tip DCs can present pathogen-derived antigens; however, this presentation is very inefficient when compared to cDCs, and does not seem to be required for the initial activation of naïve T cells.

Probing the notion that DC subsets exhibit cellular specialization in priming T cells has uncovered consistent themes in our understanding of which populations of DCs are the critical cells that initiate activation of T cell populations. Several parameters are likely to play important roles in determining which DCs perform these functions. These include anatomical localization, pathogen (or particle) size, the capacity of a virus or pathogen to invade DCs and other cell types, and the intrinsic capacity of DC subsets to take up and present antigens. Classically, tissue-derived

DCs that migrate to the regional lymph node(s) and present antigens to T cells have been thought to be the central initiators of the T cell response. Studies of the presentation of antigens derived from pathogens that infect the skin or lungs has yielded unexpected findings (Allan et al. 2003, 2006; Belz et al. 2004a, b) (A.M. Mount et al., unpublished observations). Cutaneous infection with HSV-1 demonstrated a lack of involvement of LCs, highlighting that trafficking DCs are not always able to prime naïve $CD8^+$ T cells (Allan et al. 2003). By contrast, the second population of trafficking DCs found in peripheral tissues, the dermal/interstitial DCs, in addition to the CD8α DCs, seem to have a crucial role in presentation of viral antigens in HSV-1, influenza, murine γ-herpes virus (Allan et al. 2003; Allan et al. 2006; Belz et al. 2004a, b) (A.M. Mount et al., unpublished observations). Indeed, the handling of viral antigens by the CD8α DCs appears to be a common pathway for ensuring the initiation of the T cell response immediately after infection.

3.1.2 DC Subsets and $CD4^+$ T Cell Activation

The role of different DCs in MHC class II antigen presentation promoting $CD4^+$ T cell priming in the setting of an infectious pathogen is poorly understood at this stage. Analysis of this arm of the immune response has been largely hampered by the paucity of infectious models, that allow simultaneous analysis of the $CD4^+$ and $CD8^+$ T cell responses to viral antigens. Drawing on the studies that have investigated $CD4^+$ T cell priming using both model and infectious antigens, it is possible to define a general dichotomy in the role of DC subsets in priming $CD4^+$ and $CD8^+$ T cells: amplification of $CD8^+$ T cells is largely driven by CD8α DCs, while activation of $CD4^+$ T cells relies largely on non-CD8α DC subsets.

Several studies have implicated the involvement of $CD11b^+$ tissue-derived migratory DCs in priming $CD4^+$ T cell responses (Ingulli et al. 2002; Manickasingham and Reise Sousa 2000; Zhao et al. 2003). The analysis of the model MHC class II-restricted model antigen hen egg lysozyme (HEL) administered by subcutaneous (s.c.) injection demonstrated that both CD8α DCs and $CD8\alpha^-$ (non-CD8α) could be involved in presenting HEL,but CD8α DCs were most efficient (Manickasingham and Reise Sousa 2000). Strikingly, an analysis of a second model antigen, ovalbumin (OVA), showed $CD11b^+$ DCs, but not CD8α DCs, induced OVA-specific $CD4^+$ T cell priming after s.c. administration (Ingulli et al. 2002). Itano and colleagues (Itano et al. 2003) employed fluorescently-labelled protein to trace the role of the skin-derived migratory DCs in antigen presentation to $CD4^+$ T cells. LCs and dermal DCs both trafficked to the draining lymph node and activated naïve T cells resulting in functionally effective $CD4^+$ T cells. This occurred in the apparent absence of significant involvement of CD8α DCs. Similarly, in murine models of Leishmaniasis, a parasitic infection whose control is mediated mainly by $CD4^+$ T cells (Reiner and Locksley 1995), antigen presentation appears to be restricted to CD8α DCs (Filippi et al. 2003) and $CD11b^+$ DCs, likely the dermal DCs (Lemos et al. 2004). These studies imply that tissue-derived trafficking DCs may play a more important role in activating $CD4^+$ T cells than $CD8^+$ T cells, but they do not discount the involvement of CD8α DCs in this process. More recently, we have developed an experimental system allowing simultaneous analysis of DC subsets presenting both MHC class I and II antigens from the same protein to $CD4^+$ and $CD8^+$ T cells (Mount et al. 2008). These studies reinforced our understanding that amplification of $CD8^+$ is largely driven by CD8α DCs while non-CD8α DCs are most important for activation of $CD4^+$ T cells. Extending our previous work, this study highlighted the contributions that multiple populations make in activating different T cell populations, and that the route of infection and migratory behaviour of DCs might play critical roles in determining which DC subsets present viral antigens.

3.2 The Behaviour of DCs in Persistent Viral Infection

Persistent viruses generally endeavour to establish a symbiotic relationship with the host. Often these viruses express several genes that can interfere with host cellular functions, thereby facilitating the establishment of persistent or latent infections. Despite these mechanisms, the immunocompetent host usually generates a very robust immune response during the acute phase of infection (Munks et al. 2007; Stevenson et al. 1999). However, DCs themselves are commonly infected in persistent infections and are likely to be ultimate targets of immune evasins. This suggests that immune evasion genes are generally not expressed during the early phase of infection and the virus exploits DC function during persistent or latent infection.

The survival of a persistent virus depends on balancing the seemingly contradictory processes of effective priming with efficient immune evasion. One way in which this might be achieved is that, the local draining lymph node may create a transient environment of immune privilege allowing viruses, such as human immunodeficiency virus (HIV) and hepatitis C virus (HCV), to initially elicit robust immune responses that reduce viral loads (Mellor and Munn 2008). Despite this, these responses fail to fully eradicate the virus, allowing persistent infection to establish and often to become refractory to immune mechanisms, in the long-term. Surprisingly, however, the host usually remains able to contain the virus for long periods of time following initial infection before it succumbs to the viral-mediated immune dysregulation.

In order for a virus to evade, or establish latency in its host, it may express cell autonomous viral evasion genes, which act by exploiting the immune system that recognizes pathogen invasion by tissue damage and inflammation. By targeting these pathways, the pathogen is able to damp down the immune response and facilitate its colonisation and survival. Viruses have evolved a myriad of so called 'viral evasins' and a number of examples are shown in Table 4. These molecules target many components of the cellular machinery, including (a) the regulation of MHC molecules – either down-regulation, or inhibition of induction; (b) molecules that allow recognition of 'induced-self' by natural killer (NK) cells; (c) expression of co-stimulatory molecules; (d) the IFN signalling pathway; (e) survival pathways – either induction of apoptosis, or inhibition; and (f) the Toll-like receptor

Table 4 Viruses employ multiple mechanisms to elude the immune system[a]

Virus	Gene	Target	Reference
MCMV	gp34 (*m04*), gp48 (*m06*), gp40 (*m152*)	MHC class I	Bubeck et al. (2002), Kleijnen et al. (1997), Krmpotic et al. (1999)
	m147.5	CD86	
	m36	Pro-caspase 8	Menard et al. (2003)
	m142, m143	IFN-inducible dsRNA-dependent protein kinase	Valchanova et al. (2006)
	m145, m155	Inhibit NKG2D ligands	Krmpotic et al. (2005); Lodoen et al. (2003)
	m138	Costimulation B7-1	Mintern et al. (2006)
HCMV	vIL10	Immune-cell proliferation, inflammatory cytokines, costimulation	Kotenko et al. (2000); Lockridge et al. (2000)
	US3, US11	MHC class I	Ahn et al. (1996)
KSHV	K3	MHC class I	Coscoy and Ganem (2001), Ishido et al. (2000)
	K5	Costimulation ICAM-1 and B7-2	Coscoy and Ganem (2001), Ishido et al. (2000)
Murine γ-herpesvirus 68	mK3	MHC class I	Stevenson et al. (2000), Stevenson et al. (2002)
	ORF73	Protein degradation	Bennett et al. (2005)
	M11 (v-Bcl-2) ORF (v-cyclin)	Apoptosis	Roy et al. (2000)
	M3	Chemokine binding protein	Parry et al. (2000)
Vaccinia virus	A46R, A52R	Activation/costimulation	Bowie et al. (2000), Stack et al. (2005)
Influenza	Ncr1	NKp46	Gazit et al. (2006), Mandelboim et al. (2001)
Herpes simples	ICP47	MHC class I	Fruh et al. (1995), Hill et al. (1995)
Hepatitis C virus	protease NS3/4A	IPS1	Li et al. (2005), Loo et al. (2006), Meylan et al. (2005)
Respiratory syncytial virus and measles virus		TLR7 and TLR9 IFN production	Schlender et al. (2005)

[a]A small sample, rather than an exhaustive catalogue, of some of the approaches used by viruses to manipulate the host immune system to their advantage

(TLR) system. Given that components of the antigen presentation machinery, co-stimulatory and survival molecules dominate the genes regulated by viral evasins, DCs are likely to be key cellular targets. The local control of reactivating virus depends on the capacity to produce continually the effector $CD8^+$ T cells which can quench the widespread reactivation of virus and viral spread. The dual expression of genes promoting DC survival (eg. vBcl-2) and those that interfere with immune priming provide an opportunity to limit the immunogenicity of the virus.

In some infections, such as murine γ-herpes virus (γ-HV), activation of antigen-specific $CD8^+$ T cells to lytically-expressed antigens seems to be largely dependent on a DC (Kupresanin et al. 2007) while at least one population of $CD8^+$ T cells can only be generated in B cell-sufficient mice (Stevenson et al. 1999) implying that not all viral proteins are processed in precisely the same manner. It is not clear whether latent epitopes depend exclusively on a DC, or rely on other APCs for efficient antigen presentation. In some cases, DCs may be generally poorly infected, partly through the action of IFN-α or other inflammatory mediators (Smith et al. 2007). Alternately, rather than being globally crippled by viral infection (Borrow et al. 1995; Smith et al. 2007), DCs might act as ferries to disseminate virus to other cell types and establish persistence or latency (Kushnir et al. 1998). Although antigen presentation is considered to be the major role of DCs during infection, it is clear that they can perform many diverse functions during infection that may significantly impact on the outcome of a pathogen encounter.

3.3 The Interaction of Trafficking and Resident DCs in Viral Infection

Antigen presentation during acute viral infection of peripheral tissues depends on the delivery of viral antigens to the lymph node draining the site of infection. Although persistent viral infections may have been acquired via a similar process, antigen presentation during the latent or chronic phase of the infection does not depend on the behaviour of the migratory DCs. Therefore, several scenarios must exist to ensure DCs are able to effectively deal with the viruses they encounter (Fig. 2).

A small group of viruses are able to infect DCs in the peripheral tissues without any apparent deleterious effects on the antigen presenting capacity of the DC themselves. This has been observed for model infections such as lentivirus vectors (He et al. 2006), and influenza virus (Belz et al. 2004b), despite the ability of such viruses to induce cytopathic effect. In these situations, the migratory DCs are a major subset capable of presenting endogenously produced MHC class I and II antigens in the draining lymph node.

In other cases, the migratory DCs are unable to present viral antigen themselves (due to destruction by the virus, or expression of viral evasins) but act as ferries transporting virus or viral products to the draining lymph node where these components are transferred to lymph node-resident DCs. In this setting, the CD8α DCs subset has a special ability to capture or take up virus, viral antigens and components of apoptotic cells from other cells or DCs, and to subsequently process and present these antigens on MHC class I molecules to $CD8^+$ T cells while the migratory DCs may still retain their capacity to present antigens via MHC class II molecules (Belz et al. 2004b; Zhao et al. 2003). This model may imply that the presentation of MHC class II peptides could be limited by factors specifically targeting the migratory DCs.

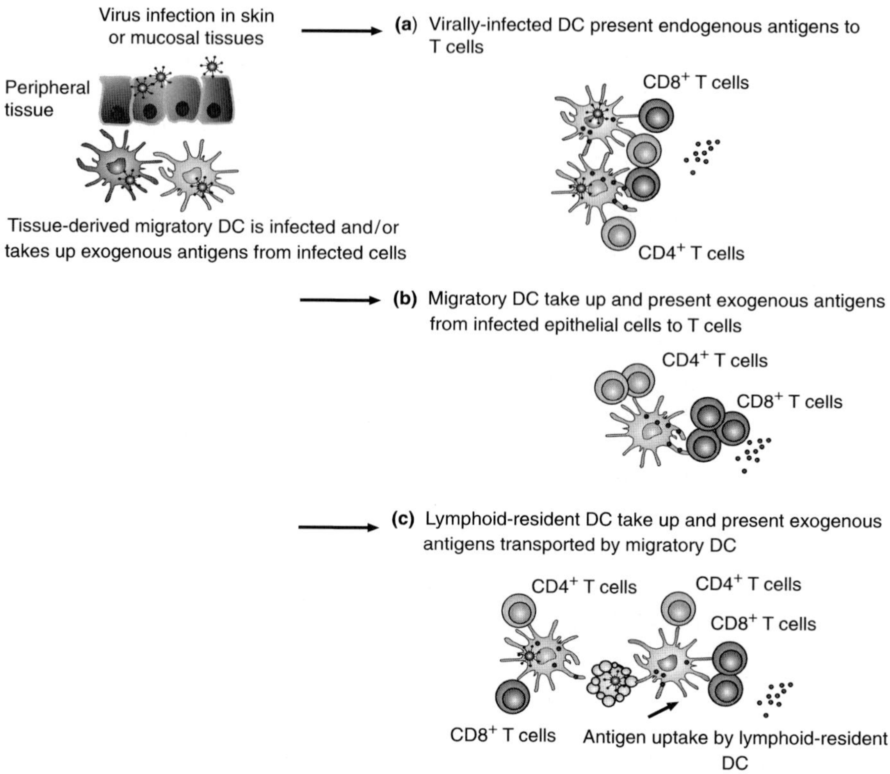

Fig. 2 The interactions between migratory and resident DCs during tissue infection. **(a)** A virus infects peripheral tissues and subsequently infects DCs but does not interfere with migration or antigen presentation capacity. These DCs are able to load endogenously-generated viral antigens into their major histocompatibility (MHC) class I and II molecules for presentation to $CD4^+$ and $CD8^+$ T cells. **(b)** At low level infections, the migratory DCs themselves may not become significantly infected, but are able to take up exogenous antigens from the infected epithelial cells, migrate to the lymph node draining the site of infection, and present the viral antigens to T cells. **(c)** In other situations, the virus infects the migratory DCs. These DCs migrate to the lymph node where they present endogenous antigens to T cells, or alternatiely, act as a source of exogenous viral antigens to lymphoid-resident CD8α DCs. The resident DCs may acquire their antigen either from live, or dying migratory DCs, or from cellular fragments of other cells carried in the afferent lymph. The migratory DCs preferentially present their antigens on MHC class II molecules to $CD4^+$ T cells, while the lymphoid-resident DC present their antigens via the MHC class I cross-presentation pathway to $CD8^+$ T cells. The relative contribution of direct (endogenous antigens) and cross-presentation (exogenous antigens) is at this stage unknown

However, our recent data demonstrate that the broader repertoire of DC subsets that present viral antigens to $CD4^+$ T cells is likely to circumvent such arising situation (Mount et al., unpublished data).

The relationship between the number of migratory DCs and lymph node-resident DCs that can present viral antigens is likely to largely reflect features of the virus itself. For example, HSV replicates poorly in the murine surrogate host resulting in relatively little infectious virus available to either infect, or be taken up by migratory DCs cells (Allan et al. 2003, 2006; Smith et al. 2003) (M. Lay et al., unpublished findings). Infections such as influenza virus, result in the generation of a large amount of virus that can infect epithelial and migrating cells and drain from the lung to the regional lymph node. This might promote the presence of a larger amount of antigen available for cross-presentation within the lymph node (Belz et al. 2004b). To further complicate these models, the contributions that the recruitment of monocyte-derived DCs might make to the overall kinetics of DCs within the lymph node and to antigen presentation, particularly after the acute phase of infection, have not yet been evaluated. As yet, however, there is no clear understanding of how the physiological transfer of antigen is mediated, although it seems likely that it is associated with an amplification step given the observed speed and tempo of the responding $CD8^+$ T cells (Belz et al. 2002). With our growing understanding of the complexity of the roles of different DCs in the immune response to viral infections, further work will be required to determine whether this model fits the physiological scenario, or requires further modification.

3.4 Activation of B Cells in Viral Infection

The lymph node is the staging ground for activation of both the T and B cell immune response to pathogens. DCs are part of the essential armoury necessary for the initial activation of T cells following viral infection, partly because T cells require the presentation of processed antigens. In contrast, naïve B cells need to see antigen in a native conformation, preferentially in the form of immune complexes, so whether B cells also depend on DCs to acquire antigen entering the lymph node in the immune response is unclear.

Soluble antigens are able to filter through the lymph node, but are channelled along a conduit system to reach the deeper portions of the node (Sixt et al. 2005). The conduits are formed by collagen fibres wrapped in a layer of fibroreticular cells. Collectively, the conduits form a three-dimensional framework that connect the interstitial space surrounding the high endothelial venules and the sinuses of the lymph node, but the network is relatively sparse surrounding lymphoid follicles compared to the T cell area. This network has been thought to be integral in facilitating the migration of DCs in the lymph node to activate T cells.

The delivery of antigens to naïve B cells is likely to occur via several potential routes. Passive diffusion of antigens carried in the blood or in the afferent lymph into B cell follicles, through which most naïve B cells circulate, is likely to provide only limited access to small molecules due to the structural constraints imposed by the reticular network (Pape et al. 2007). Immunoglobulin-mediated endocytosis provides a mechanism for the uptake of these antigens. During inflammation, flux of soluble antigens via this route may increase due to the increased permeability of the subcapsular sinus endothelial lining in response to toxins, adjuvants and cytokines. DCs have been shown to interact with B cells by positioning themselves adjacent to high endothelial venules to access naïve B cells as they enter the lymph node; by migrating across T cell areas from conduits or sinuses or by migrating into B cell follicles potentially carrying antigen to antigen-specific B cells (Pape et al. 2007; Qi et al. 2006). Alternately, circulating B cells may acquire soluble antigens directly from the blood prior to their entry to the lymph node (Pape et al. 2007).

Soluble antigens of small molecular size can access the follicle, but particulate antigens entering via the lymph require active transport within the lymph node to enable the close location of antigen to responding B lymphocytes. Although at first, it might be assumed that DCs are involved in this pathway, but recent studies have identified that macrophages positioned at the boundary between the subcapsular sinus of the lymph node and the follicle are the cellular critical link (Carrasco and Batista 2007; Junt et al. 2007; Phan et al. 2007). These macrophages, which characteristically express the lectin-like receptor sialoadhesin (CD169), act to capture rapidly the viral particles and particulate antigens, and present them to B cells in the underlying follicles (Junt et al. 2007; Norbury et al. 2002; Taylor et al. 2005). These subcapsular sinus macrophages are distinct from other macrophages in the lymph node, such as the medullary cord macrophages, as they have a reduced phagocytic ability, lack expression of the mannose receptor but express sulphated glycoproteins recognized by the mannose receptor (Taylor et al. 2005). In sequestering virus and viral particles during the immune response, these subcapsular sinus macrophages may also limit systemic spread of virus and thus act as critical gate-keepers at the lymph-tissue interface (Junt et al. 2007). These studies highlight the contrasting roles of different professional APCs in activating divergent arms of the immune response.

4 Cooperation Between DCs and Other Immune Cells

Although viruses, particularly but not exclusively, persistent viruses can encode viral evasion genes that allow interference with the generation of the immune response in a cell autonomous manner, cooperation between DCs and other lymphoid cell types, such as NK cells and regulatory T (T_{reg}) cells, also play essential roles in antiviral responses.

4.1 Regulatory T Cells

The local environment of the lymph node provides the APCs, responding lymphoid cells such as T cells and the local milieu of cytokines to promote either potent T cell activation, or alternately, a state of immunological suppression. As outlined above, immature DCs exhibit weak T cell stimulatory capacity, suggesting that they may induce tolerance (Hawiger et al. 2001; Probst et al. 2002). Mature DCs classically activate robust responses, but these attributes alone are not necessarily sufficient to induce T cell priming; highly mature DCs that express abundant costimulatory molecules are paradoxically sometimes immunosuppressive (Reise Sousa 2006). The molecular mechanisms underlying such influences of DCs are poorly defined but include the regulatory effects of cytokines such as interleukin (IL)-10, transforming growth factor (TGF)-β, inhibitory molecules program death receptor (PD)-1 and PDL-2, and enzymes such as indoleamine 2,3-dioxygenase, arginase or iNOS (Bronte and Zanovello 2005; Ferguson and Griffith 2006; Keir et al. 2007; Mellor and Munn 2004; Okazaki and Honjo 2006). In certain settings, these regulators can act in a cell autonomous manner, or function as potent inducers of T_{reg} cells. Chronic infections, such as with *L. major*, are characterised by a dominance of T_{reg} cells. In viral infections, the suppressive role of T_{reg} cells has been demonstrated in limiting the expansion of effector $CD8^+$ T cells in HSV infection although whether they mediate their effects by direct interaction with T cells, or by collaboration with a DC intermediary, has not been fully investigated (Belkaid and Rouse 2005; Suvas et al. 2003). The molecular mechanisms by which DCs can preferentially activate T_{reg} cells are poorly elucidated. It may reflect specific interactions with individual DC subsets such as pDCs (Tang et al. 2006; Tang and Bluestone 2006), or alternately, the response of DCs to the local cytokine milieu. Irregardless, it is clear that a small population of DCs can create potent immunosuppression by activating T_{reg} cells.

4.2 Natural Killer Cells

As we begin to decipher how the immune system responds to infectious insults, and the close collaboration that must occur between different cell types to effect protective immunity, it has become clear that cooperation between NK cells and DCs is critical in several infections. NK cells are specialized lymphocytes that provide a first line of defence against pathogens and tumours. Their behaviour is tightly regulated by NK-specific surface molecules that transmit inhibitory and activatory signals to the cells (Ferguson and Griffith 2006). The central role of NK cells was initially highlighted in depletion experiments in mice that were normally highly resistant to murine cytomegalovirus (MCMV) (Bancroft et al. 1981; Biron 1999). In the absence of NK cells, either by removal using the monoclonal antibody NK1.1 or by anti-asialo-GM1 antibody, mice became highly susceptible to infection. It was later determined that the viral gene *m157*, a distant homologue of MHC class I proteins, bound to the NK cell activating receptor Ly49H provided a mechanism for direct recognition of infection (Arase et al. 2002; Smith et al. 2002). Despite the importance of NK cells in protection from infection, activation of NK cells coordinating the response appears predominantly to depend on signals that originate from the DCs (Andrews et al. 2005; Barr et al. 2007; Degli-Esposti and Smyth 2005). Compelling evidence about how this DC–NK cell crosstalk is mediated, has been investigated in MCMV infection in mice (Andoniou et al. 2005; Andrews et al. 2003). One of the characteristic of mice, which are susceptible to MCMV infection, is that they fail to amplify the NK cell subset in late infection and therefore fail to limit viral replication. DCs, specifically CD8α DCs, are a major target of MCMV infection and develop functional impairment in response to this infection. The presence of Ly49H$^+$ NK cells allows maintenance of CD8α DCs in the spleen during infection (Andrews et al. 2003). The initial activation of NK cells that results in IFN-γ production following infection depends critically on the production of IL-18, and to a lesser extent, IL-12. Following stimulation, several DC populations can secrete these cytokines in addition to IL-2 and type I IFN (IFN-α and IFN-β) to promote NK cell IFN-γ production and enhance cytotoxic function (Gerosa et al. 2002; Granucci et al. 2004; Orange and Biron 1996). pDCs, however, secrete large amounts of IL-12, IL-18, IFN-α, and TNF that can activate NK cell cytotoxicity and IFN-γ production in vitro. Depletion of IL-12, either in MCMV or HSV infection, does not appear to significantly alter the capacity of NK cells to produce IFN-γ, while removal of IL-18 diminished the capacity of cDCs to stimulate NK cells, and almost completely abrogated the ability of CD11b$^+$ cDCs and pDCs to secrete this cytokine (Andoniou et al. 2005; Barr et al. 2007). Regulation of this function for pDCs, but not cDCs, is through the TLR9 (Andoniou et al. 2005). Other mutations that affect sensing of viral infection by TLR3, MyD88, TRIF or UNC93B also significantly impair the type I IFN response to infection with MCMV *in vivo*, but deficiencies incurred by the loss of these receptors may be compensated by the ability of CD8α DCs to produce both IL-12 and IL-18 (Hoebe et al. 2003; Tabeta et al. 2004, 2006).

5 Conclusions and Future Directions

The importance of the heterogeneity of the DC network and the distinct, non-overlapping functions that individual DC populations perform are only beginning to be unravelled. The systematic dissection of phenotype and function of these populations is contributing to the wealth of knowledge about this system and helping us to understand how this type of integration between related cell types works to generate immunity or tolerance. It is clear that by understanding such features of the DCs, it should help us develop targeting strategies for vaccination and other immunotherapeutic applications. Expanding these studies to further understand the interplay between different DC populations, and between DCs and other lymphoid cells, will be essential in elucidating the dynamic regulation of the generation of the immune response by these cells. The majority of studies of the heterogeneity of DCs have been carried out in the mouse, a system that still holds many surprises, but is now relatively well-defined. Unfortunately, our knowledge of human DC subsets, particularly in secondary lymphoid organs such as lymph nodes, is much poorer, and often derived from DCs extracted from diseased tissues. Defining the phenotype and function of the DC populations in both normal and pathological tissues should be a priority for the future. Moreover, the development of consistent 'humanized' mouse models will greatly facilitate our capacity to draw parallels between experimental systems and our ultimate goal of developing treatments for humans. To complement these approaches, new tools which enable the measurement of antigen uptake and allow simultaneous analysis of MHC class I and II presentation, both *in vitro* and *in vivo* will be required. These types of tools will allow us to determine whether different DC subsets, indeed can drive different outcomes for T cells. In the viral setting, reagents such as antibodies, that specifically detect lytically and latently infected cells will be essential in discriminating which cells are infected, how the type of infection influences the capacity of DCs to facilitate or impair an immune response, and what contribution processes, such as cross-presentation, make in generating effective protective immunity.

Acknowledgements Our work is supported by grants from the National Health and Medical Research Council (Aust)(G.T.B) and the Wellcome Trust Foundation (UK) (G.T.B). G.T.B. is a Wellcome Trust Senior Overseas Fellow and a Howard Hughes International Scholar. F.M is supported by a fellowship from the Swiss National Science Foundation. A.M is supported by a University of Melbourne Postgraduate Award.

References

Ackerman AL, Cresswell P (2004) Cellular mechanisms governing cross-presentation of exogenous antigens. Nat Immunol 5:678–684

Ahn K et al (1996) Human cytomegalovirus inhibits antigen presentation by a sequential multistep process. Proc Natl Acad Sci USA 93:10990–10995

Akashi K et al (2000) A clonogenic common myeloid progenitor that gives rise to all myeloid lineages. Nature 404:193–197

Albert ML et al (1998a) Immature dendritic cells phagocytose apoptotic cells via alphavbeta5 and CD36, and cross-present antigens to cytotoxic T lymphocytes. J Exp Med 188:1359–1368

Albert ML et al (1998b) Dendritic cells acquire antigen from apoptotic cells and induce class I-restricted CTLs. Nature 392:86–89

Allan RS et al (2003) Epidermal viral immunity induced by CD8α^+ dendritic cells but not by Langerhans cells. Science 301:1925–1928

Allan RS et al (2006) Migratory dendritic cells transfer antigen to a lymph node-resident dendritic cell population for efficient CTL priming. Immunity 25:153–162

Andoniou CE et al (2005) Interaction between conventional dendritic cells and natural killer cells is integral to the activation of effective antiviral immunity. Nat Immunol 6:1011–1019

Andrews DM et al (2005) Cross-talk between dendritic cells and natural killer cells in viral infection. Mol Immunol 42:547–555

Andrews DM et al (2003) Functional interactions between dendritic cells and NK cells during viral infection. Nat Immunol 4:175–181

Arase H et al (2002) Direct recognition of cytomegalovirus by activating and inhibitory NK cell receptors. Science 296:1323–1326

Asselin-Paturel C et al (2001) Mouse type I IFN-producing cells are immature APCs with plasmacytoid morphology. Nat Immunol 2:1144–1150

Banchereau J et al (2000) Immunobiology of dendritic cells. Annu Rev Immunol 18:767–811

Banchereau J and Steinman RM (1998) Dendritic cells and the control of immunity. Nature 392:245–252

Bancroft GJ et al (1981) Genetic influences on the augmentation of natural killer (NK) cells during murine cytomegalovirus infection: correlation with patterns of resistance. J Immunol 126: 988–994

Barchet W et al (2005) Plasmacytoid dendritic cells–virus experts of innate immunity. Semin Immunol 17:253–261

Barr DP et al (2007) A role for plasmacytoid dendritic cells in the rapid IL-18-dependent activation of NK cells following HSV-1 infection. Eur J Immunol 37:1334–1342

Basta S, Alatery A (2007) The cross-priming pathway: a portrait of an intricate immune system. Scand J Immunol 65:311–319

Belkaid Y and Rouse BT (2005) Natural regulatory T cells in infectious disease. Nat Immunol 6:353–360

Bell D et al (1999) Dendritic cells. Advances in Immunology 72:255–324

Belz GT et al (2002) Cross-presentation of antigens by dendritic cells. Crit Rev Immunol 22: 439–448

Belz GT et al (2005) CD8α^+ dendritic cells selectively present MHC class I-restricted noncytolytic viral and intracellular bacterial antigens in vivo. J Immunol 175:196–200

Belz GT et al (2004a) Cutting Edge: Conventional CD8α^+ dendritic cells are generally involved in priming CTL immunity to viruses. J Immunol 172:1996–2000

Belz GT et al (2004b) Distinct migrating and nonmigrating dendritic cell populations are involved in MHC class I-restricted antigen presentation after lung infection with virus. Proc Natl Acad Sci USA 101:8670–8675

Belz GT et al (2007) Shaping naive and memory CD8$^+$ T cell responses in pathogen infections through antigen presentation. Adv Exp Med Biol 590:31–42

Belz GT et al (2006) Bone marrow-derived cells expand memory CD8$^+$ T cells in response to viral infections of the lung and skin. Eur J Immunol 36:327–335

Bennett NJ et al (2005) Gamma-herpesvirus latency requires T cell evasion during episome maintenance. PLoS Biol 3:e120

Bevan MJ (1976) Cross-priming for a secondary cytotoxic response to minor H antigens with H-2 congenic cells which do not cross-react in the cytotoxic assay. J Exp Med 143:1283–1288

Bhardwaj N et al (1994) Influenza virus-infected dendritic cells stimulate strong proliferative and cytolytic responses from human CD8$^+$ T cells. J Clin Investig 94:797–807

Biron CA (1999) Initial and innate responses to viral infections – pattern setting in immunity or disease. Curr Opin Microbiol 2:374–381

Boname JM et al (2004) Viral degradation of the MHC class I peptide loading complex. Immunity 20:305–317

Borrow P et al (1995) Virus-induced immunosuppression: immune system-mediated destruction of virus-infected dendritic cells results in generalized immune suppression. J Virol 69:1059–1070

Bowie A et al (2000) A46R and A52R from vaccinia virus are antagonists of host IL-1 and toll-like receptor signaling. Proc Natl Acad Sci USA 97:10162–10167

Bronte V, Zanovello P (2005) Regulation of immune responses by L-arginine metabolism. Nat Rev Immunol 5:641–654

Bubeck A et al (2002) The glycoprotein gp48 of murine cytomegalovirusL proteasome-dependent cytosolic dislocation and degradation. J Biol Chem 277:2216–2224

Carrasco YR, Batista FD (2007) B cells acquire particulate antigen in a macrophage-rich area at the boundary between the follicle and the subcapsular sinus of the lymph node. Immunity 27:160–171

Caux C et al (1994) B70/B7–2 is identical to CD86 and is the major functional ligand for CD28 expressed on human dendritic cells. J Exp Med 180:1841–1847

Cella M et al (1999) Plasmacytoid monocytes migrate to inflamed lymph nodes and produce large amounts of type I interferon. Nat Med 5:919–923

Coscoy L, Ganem D (2001) A viral protein that selectively downregulates ICAM-1 and B7–2 and modulates T cell costimulation. J Clin Investig 107:1599–1606

D'Amico A, Wu L (2003) The early progenitors of mouse dendritic cells and plasmacytoid predendritic cells are within the bone marrow hemopoietic precursors expressing Flt3. J Exp Med 198:293–303

Degli-Esposti MA, Smyth MJ (2005) Close encounters of different kinds: dendritic cells and NK cells take centre stage. Nat Rev Immunol 5:112–124 den Haan JM et al (2000) $CD8^+$ but not $CD8^-$ dendritic cells cross-prime cytotoxic T cells in vivo. J Exp Med 192:1685–1696

Ferguson TA, Griffith TS (2006) A vision of cell death: Fas ligand and immune privilege 10 years later. Immunol Rev 213:228–238

Filippi C et al (2003) $CD4^+$ T cell polarization in mice is modulated by strain-specific major histocompatibility complex-independent differences within dendritic cells. J Exp Med 198:201–209

Fleeton MN et al (2004) Peyer's patch dendritic cells process viral antigen from apoptotic epithelial cells in the intestine of reovirus-infected mice. J Exp Med 200:235–245

Fruh K et al (1995) A viral inhibitor of peptide transporters for antigen presentation. Nature 375:415–418

Gazit R et al (2006) Lethal influenza infection in the absence of the natural killer cell receptor gene Ncr1. Nat Immunol 7:517–523

Geissmann F et al (2003) Blood monocytes consist of two principal subsets with distinct migratory properties. Immunity 19:71–82

Gerosa F et al (2002) Reciprocal activating interaction between natural killer cells and dendritic cells. J Exp Med 195:327–333

Ginhoux F et al (2006) Langerhans cells arise from monocytes in vivo. Nat Immunol 7:265–273

Granucci F et al (2004) A contribution of mouse dendritic cell-derived IL-2 for NK cell activation. J Exp Med 200:287–295

Guermonprez P et al (2002) Antigen presentation and T cell stimulation by dendritic cells. Annu Rev Immunol 20:621–667

Harshyne LA et al (2001) Dendritic cells acquire antigens from live cells for cross-presentation to CTL. J Immunol 166:3717–3723

Hawiger D et al (2001) Dendritic cells induce peripheral T cell unresponsiveness under steady state conditions in vivo. J Exp Med 194:769–779

He Y et al (2006) Skin-derived dendritic cells induce potent $CD8^+$ T cell immunity in recombinant lentivector-mediated genetic immunization. Immunity 24:643–656

Heath WR et al (2004) Cross-presentation, dendritic cell subsets, and the generation of immunity to cellular antigens. Immunol Rev 199:9–26

Henri S et al (2001) The dendritic cell populations of mouse lymph nodes. J Immunol 167:741–748

Hill A et al (1995) Herpes simplex virus turns off the TAP to evade host immunity. Nature 375: 411–415

Hoebe K et al (2003) Identification of Lps2 as a key transducer of MyD88-independent TIR signalling. Nature 424:743–748

Inaba K et al (1992) Generation of large numbers of dendritic cells from mouse bone marrow cultures supplemented with granulocyte/macrophage colony-stimulating factor. J Exp Med 176:1693–1702

Inaba K et al (2000) The formation of immunogenic major histocompatibility complex class II-peptide ligands in lysosomal compartments of dendritic cells is regulated by inflammatory stimuli. J Exp Med 191:927–936

Ingulli E et al (2002) In situ analysis reveals physical interactions between $CD11b^+$ dendritic cells and antigen-specific CD4 T cells after subcutaneous injection of antigen. J Immunol 169: 2247–2252

Ishido S et al (2000) Downregulation of major histocompatibility complex class I molecules by Kaposi's sarcoma-associated herpesvirus K3 and K5 proteins. J Virol 74:5300–5309

Itano AA et al (2003) Distinct dendritic cell populations sequentially present antigen to CD4 T cells and stimulate different aspects of cell-mediated immunity. Immunity 19:47–57

Iyoda T et al (2002) The $CD8^+$ dendritic cell subset selectively endocytoses dying cells in culture and in vivo. J Exp Med 195:1289–1302

Jung S et al (2002) In vivo depletion of $CD11c^+$ dendritic cells abrogates priming of $CD8^+$ T cells by exogenous cell-associated antigens. Immunity 17:211–220

Junt T et al (2007) Subcapsular sinus macrophages in lymph nodes clear lymph-borne viruses and present them to antiviral B cells. Nature 450:110–114

Karsunky H et al (2003) Flt3 ligand regulates dendritic cell development from $Flt3^+$ lymphoid and myeloid-committed progenitors to $Flt3^+$ dendritic cells in vivo. J Exp Med 198:305–313
Keir ME et al (2007) PD-1 and its ligands in T-cell immunity. Curr Opin Immunol 19:309–314
Kleijnen MF et al (1997) A mouse cytomegalovirus glycoprotein, gp34, forms a complex with folded class I MHC molecules in the ER which is not retained but is transported to the cell surface. Embo J 16:685–694
Kondo M et al (1997) Identification of clonogenic common lymphoid progenitors in mouse bone marrow. Cell 91:661–672
Kotenko SV et al (2000) Human cytomegalovirus harbors its own unique IL-10 homolog (cmvIL-10). Proc Natl Acad Sci USA 97:1695–1700
Krmpotic A et al (2005) NK cell activation through the NKG2D ligand MULT-1 is selectively prevented by the glycoprotein encoded by mouse cytomegalovirus gene m145. J Exp Med 201:211–220
Krmpotic A et al (1999) The immunoevasive function encoded by the mouse cytomegalovirus gene m152 protects the virus against T cell control in vivo. J Exp Med 190:1285–1296
Krutzik SR et al (2005) TLR activation triggers the rapid differentiation of monocytes into macrophages and dendritic cells. Nat Med 11:653–660
Kupresanin F et al (2007) Dendritic cells present lytic antigens and maintain function throughout persistent γ-herpesvirus infection. J Immunol 179:7506–7513
Kushnir N et al (1998) Dendritic cells and resting B cells form clusters in vitro and in vivo: T cell independence, partial LFA-1 dependence, and regulation by cross-linking surface molecules. J Immunol 160:1774–1781
Legge KL, Braciale TJ (2003) Accelerated migration of respiratory dendritic cells to the regional lymph nodes is limited to the early phase of pulmonary infection. Immunity 18:265–277
Lemos MP et al (2004) MHC class II expression restricted to $CD8\alpha^+$ and $CD11b^+$ dendritic cells is sufficient for control of Leishmania major. J Exp Med 199:725–730
Leon B et al (2007) Monocyte-derived dendritic cells formed at the infection site control the induction of protective T helper 1 responses against Leishmania. Immunity 26:519–531
Li K et al (2005) Immune evasion by hepatitis C virus NS3/4A protease-mediated cleavage of the Toll-like receptor 3 adaptor protein TRIF. Proc Natl Acad Sci USA 102:2992–2997
Lilley BN, Ploegh HL (2005) Viral modulation of antigen presentation: manipulation of cellular targets in the ER and beyond. Immunol Rev 207:126–144
Liu YJ (2005) IPC: professional type 1 interferon-producing cells and plasmacytoid dendritic cell precursors. Annu Rev Immunol 23:275–306
Lockridge KM et al (2000) Primate cytomegaloviruses encode and express an IL-10-like protein. Virology 268:272–280
Lodoen M et al (2003) NKG2D-mediated natural killer cell protection against cytomegalovirus is impaired by viral gp40 modulation of retinoic acid early inducible 1 gene molecules. J Exp Med 197:1245–1253
Loo YM et al (2006) Viral and therapeutic control of IFN-beta promoter stimulator 1 during hepatitis C virus infection. Proc Natl Acad Sci USA 103:6001–6006
Loureiro J, Ploegh HL (2006) Antigen presentation and the ubiquitin-proteasome system in host-pathogen interactions. Adv Immunol 92:225–305
Macatonia SE et al (1987) Localization of antigen on lymph node dendritic cells after exposure to the contact sensitizer fluorescein isothiocyanate. Functional and morphological studies. J Exp Med 166:1654–1667
Mandelboim O et al (2001) Recognition of haemagglutinins on virus-infected cells by NKp46 activates lysis by human NK cells. Nature 409:1055–1060
Manickasingham S, Reise Sousa C (2000) Microbial and T cell-derived stimuli regulate antigen presentation by dendritic cells in vivo. J Immunol 165:5027–5034
Mellman I, Steinman RM (2001) Dendritic cells: specialized and regulated antigen processing machines. Cell 106:255–258
Mellor AL, Munn DH (2004) IDO expression by dendritic cells: tolerance and tryptophan catabolism. Nat Rev Immunol 4:762–774

Mellor AL, Munn DH (2008) Creating immune privilege: active local suppression that benefits friends, but protects foes. Nat Rev Immunol 8(1):74–80
Menard C et al (2003) Role of murine cytomegalovirus US22 gene family members in replication in macrophages. J Virol 77:5557–5570
Merad M (2002) Langerhans cells renew in the skin throughout life under steady-state conditions. Nat Immunol 3:1135–1141
Meylan E et al (2005) Cardif is an adaptor protein in the RIG-I antiviral pathway and is targeted by hepatitis C virus. Nature 437:1167–1172
Mintern JD et al (2006) Viral interference with B7–1 costimulation: a new role for murine cytomegalovirus fc receptor-1. J Immunol 177:8422–8431
Mount AM, Smith CM, Kupresanin F, Stoermer K, Heath WR et al (2008) Multiple dendritic cell populations activate CD4+ T cells after viral stimulation. PLoS ONE 3:: e1691
Munks MW et al (2007) Viral interference with antigen presentation does not alter acute or chronic CD8 T cell immunodominance in murine cytomegalovirus infection. J Immunol 178: 7235–7241
Naik SH et al (2006) Intrasplenic steady-state dendritic cell precursors that are distinct from monocytes. Nat Immunol 7:663–671
Norbury CC et al (2002) Visualizing priming of virus-specific $CD8^+$ T cells by infected dendritic cells in vivo. Nat Immunol 3:265–271
Norbury CC et al (2001) Multiple antigen-specific processing pathways for activating naive $CD8^+$ T cells in vivo. J Immunol 166:4355–4362
O'Keeffe M et al (2002) Mouse plasmacytoid cells: long-lived cells, heterogeneous in surface phenotype and function, that differentiate into $CD8^+$ dendritic cells only after microbial stimulus. J Exp Med 196:1307–1319
Odermatt B et al (1991) Virus-triggered acquired immunodeficiency by cytotoxic T-cell-dependent destruction of antigen-presenting cells and lymph follicle structure. Proc Natl Acad Sci USA 88:8252–8256
Okazaki T, Honjo T (2006) The PD-1-PD-L pathway in immunological tolerance. Trends Immunol 27:195–201
Orange JS, Biron CA (1996) Characterization of early IL-12, IFN-alphabeta, and TNF effects on antiviral state and NK cell responses during murine cytomegalovirus infection. J Immunol 156:4746–4756
Pape KA et al (2007) The humoral immune response is initiated in lymph nodes by B cells that acquire soluble antigen directly in the follicles. Immunity 26:491–502
Parry CM et al (2000) A broad spectrum secreted chemokine binding protein encoded by a herpesvirus. J Exp Med 191:573–578
Phan TG et al (2007) Subcapsular encounter and complement-dependent transport of immune complexes by lymph node B cells. Nat Immunol 8:992–1000
Pierre P et al (1997) Developmental regulation of MHC class II transport in mouse dendritic cells. Nature 388:787–792
Ploegh HL (1998) Viral strategies of immune evasion. Science 280:248–253
Pooley JL et al (2001) Cutting edge: intravenous soluble antigen is presented to CD4 T cells by $CD8_-$ dendritic cells, but cross-presented to CD8 T cells by $CD8^+$ dendritic cells. J Immunol 166:5327–5330
Probst HC et al (2002) Cutting edge: competition for APC by CTLs of different specificities is not functionally important during induction of antiviral responses. J Immunol 168:5387–5391
Pulendran B et al (1997) Developmental pathways of dendritic cells in vivo: distinct function, phenotype, and localization of dendritic cell subsets in FLT3 ligand- treated mice. J Immunol 159:2222–2231
Qi H et al (2006) Extrafollicular activation of lymph node B cells by antigen-bearing dendritic cells. Science 312:1672–1676
Reiner SL, Locksley RM (1995) The regulation of immunity to Leishmania major. Annu Rev Immunol 13:151–177
Reise Sousa C (2006) Dendritic cells in a mature age. Nat Rev Immunol 6:476–483

Romani N et al (1989) Presentation of exogenous protein antigens by dendritic cells to T cell clones. Intact protein is presented best by immature, epidermal Langerhans cells. J Exp Med 169:1169–1178

Roy DJ et al (2000) Murine gammaherpesvirus M11 gene product inhibits apoptosis and is expressed during virus persistence. Arch Virol 145:2411–2420

Salomon B et al. (1998) Three populations of mouse lymph node dendritic cells with different origins and dynamics. J Immunol 160:708–717

Schlender J et al (2005) Inhibition of toll-like receptor 7- and 9-mediated alpha/beta interferon production in human plasmacytoid dendritic cells by respiratory syncytial virus and measles virus. J Virol 79:5507–5515

Schnorrer P et al (2006) The dominant role of $CD8^+$ dendritic cells in cross-presentation is not dictated by antigen capture. Proc Natl Acad Sci USA 103:10729–10734

Schuler G, Steinman RM (1985) Murine epidermal Langerhans cells mature into potent immunostimulatory dendritic cells in vitro. J Exp Med 161:526–546

Schulz O, Reise Sousa C (2002) Cross-presentation of cell-associated antigens by $CD8\alpha^+$ dendritic cells is attributable to their ability to internalize dead cells. Immunology 107:183–189

Serbina NV et al (2003a) Sequential MyD88-independent and -dependent activation of innate immune responses to intracellular bacterial infection. Immunity 19:891–901

Serbina NV et al (2003b) TNF/iNOS-producing dendritic cells mediate innate immune defense against bacterial infection. Immunity 19:59–70

Sharpe AH, Freeman GJ (2002) The B7-CD28 superfamily. Nat Rev Immunol 2:116–126

Shortman K, Naik SH (2007) Steady-state and inflammatory dendritic-cell development. Nat Rev Immunol 7:19–30

Sigal LJ et al (1999) Cytotoxic T-cell immunity to virus-infected non-haematopoietic cells requires presentation of exogenous antigen [see comments]. Nature 398:77–80

Sixt M et al (2005) The conduit system transports soluble antigens from the afferent lymph to resident dendritic cells in the T cell area of the lymph node. Immunity 22:19–29

Smith CM et al (2003) Cutting Edge: Conventional $CD8\alpha^+$ dendritic cells are preferentially involved in CTL priming after footpad infection with herpes simplex virus-1. J Immunol 170:4437–4440

Smith CM et al (2007) Murine gammaherpesvirus-68 inhibits antigen presentation by dendritic cells. PLoS ONE 2:e1048

Smith HR et al (2002) Recognition of a virus-encoded ligand by a natural killer cell activation receptor. Proc Natl Acad Sci USA 99:8826–8831

Stack J et al (2005) Vaccinia virus protein A46R targets multiple Toll-like-interleukin-1 receptor adaptors and contributes to virulence. J Exp Med 201:1007–1018

Steinman RM (1991) The dendritic cell system and its role in immunogenicity. Annu Rev Immunol 9:271–296

Steinman RM, Cohn ZA (1973) Identification of a novel cell type in peripheral lymphoid organs of mice. I. Morphology, quantitation, tissue distribution. J. Exp. Med. 137:1142–1162

Stevenson PG et al (1999) Changing patterns of dominance in the $CD8^+$ T cell response during acute and persistent murine gamma-herpesvirus infection. Eur J Immunol 29:1059–1067

Stevenson PG et al (2000) Inhibition of MHC class I-restricted antigen presentation by gamma 2-herpesviruses. Proc Natl Acad Sci USA 97:8455–8460

Stevenson PG et al (2002) K3-mediated evasion of CD8 + T cells aids amplification of a latent gamma-herpesvirus. Nat Immunol 3:733–740

Stoitzner P et al (2003) Visualization and characterization of migratory Langerhans cells in murine skin and lymph nodes by antibodies against Langerin/CD207. J Investig Dermatol 120:266–274

Suvas S et al (2003) CD4 + CD25 + T cells regulate virus-specific primary and memory $CD8^+$ T cell responses. J Exp Med 198:889–901

Tabeta K et al (2004) Toll-like receptors 9 and 3 as essential components of innate immune defense against mouse cytomegalovirus infection. Proc Natl Acad Sci USA 101:3516–3521

Tabeta K et al (2006) The Unc93b1 mutation 3d disrupts exogenous antigen presentation and signaling via Toll-like receptors 3, 7 and 9. Nat Immunol 7:156–164

Tang Q et al (2006) Visualizing regulatory T cell control of autoimmune responses in nonobese diabetic mice. Nat Immunol 7:83–92
Tang Q, Bluestone JA (2006) Plasmacytoid DCs and T(reg) cells: casual acquaintance or monogamous relationship? Nat Immunol 7:551–553
Taylor PR et al (2005) Macrophage receptors and immune recognition. Annu Rev Immunol 23:901–944
Thomas S et al (2007) Antigen presentation by nonhemopoietic cells amplifies clonal expansion of effector CD8 T cells in a pathogen-specific manner. J Immunol 178:5802–5811
Turley SJ et al (2000) Transport of peptide-MHC class II complexes in developing dendritic cells. Science 288:522–527
Valchanova RS et al (2006) Murine cytomegalovirus m142 and m143 are both required to block protein kinase R-mediated shutdown of protein synthesis. J Virol 80:10181–10190
Vermaelen KY et al (2001) Specific migratory dendritic cells rapidly transport antigen from the airways to the thoracic lymph nodes. J Exp Med 193:51–60
Vremec D et al (2000) CD4 and CD8 expression by dendritic cell subtypes in mouse thymus and spleen. J Immunol 164:2978–2986
Vremec D, Shortman K (1997) Dendritic cell subtypes in mouse lymphoid organs: cross-correlation of surface markers, changes with incubation, and differences among thymus, spleen, and lymph nodes. J Immunol 159:565–573
Vremec D et al (1992) The surface phenotype of dendritic cells purified from mouse thymus and spleen: investigation of the CD8 expression by a subpopulation of dendritic cells. J Exp Med 176:47–58
West MA et al. (2004) Enhanced dendritic cell antigen capture via toll-like receptor-induced actin remodeling. Science 305:1153–1157
Wilson NS et al (2003) Most lymphoid organ dendritic cell types are phenotypically and functionally immature. Blood 102:2187–2194
Wilson NS, Villadangos JA (2004) Lymphoid organ dendritic cells: beyond the Langerhans cells paradigm. Immunol Cell Biol 82:91–98
Wilson NS et al (2008) Normal proportion and expression of maturation markers in migratory dendritic cells in the absence of germs or Toll-like receptor signaling. Immunol Cell Biol 86: 200–205
Winzler C et al (1997) Maturation stages of mouse dendritic cells in growth factor-dependent long-term cultures. J Exp Med 185:317–328
Witmer-Pack MD et al (1993) Identification of macrophages and dendritic cells in the osteopetrotic (op/op) mouse. J Cell Sci 104:1021–1029
Yewdell JW, Haeryfar SM (2005) Understanding presentation of viral antigens to CD8 + T cells in vivo: the key to rational vaccine design. Annu Rev Immunol 23:651–682
Yewdell JW, Hill AB (2002) Viral interference with antigen presentation. Nat Immunol 3: 1019–1025
Yewdell JW et al (1999) Mechanisms of exogenous antigen presentation by MHC class I molecules in vitro and in vivo: implications for generating $CD8^+$ T cell responses to infectious agents, tumors, transplants, and vaccines. Adv Immunol 73:1–77
Zammit DJ et al (2005) Dendritic cells maximize the memory CD8 T cell response to infection. Immunity 22:561–570
Zhao X et al (2003) Vaginal submucosal dendritic cells, but not Langerhans cells, induce protective Th1 responses to herpes simplex virus-2. J Exp Med 197:153–162
Zuniga EI et al (2004) Bone marrow plasmacytoid dendritic cells can differentiate into myeloid dendritic cells upon virus infection. Nat Immunol 5:1227–1234

Part II
Role of Dendritic Cells in Disease

Dendritic Cells and their Potential Implication in Pathology and Treatment of Rheumatoid Arthritis

M.H. Wenink, W. Han, R.E.M. Toes, and T.R.D.J. Radstake

Contents

Abstract Dendritic cells (DC) are the professional antigen presenting cells that protect us against invading organisms. On the other hand, they uphold tolerance thereby avoiding the initiation of autoimmunity. In performing these contrasting but essential tasks DC are unique and divide these processes in time and space. It is often thought that a loss of separation of these tasks underlies the breakthrough of tolerance leading to autoimmune conditions such as rheumatoid arthritis. In this review, we will focus on the evidence which points towards the implication of DC in the inflammatory process observed in RA and in experimental models of arthritis. Finally, we will conclude on future programs exploiting the capacity of DC to cure conditions such as RA.

1 Introduction

Dendritic cells (DC) are generally accepted as the professional antigen presenting cells of our immune system, perfectly adept for antigen uptake and subsequent

T.R.D.J. Radstake (✉)
Department of Rheumatology, Radboud University Nijmegen Medical Centre, Nijmegen, The Netherlands
t.radstake@reuma.umcn.nl

G. Lombardi, Y. Riffo-Vasquez (eds.), *Dendritic Cells,* Handbook of Experimental Pharmacology 188,

presentation to T cells. DC are key regulators of T- and B-cell immunity owing to their superior ability to present antigens compared with other antigen presenting cells (APC). By these means, DC are able to evoke any desired immune response that is essential to protect the host from invading microorganisms and uphold tolerance to self proteins. A failure in one of these critical processes would indefinitely have detrimental effects on the host, either by massive invasion of harmful microorganisms or by destruction of various organs due to auto-reactivity. Recently, many researchers have elegantly reviewed the biological features of DC (Banchereau et al. 2003; Banchereau and Steinman 1998; Steinman and Banchereau 2007; Steinman and Nussenzweig 2002; Tacken et al. 2007). In this review, we discuss the general biology of these fascinating cells with special emphasis on the role played potentially in rheumatoid arthritis (RA), one of the commonest autoimmune diseases worldwide. We will centralize the role of DC in this condition knowing that other immune cells can not be excluded as being essential in the disease process. Finally we will conclude on potential options in which DC can be harnessed to treat RA, which despite enormous advances in our therapeutic armamentarium still is accountable for severe disability and premature death.

2 Dendritic Cell Biology in General

2.1 Dendritic Cells; A Stunning Machinery Divided in Time and Space

As sentinels of the immune system, DC scavenge all compartments of the body residing at the interface between innate and adaptive immunity. DC are pivotal for the recognition of an universe of antigens and control a plethora of immune responses. The name of these fascinating cells is derived from the Greek 'dendron' meaning tree and resembling its phenomenon structures as witnessed through the microscope (Steinman and Cohn 1973). DC can have a clear distinct function depending upon the state of maturation. As immature DC, they are distributed in the peripheral tissues where they sample the environment for so-called 'danger signals' which can be of exogenous and endogenous nature. For this crucial task, DC contain a specialized endocytic system having many uptake receptors designed to deliver antigen to their compartments of processing (Dudziak et al. 2007; Gil-Torregrosa et al. 2004; Guermonprez and Amigorena 2005; Guermonprez et al. 2002; Trombetta and Mellman 2005). From the plethora of antigen uptake receptors on DC, Toll-like receptors, Fc gamma receptors and lectins are probably the most intensively investigated in autoimmune diseases such as RA (Bax et al. 2007; Duez et al. 2006; Herrada et al. 2007; Laborde et al. 2007; Reis and Sousa 2004a, b; van Vliet et al. 2007). Upon encountering danger signals DC commence a complex process generally termed as "maturation", which involves numerous pathways and greatly enhances their capacity for antigen processing, presentation to naïve T cells and eventually, priming of T cell responses (Guermonprez et al. 2002; Mellman 2005;

Zwickey et al. 2006). In contrast to immature DC, mature DC home to the lymph-nodes or secondary lymphoid organs guided by specific chemokine receptors such as CCR7, the expression of which is initiated by the maturation process (Randolph et al. 2005). Next to the change in chemokine-receptor expression and chemokine secretion, the general features encompassing DC maturation are well understood and include the upregulation of co-stimulatory molecules CD80/CD86, the translocation of MHC molecules to the cell surface and production of pro-inflammatory mediators which latter is particularly dependent on the nature of the stimulus encountered (Langenkamp et al. 2002; Lanzavecchia and Sallusto 2001a, b, c; Mellman and Steinman 2001; Trombetta and Mellman 2005). The essence of DC behavior is that these complex processes take place divided in time and space, probably to ensure that antigen uptake and subsequent presentation to T cells takes place in a well controlled but different environment and/or location. It is therefore often suggested that the initiation of autoimmune diseases might be hidden in an aberrant separation of these processes perhaps leading to the breakthrough of tolerance, which latter is considered obligatory for the initiation of autoimmunity.

2.2 *Receptors that DC Utilize to Act upon the 'Milieu Interior'*

Following the engagement of a specific receptor, antigen presentation will also be affected by intracellular routing of the targeted receptor. Currently there are three large groups of receptors that are the most well characterized regarding their role in DC activation. At first, Toll-like receptors (TLR) are perhaps the pattern-recognition receptors which are studied most extensively and now widely accepted as potent initiators of DC activation or maturation. At present, 11 TLR subtypes have been identified in humans each having its specific ligands, cellular localization and expression profiles. TLR2 (as heterodimer in combination with TLR1 or TLR6) and TLR4 are extracellular receptors that are designed to recognize lipid-based structures both from gram-positive and gram-negative bacteria, including lipopeptides and lipopolysaccharides (LPS) (Hoshino et al. 2006; Lien et al. 1999; Takeuchi et al. 2001). Although TLR3 was suggested to be located on the cell surface, at least in some cell types, TLR3, TLR7, TLR8 and TLR9 are generally addressed as intracellular receptors located in the endosomal compartments and involved in the recognition of nucleic acids derived from viruses, bacteria and the host including single stranded RNA, double stranded RNA and CpG DNA motifs (Alexopoulou et al. 2001; Diebold et al. 2004; Takeuchi et al. 2001). TLR10, which is believed to originate from the TLR1/TLR6 precursor, has only been identified in human and no specific ligands have been described thus far. TLR5 is a subtype that is studied less extensively, which is perhaps explained by the fact that only one ligand has been identified thus far namely flagellin (Hayashi et al. 2001) and although profilin has been described as a ligand for mouse TLR11 (Zhang et al. 2006), human TLR11 has not been identified. Downstream TLR signaling involves a family of five adaptor (MyD88, Mal, TRIF, TRAM, and SARM) proteins that couple protein kinases ultimately leading to activation of transcription factors among which, nuclear factor κB (NF-κB) and members of the interferon regulatory factor (IRF) family are the most thoroughly investigated nowadays (reviewed in (O'Neill et al. 2003; Roelofs et al. 2008)). In contrast to the expectation in the first year after its discovery, the TLR system is highly specific in which, multiple cellular responses are observed depending upon the ligands used. Much of this specificity is likely to come forth from the use of various co-molecules and down-stream adaptor pathways by various TLR.

Secondly, Fc gamma receptors (FcγR) are expressed on the cell surface of various hematopoietic cell types. They recognize IgG and IgG containing IC and as a result constitute the link between humoral and cell-mediated immunity (Nimmerjahn and Ravetch 2006). In man, the FcγR system comprises two opposing families, the activating FcγRs I, IIa and III and the inhibitory FcγRIIb, the balance of which determines the outcome of IC mediated inflammation (Dijstelbloem et al. 2001; Nimmerjahn and Ravetch 2006; 2007; Ravetch and Bolland 2001). Both activating as well inhibiting FcγR are expressed on immature DC and complete maturation of DC results in a down regulation of FcγR expression, again highlighting the deprived capacity of antigen uptake of mature DC. Nowadays, substantial evidence indicates that the balance between activating and inhibitory FcγR determines DC behavior (Boruchov et al. 2005; Dhodapkar et al. 2007; Radstake et al. 2004a, 2006). In fact, the balance between activating and inhibitory FcγR has been shown to be crucial in the susceptibility to and phenotype of various inflammatory conditions. The activating FcγR mediates its effect through an immunoreceptor tyrosine-based activation motif (ITAM). In contrast, the inhibitory FcγRIIb signals through an immunoreceptor tyrosine-based inhibitory motif (ITIM). It is the phosphorylation of the 5'phosphoinositol phosphatase SHIP by ITIM which inhibits the ITAM regulating signaling pathways so that the balance between these FcγR systems determines cell fate.

Finally, DCs express a wide variety of C-type Lectins (CLRs), molecules that bind the carbohydrate moiety of glycoproteins (Figdor et al. 2002). Similar to TLR, distinct DC subsets express different CLRs. CLRs act as anchors for a large number of microbes including viruses, bacteria, parasites and fungi. Besides, CLRs appear to carry multiple functions, for example, adhesion molecules between DCs and other cell-types. Interestingly, these CLRs signal through ITAM (DC-SIGN (Geijtenbeek et al. 2000), Dectin-1 (Brown 2006)) or ITIM (DCIR (Bates et al. 1999), MICL (Marshall et al. 2004)) indicating that signaling via FcγRs by IgG containing immune complexes could affect many more pathways than that of FcγR itself.

2.3 The Balance between Tolerance and Immunity is Critically Tuned by DC

As mentioned previously, DC not only play a role in the initiation of immunity but are also indispensable for the preservation of tolerance. For this aim, DC capture antigens, even in the absence of overt infection or inflammation. Taking this into account, Matzinger et al. postulated an intriguing danger model, in which the immune system is more concerned with damage than with foreignness and is called into action by danger signals that derive from injured tissues (Matzinger 2002). The observation that lysates of dying cells induce maturation of in-vitro derived DCs first indicated that components from dying cells can activate DCs (Gallucci et al. 1999). These endogenous activating molecules are collectively called damage associated molecular patterns (DAMPs) which includes heat shock proteins (HSP) (Srivastava and Maki 1991), high-mobility box protein 1 (HMGB-1) (Lotze and Tracey 2005), β-defensin (Biragyn et al. 2002), hyaluronic acid (Termeer et al. 2002) and fibronectin (Okamura et al. 2001). In line with this model it became evident that TLR play a pivotal role in scavenging of such endogenous ligands. Besides TLR, FcγR and lectins might also be implicated in such a model since FcγR have been demonstrated to cooperate with TLR (Bave et al. 2003) and lectins also recognize endogenous as well as exogenous ligands.

With all these tools, the DC system is designed to control the T cell pool consisting of billions of different lymphocytes, which if left uncontrolled, will lead to severe disease conditions (reviewed in (Steinman and Banchereau 2007)). Therefore, DC are often referred to as the 'generals' of the immune system controlling several immunological checkpoints both centrally as well as peripherally. In this light, DC control many T cell responses. Whereas clones of lymphocytes are subject to silencing or tolerance by so-called 'tolerogenic DC', which either delete or suppress T cells under steady-state conditions or after the resolution of infections (Hawiger et al. 2001; Luo et al. 2007; Probst et al. 2005). In situations which require an immune response, T helper cells acquire the capacity to produce the desired combination of potent cytokines under direct supervision of DC. To battle intracellular pathogen infections a Th1 response is initiated characterized by IFNγ and IL-12 production (Napolitani et al. 2005; Pulendran et al. 1999). In contrast, to resist helminths Th2 responses are called into action that are driven by cytokines such as IL-4 and IL-13 (Seder et al. 1992). More recently, it became evident that in order to mobilize phagocytes to body surfaces to resist extra-cellular organisms a Th17 subset of T cells producing IL-17 is crucial, which is driven by IL-1, IL-6 and IL-23 made by DC (Annunziato et al. 2007; Wilson et al. 2007). In fact, this variety in immune deviation perfectly illustrates the necessity of the DC driven immune response for survival of the host. However, a failure to control or counter-act these pathways would lead to the opposite. Namely, an uncontrolled Th1 response leads to sepsis, shock and possibly a breakthrough of tolerance initiating auto-immunity. In turn, an exaggerated Th2 response leads to asthma and fibrosis, whereas a dominant IL-17 production ignites an autoimmune reaction. Altogether, DC are crucial in keeping the immune homeostasis, upholding tolerance at the one hand and eliminating infections at the other hand. The next chapter will deal with the potential roles DC play in arthritis and will highlight on the fact that this role is probably based on a, at least partly disappeared separation of DC functions.

3 Dendritic Cells and Their Potential Role in Rheumatoid Arthritis (RA)

Inappropriate responses to self-constituents can lead to chronic inflammatory conditions, termed autoimmune diseases. It is increasingly appreciated that a pivotal step leading to the breakthrough of tolerance as an initiating event of autoimmunity is directed by the abundant production of cytokines. In this light, DC can be hypothetically implicated in various autoimmune diseases in general and altering the behavior of these cells could be regarded as clinically beneficial (Box 1). Rheumatoid arthritis (RA) is one of the commonest autoimmune diseases affecting approximately 1% of the population worldwide. Despite a huge effort to decipher the underlying pathways which explain its pathology, it is far from being fully elucidated. RA is a multi-factorial disease, in which both environmental as well genetic factors are implicated. Nowadays, it is generally accepted that the influx of a myriad of inflammatory immune cells including monocytes, macrophages, T cells, B cells, neutrophils, NK cells and DC into the synovial compartment underlies a substantial part of the pathology that is still observed in daily clinical practice of the rheumatologist. The first evidence that highlighted the potential role of DC in RA came from the observation that DC are able to infiltrate the synovial tissue and fluid potentially contributing to the disease initiation and or perpetuation by mediating T cell activation (Thomas et al. 1994; Thomas and Lipsky 1996a, b; Thomas and Quinn 1996). Next to this, histopathological evidence from combined analysis of RA synovial sections and RA experimental models indicate that DCs drive the formation of ectopic lymphoid organs often observed in RA synovium (Page et al. 2002; Weyand and Goronzy 2003). In the synovium, DC are located in the perivascular regions. Whether they mature locally or are attracted both as immature and mature cell types remains a matter of debate. However, based upon the markers found in the synovial tissue compared with that seen in draining lymphnodes local maturation and subsequent migration to the lymphoid system seems to gain the upper hand (Page and Miossec 2004). In any case both immature and mature DC are present in the synovial tissue and closely related in time and space. Perhaps this breach in separation in these latter dimensions, which is probably essential for the function of the DC compartment as discussed before, underlies the initiation of autoimmunity. Next to their local (synovial) appearance, the potential altered behavior of ex vivo and in vitro derived DC in RA have been studied extensively. At first, since FcγR expression and balances between activating or inhibiting subtypes was shown to be pivotal for the onset and outcome of experimental arthritis, the expression of FcγR subtypes on DC was investigated. Interestingly, DC from RA patients with high levels of disease activity displayed a distinct pattern of FcγR expression compared to those with disease in remission and healthy counterparts, a finding that clearly reflects the level of cytokine production by these cells upon stimulation with IgG containing immune complexes (Liu et al. 2006, 2005; Pricop et al. 2001; Radstake et al. 2004a, 2004c, 2005; Salmon and Pricop 2001). Next to this, DC from RA patients with a highly active disease demonstrated a clearly potentiated response to purified ligands for TLR2 and TLR4 whereas TLR3/TLR7 responses were comparable between patients and controls (Radstake et al. 2004b; Roelofs et al. 2006, 2005). Intriguingly, the combination of various TLR ligands resulted in a synergistic effect with regard to the level of cytokine production (Roelofs et al. 2005). This latter phenomenon is of special interest since the combination of different TLR ligands with that of non-TLR ligands has been suggested to be involved in the breakthrough of tolerance (Hamilton-Williams et al. 2005; Waldner et al. 2004). Further exploration into the mechanisms behind TLR signaling in RA pathogenesis revealed that both TLR as well as their ligands are abundantly expressed in the synovial compartment. In this light, endogenous ligands for TLR4 (HSPB8) and TLR3 (host RNA) are highly expressed and potentially released upon an initiating event that might be as trivial as a small trauma (Brentano et al. 2005; Roelofs et al. 2006). The potential implication of TLR signaling in arthritis was recently highlighted by the observation that the inhibition of TLR4 signaling and expression of TLR2/TLR4 in a interleukin 1 receptor antagonist knockout mice has clear consequences for the phenotype and occurrence of experimental arthritis (Abdollahi-Roodsaz et al. 2007a, b). Although the role of DC has not been completely unraveled, the clear type I of interferon signature that is observed in at least a substantial part of the RA patients suggests the involvement of plasmacytoid DC since these cells are still considered as the major producers of this cytokine (Ronnblom and Alm 2002; van der Pouw Kraan et al. 2007). The finding that the pDC/mDC ratio in synovial fluid from RA exceeds that of that seen in peripheral blood further substantiated the role of these plasmacytoid DC. Furthermore, the number of circulating DC subsets was lower in RA patients suggesting that pDC/mDC are selectively homed to the inflamed joint (Jongbloed et al. 2006). Since DC play a crucial role in the direction of T cells, it is tempting to speculate that dendritic cells are implicated in the pronounced presence of Th1 and Th17 as observed in the synovial compartment of RA patients (reviewed in (Lubberts 2007)).

4 Dendritic Cells in Experimental Animal Models of RA, the Proof is in the Eating

As discussed before, the immune system is constantly confronted with antigens (Ags) and proteins that have not been encountered previously. Such new Ags can be found intracellularly (for example viruses and certain bacteria), or extracellularly (for example protozoa and helminthes). In order to combat these different sets of pathogens, the immune system has to mount different immune responses. Th1-lymphocytes and cytotoxic T lymphocytes (CTLs) will be effective against intracellular pathogens, but not against extracellular pathogens, whereas Th2-lymphocytes and IgE-secreting B cells are crucial in the defense against extracellular parasites. Moreover, the immune system is also facing a third set of Ags on a regular basis to which no "conventional" immune reaction (i.e.: Th1/Th2-reaction) should be mounted as this would be harmful to the host. These novel Ags can enter the organism via food intake or via the airway epithelium. The important role of the environment (exogenous antigens) was recently clearly underscored by the fact that IL-1ra knockout mice that are held under sterile conditions do not develop arthritis. In contrast, upon a breach of sterile conditions, severe arthritis develops (Abdollahi-Roodsaz et al. 2007a). For this reason, it is of high importance that the immune system is able to modulate the immune response into the proper direction in order to avoid unwanted, and possibly harmful immune responses. The refined methods adapted by DC to steer the outcome of immune responses can also be taken to our advantage by using them in the treatment of autoimmunity. The first direct evidence for the involvement of DC in experimental arthritis originated probably from the experiments performed by Leung et al. (Leung et al. 2002) Here, the transfer of collagen-pulsed DC induced arthritis that was both DC as well antigen specific since the transfer of T cells and/or non-pulsed DC had no effect. Only very recently, an adoptive transfer model in adjuvant induced arthritis showed that the influx of CD45 + MHCII+ (DC like cells) was already apparent at day 3 far before the influx of PMNs that usually occurs at day 12–14 (Moghaddami et al. 2007). Interestingly, by day 14, the CD45 + MHC-II+ cells constituted approximately half of all CD45+ cells in the synovial compartment suggesting the implication of these cells as early as the initiation of the inflammatory circle.

Another well-defined mouse model for RA is collagen-induced arthritis (CIA). CIA is a multifaceted, immunologically mediated disease involving T cells, B cells and populations of inflammatory cells that infiltrate the joint tissue and induce pathology (Luross and Williams 2001). CIA is induced through immunization with bovine type II collagen (CII) emulsified in CFA. DC will present the CII to T cells leading to T helper cell (Th) activation. Type II collagen (CII)-specific Th cells are necessary to help the B cells to produce anti-CII specific antibodies. These antibodies, in their turn, can efficiently activate the complement-system in the joints. This complement activation will lead to endothelial cell activation and the release of chemo-attractants like C5a that allow inflammatory cells to migrate into the joint. Here, they will be activated through FcγRs and start to produce lots of cytokines, such as TNF and IL-1, eventually leading to tissue-destruction. The presence of CII-specific antibodies is crucial for the disease induction, as B cell-deficient mice are not able to develop arthritis (Svensson et al. 1998) and as transfer of CII-specific antibodies is already sufficient to induce arthritis (Holmdahl et al. 1990; Terato et al. 1992). The main CII-specific antibodies that are produced are of the IgG2a isotype, which are produced with the help of Th1 cells.

Immunomodulation could be achieved by using DC that instruct Th2 and or a Treg response in case of Th1/Th17-dependent autoimmunity. Treatment of DC with pharmacological agents such as TNF, IL-10, dexamethason, vitamin D and vasoactive intestinal peptide, give rise to semi-mature DC with immunomodulatory capacities (Barrat et al. 2002; Delgado et al. 2005; Kim et al. 2006, 2005; Matyszak et al. 2000; Menges et al. 2002; Penna and Adorini 2000; Steinbrink et al. 1997; Wakkach et al. 2003). Intriguingly, TNF-, IL-10- or dexamethasone (Dex)-treated DC are all able to inhibit CIA (van Duivenvoorde et al. 2004, 2007). However, they seem to employ different mechanisms to achieve this clinical effect. TNF and IL-10 modulated DCs skew the immune response towards a Th2-like phenotype, as they were well capable of activating Th2 cells. Dex-treated DCs can inhibit the pathogenic Th1 responses by the induction of IL-10-producing T cells. However, upon re-stimulation with fully mature DC, the responding T cells can also produce both Th1 and Th2 cytokines (IFN-γ and IL-5, respectively), indicating that Dex-treated DC do not permanently redirect the immune response, but only temporarily suppress the (ongoing) immune response. Another approach to generate immunomodulatory DC is by genetic modification. DC genetically engineered to express IL-4 are able to inhibit and suppress established CIA (Kim et al. 2001; Morita et al. 2001), presumably by promoting the Th2-axis. Also unmodulated immature DC exhibit tolerogenic properties (Dhodapkar et al. 2001; Jonuleit et al. 2000). Repetitive injections of immature DC are able to suppress CIA. This suppression was mediated by expansion of regulatory T cells with high immunosuppressive potential (Charbonnier et al. 2006).

Another approach to steer immune responses via DC could be the specific targeting of immature DC in vivo. Several groups showed that they were able to effectively target immature DC through antibody-mediated Ag routing via the DEC-205 receptor (Bonifaz et al. 2002; Mahnke et al. 2000). The DEC-205 receptor is one of a number of potential receptors for antigen uptake, expressed on DC. Ags can be introduced onto anti-DEC-205 antibodies for selectively targeting DC, and because DEC-205 targets ligands in DC to late endosomal compartments that contain lysosome-associated membrane protein (LAMP) and MHC class II, the Ags are processed and presented efficiently to responding T cells. When autoantigens are known, it would be a challenge to attach them to such antibodies for selective targeting to immature DC. In this way induction of CD4 + CD25+ regulatory T cells or deletion of pathogenic T cells can be achieved (Mahnke et al. 2003).

Although most of the effects derived by DC are thought to be moderated by interaction of T cells, B cells or other immune cells, an interesting hypothesis came from the observation that exosomes derived from DC have therapeutic potential as well. Exosomes are non-nucleated nano-sized particles actively secreted by various immune cells including DC that contain multiple proteins with immune modulating capacity. Nowadays, various studies have demonstrated that the use of such DC derived exosomes exert beneficial therapeutic responses in animal models of arthritis (Bianco et al. 2007; Kim et al. 2007). Since these exosomes are very stable vesicles, they may provide a good approach for the future treatment of arthritis.

Most autoimmune patients are, nowadays, still treated with immunosuppressive agents, like glucocorticosteroids. As these treatment modalities suppress the immune activation in a non-specific fashion, they also have a lot of side effects and patients sometimes need to stop their medication when they develop an infection. Therefore, modulating the immune system in an Ag-specific manner with DC to prevent or treat autoimmunity might be a very advantageous intervention, as this will probably lead to fewer side effects. An obvious disadvantage for the usage of DC for immunomodulation is the necessity to culture DC populations on an individual basis, thereby preventing the large-scale use of DC-based intervention strategies. Nonetheless, this “ex vivo” approach appears to be valuable because DC can be loaded with a large range of Ags, and more importantly, DC maturation can be regulated. This could bypass the potential hazard associated with nasal tolerance induction in cases in which the "tolerogen" would be given around the time of a sub-clinical upper respiratory tract infection. This situation could result in DC activation and, as a consequence, induce immunity rather than tolerance (Unger et al. 2003). The tolerizing effects of DC have also been studied in humans. In one study, immature DC pulsed with an influenza matrix peptide were injected into healthy volunteers (Dhodapkar et al. 2001). As a result influenza-specific IFN-γ producing CD8$^+$ T cells initially disappeared from the blood, and in their place, peptide-specific IL-10-secreting T cells emerged. In contrast, injection of fully activated DC, loaded with the same peptide expanded the influenza-specific immunity. These findings indicate that DC in different activation states can be used safely in humans to modulate the outcome of immune responses.

5 Exploiting DC for Future Treatment of RA

In the previous sections we have distilled ideas from the current literature that describe the potential implications of DC in Rheumatoid Arthritis and the empowerment of these cells to battle this condition. As discussed before, DC play a central role in directing the outcome of immune responses and are therefore a powerful tool to use as a therapy for tumors, infectious diseases as well as for autoimmune diseases. Broadly, two approaches to DC-based vaccine therapies are being developed namely ex vivo and in vivo DC-based vaccines (reviewed in (Ueno et al. 2007)). However, before we begin the battle against these diseases, various obstacles remain. First, we are only beginning to understand the signaling pathways that turn on DC maturation and activation pathways resulting in the myriad of DC-mediated immune responses. Further deciphering of such pathways is vital for the implementation of DC-based therapies to battle autoimmunity. Second, the discussion on the therapeutic efficacy is hampered by the lack of knowledge regarding the auto-antigen. However, antigenic specificity may not be needed at all. Considerable evidence nowadays shows that DC act in a disease specific manner rather than an antigen specific one. Therefore, one-way to circumvent this latter discussion is to go forth from the tantalizing hypothesis that DC are defective (have an aberrant function) in RA. If so, the utilization of such knowledge would enable investigators to create DC that are functional and able to restore tolerance. Interestingly, preliminary data from our group looking at gene expression of stimulated and unstimulated DC from RA patients and their healthy counterparts has revealed results that at least suggest abnormalities in DC function that are specific for RA (unpublished results). Third, in mice the current research emphasis has been modeled on highly enriched DC and T cell populations. Instead, research on DC needs to be directed to the control of immune responses using, for example animals with a natural immune repertoire that act to clinically relevant auto-antigens and with the use of novel immune enhancers or inhibitors that have well-defined effects on DC behavior. Even so, the immune system of mice and man differs substantially in many aspects so that real progression into research should come forth from the development of mice with immune systems derived from human sources. Next to this, more research needs to be done on humans. It is clear, the patient and not mice or other animals sets the standard for the quality of knowledge that is a necessity to fully understand many aspects of the disease and thus treatment. However, the first studies are underway and will hopefully enlighten the scientific community to move forward from here. Inspired by the success in Oncology, the biology of DC is ready to be extended to dissect pathways and directs its prevention and treatment. And as Steinman and Banchereau recently stated "DC are an early player in disease development and an unavoidable target in the design of treatments" (Steinman and Banchereau 2007). Hopefully we will soon learn whether this promise is true for the battle against autoimmune diseases as it has been proven to be very promising in the fight against cancer (Bellone et al. 2007; Kawakami et al. 2008; Tacken et al. 2007).

Box 1. Overproduction **of cytokines by DC as initiator of autoimmunity.**

Type I Interferon

Type I interferons (IFN) are mainly secreted by a specific subtype of DC namely plasmacytoid DC. pDC respond to viral nucleic acids as well as to self nucleoproteins internalized in the form of immune complexes (Marshak-Rothstein et al. 2004; Marshak-Rothstein and Rifkin 2007). Type I IFN actively attracts activated granulocytes and differentiates monocytes into dendritic cells. Type I IFN has recently been proposed to be involved in a number of autoimmune disease among which Systemic lupus erythematosus, poly- and dermatomyositis, Sjogren's syndrome and RA are the best described

IL-23

In humans, IL-23 has recently been demonstrated to be involved in the initiation of the Th17 lineage. Although the exact role of IL-23 herein remains to be determined completely, IL-23 is generally regarded to switch naive T cells to undergo differentiation into IL-17 producing T cells. Since, the IL-23/IL-17 axis is thought to be implicated in many autoimmune disease including psoriasis, inflammatory bowel diseases and RA overproduction of IL-23 might be pathogenic.

TNF-a, IL-6 and IL-12

TNF-a and IL-6 are key inflammatory cytokines in RA. This assumption has been facilitated by the observation that the neutralization of these inflammatory mediators has greatly advanced our therapeutic armamentarium for RA. Although TNFa and IL-6 are not made exclusively by DC, inhibition of these cells would lower circulating levels of these mediators substantially. IL-12 production is greatly enhanced upon activation of DC via numerous pathways. The clinical efficacy of IL-12 neutralization is currently being investigated in many autoimmune conditions

References

Abdollahi-Roodsaz S, Joosten LA, Koenders MI, Devesa I, Roelofs MF, Radstake TR, Heuvelmans-Jacobs M, Akira S, Nicklin MJ, Ribeiro-Dias F, van den Berg WB (2007a) Stimulation of TLR2 and TLR4 differentially skews the balance of T cells in a mouse model of arthritis. J Clin Invest 118:205–216

Abdollahi-Roodsaz S, Joosten LA, Roelofs MF, Radstake TR, Matera G, Popa C, van der Meer JW, Netea MG, van den Berg WB (2007b) Inhibition of Toll-like receptor 4 breaks the inflammatory loop in autoimmune destructive arthritis. Arthritis Rheum 56:2957–2967

Alexopoulou L, Holt AC, Medzhitov R, Flavell RA (2001) Recognition of double-stranded RNA and activation of NF-kappaB by Toll-like receptor 3. Nature 413:732–738

Annunziato F, Cosmi L, Santarlasci V, Maggi L, Liotta F, Mazzinghi B, Parente E, Fili L, Ferri S, Frosali F, Giudici F, Romagnani P, Parronchi P, Tonelli F, Maggi E, Romagnani S (2007) Phenotypic and functional features of human Th17 cells. J Exp Med 204:1849–1861

Banchereau J, Steinman RM (1998) Dendritic cells and the control of immunity. Nature 392: 245–252

Banchereau J, Fay J, Pascual V, Palucka AK (2003) Dendritic cells: controllers of the immune system and a new promise for immunotherapy. Novartis Found Symp 252:226–235; discussion 235–8, 257–67

Barrat FJ, Cua DJ, Boonstra A, Richards DF, Crain C, Savelkoul HF, de Waal-Malefyt R, Coffman RL, Hawrylowicz CM, O'Garra A (2002) In vitro generation of interleukin 10-producing regulatory CD4(+) T cells is induced by immunosuppressive drugs and inhibited by T helper type 1 (Th1)- and Th2-inducing cytokines. J Exp Med 195:603–616

Bates EE, Fournier N, Garcia E, Valladeau J, Durand I, Pin JJ, Zurawski SM, Patel S, Abrams JS, Lebecque S, Garrone P, Saeland S (1999) APCs express DCIR, a novel C-type lectin surface receptor containing an immunoreceptor tyrosine-based inhibitory motif. J Immunol 163: 1973–1983

Bave U, Magnusson M, Eloranta ML, Perers A, Alm GV, Ronnblom L (2003) Fc gamma RIIa is expressed on natural IFN-alpha-producing cells (plasmacytoid dendritic cells) and is required for the IFN-alpha production induced by apoptotic cells combined with lupus IgG. J Immunol 171:3296–3302

Bax M, Garcia-Vallejo JJ, Jang-Lee J, North SJ, Gilmartin TJ, Hernandez G, Crocker PR, Leffler H, Head SR, Haslam SM, Dell A, van Kooyk Y (2007) Dendritic cell maturation results in pronounced changes in glycan expression affecting recognition by siglecs and galectins. J Immunol 179:8216–8224

Bellone S, Pecorelli S, Cannon MJ, Santin AD (2007) Advances in dendritic-cell-based therapeutic vaccines for cervical cancer. Expert Rev Anticancer Ther 7:1473–1486

Bianco NR, Kim SH, Morelli AE, Robbins PD (2007) Modulation of the immune response using dendritic cell-derived exosomes. Methods Mol Biol 380:443–456

Biragyn A, Ruffini PA, Leifer CA, Klyushnenkova E, Shakhov A, Chertov O, Shirakawa AK, Farber JM, Segal DM, Oppenheim JJ, Kwak LW (2002) Toll-like receptor 4-dependent activation of dendritic cells by beta-defensin 2. Science 298:1025–1029

Bonifaz L, Bonnyay D, Mahnke K, Rivera M, Nussenzweig MC, Steinman RM (2002) Efficient targeting of protein antigen to the dendritic cell receptor DEC-205 in the steady state leads to antigen presentation on major histocompatibility complex class I products and peripheral CD8+ T cell tolerance. J Exp Med 196:1627–1638

Boruchov AM, Heller G, Veri MC, Bonvini E, Ravetch JV, Young JW (2005) Activating and inhibitory IgG Fc receptors on human DCs mediate opposing functions. J Clin Invest 115:2914–2923

Brentano F, Schorr O, Gay RE, Gay S, Kyburz D (2005) RNA released from necrotic synovial fluid cells activates rheumatoid arthritis synovial fibroblasts via Toll-like receptor 3. Arthritis Rheum 52:2656–2665

Brown GD (2006) Dectin-1: a signalling non-TLR pattern-recognition receptor. Nat Rev Immunol 6:33–43

Charbonnier LM, van Duivenvoorde LM, Apparailly F, Cantos C, Han WG, Noel D, Duperray C, Huizinga TW, Toes RE, Jorgensen C, Louis-Plence P (2006) Immature dendritic cells suppress collagen-induced arthritis by in vivo expansion of CD49b+ regulatory T cells. J Immunol 177:3806–3813

Delgado M, Chorny A, Gonzalez-Rey E, Ganea D (2005) Vasoactive intestinal peptide generates CD4 + CD25+ regulatory T cells in vivo. J Leukoc Biol 78:1327–1338

Dhodapkar KM, Banerjee D, Connolly J, Kukreja A, Matayeva E, Veri MC, Ravetch JV, Steinman RM, Dhodapkar MV (2007) Selective blockade of the inhibitory Fcgamma receptor (FcgammaRIIB) in human dendritic cells and monocytes induces a type I interferon response program. J Exp Med 204:1359–1369

Dhodapkar MV, Steinman RM, Krasovsky J, Munz C, Bhardwaj N (2001) Antigen-specific inhibition of effector T cell function in humans after injection of immature dendritic cells. J Exp Med 193:233–238

Diebold SS, Kaisho T, Hemmi H, Akira S, Reise Sousa C (2004) Innate antiviral responses by means of TLR7-mediated recognition of single-stranded RNA. Science 303:1529–1531

Dijstelbloem HM, van de Winkel JG, Kallenberg CG (2001) Inflammation in autoimmunity: receptors for IgG revisited. Trends Immunol 22:510–516

Dudziak D, Kamphorst AO, Heidkamp GF, Buchholz VR, Trumpfheller C, Yamazaki S, Cheong C, Liu K, Lee HW, Park CG, Steinman RM, Nussenzweig MC (2007) Differential antigen processing by dendritic cell subsets in vivo. Science 315:107–111

Duez C, Gosset P, Tonnel AB (2006) Dendritic cells and toll-like receptors in allergy and asthma. Eur J Dermatol 16:12–16

Figdor CG, van Kooyk Y, Adema GJ (2002) C-type lectin receptors on dendritic cells and Langerhans cells. Nat Rev Immunol 2:77–84

Gallucci S, Lolkema M, Matzinger P (1999) Natural adjuvants: endogenous activators of dendritic cells. Nat Med 5:1249–1255

Geijtenbeek TB, Torensma R, van Vliet SJ, van Duijnhoven GC, Adema GJ, van Kooyk Y, Figdor CG (2000) Identification of DC-SIGN, a novel dendritic cell-specific ICAM-3 receptor that supports primary immune responses. Cell 100:575–585

Gil-Torregrosa BC, Lennon-Dumenil AM, Kessler B, Guermonprez P, Ploegh HL, Fruci D, van Endert P, Amigorena S (2004) Control of cross-presentation during dendritic cell maturation. Eur J Immunol 34:398–407

Guermonprez P, Amigorena S (2005) Pathways for antigen cross presentation. Springer Semin Immunopathol 26:257–271

Guermonprez P, Valladeau J, Zitvogel L, Thery C, Amigorena S (2002) Antigen presentation and T cell stimulation by dendritic cells. Annu Rev Immunol 20:621–667

Hamilton-Williams EE, Lang A, Benke D, Davey GM, Wiesmuller KH, Kurts C (2005) Cutting edge: TLR ligands are not sufficient to break cross-tolerance to self-antigens. J Immunol 174:1159–1163

Hawiger D, Inaba K, Dorsett Y, Guo M, Mahnke K, Rivera M, Ravetch JV, Steinman RM, Nussenzweig MC (2001) Dendritic cells induce peripheral T cell unresponsiveness under steady state conditions in vivo. J Exp Med 194:769–779

Hayashi F, Smith KD, Ozinsky A, Hawn TR, Yi EC, Goodlett DR, Eng JK, Akira S, Underhill DM, Aderem A (2001) The innate immune response to bacterial flagellin is mediated by Toll-like receptor 5. Nature 410:1099–1103

Herrada AA, Contreras FJ, Tobar JA, Pacheco R, Kalergis AM (2007) Immune complex-induced enhancement of bacterial antigen presentation requires Fcgamma receptor III expression on dendritic cells. Proc Natl Acad Sci USA 104:13402–13407

Holmdahl R, Andersson M, Goldschmidt TJ, Gustafsson K, Jansson L, Mo JA (1990) Type II collagen autoimmunity in animals and provocations leading to arthritis. Immunol Rev 118: 193–232

Hoshino K, Sugiyama T, Matsumoto M, Tanaka T, Saito M, Hemmi H, Ohara O, Akira S, Kaisho T (2006) IkappaB kinase-alpha is critical for interferon-alpha production induced by Toll-like receptors 7 and 9. Nature 440:949–953

Jongbloed SL, Lebre MC, Fraser AR, Gracie JA, Sturrock RD, Tak PP, McInnes IB (2006) Enumeration and phenotypical analysis of distinct dendritic cell subsets in psoriatic arthritis and rheumatoid arthritis. Arthritis Res Ther 8:R15

Jonuleit H, Schmitt E, Schuler G, Knop J, Enk AH (2000) Induction of interleukin 10-producing, nonproliferating CD4(+) T cells with regulatory properties by repetitive stimulation with allogeneic immature human dendritic cells. J Exp Med 192:1213–1222

Kawakami Y, Fujita T, Kudo C, Sakurai T, Udagawa M, Yaguchi T, Hasegawa G, Hayashi E, Ueda Y, Iwata T, Wang Q, Okada S, Tsukamoto N, Matsuzaki Y, Sumimoto H (2008) Dendritic cell based personalized immunotherapy based on cancer antigen research. Front Biosci 13:1952–1958

Kim SH, Kim S, Evans CH, Ghivizzani SC, Oligino T, Robbins PD (2001) Effective treatment of established murine collagen-induced arthritis by systemic administration of dendritic cells genetically modified to express IL-4. J Immunol 166:3499–3505

Kim SH, Lechman ER, Bianco N, Menon R, Keravala A, Nash J, Mi Z, Watkins SC, Gambotto A, Robbins PD (2005) Exosomes derived from IL-10-treated dendritic cells can suppress inflammation and collagen-induced arthritis. J Immunol 174:6440–6448

Kim SH, Bianco N, Menon R, Lechman ER, Shufesky WJ, Morelli AE, Robbins PD (2006) Exosomes derived from genetically modified DC expressing FasL are anti-inflammatory and immunosuppressive. Mol Ther 13:289–300

Kim SH, Bianco NR, Shufesky WJ, Morelli AE, Robbins PD (2007) Effective treatment of inflammatory disease models with exosomes derived from dendritic cells genetically modified to express IL-4. J Immunol 179:2242–2249

Laborde EA, Vanzulli S, Beigier-Bompadre M, Isturiz MA, Ruggiero RA, Fourcade MG, Catalan Pellet AC, Sozzani S, Vulcano M (2007) Immune complexes inhibit differentiation, maturation, and function of human monocyte-derived dendritic cells. J Immunol 179:673–681

Langenkamp A, Casorati G, Garavaglia C, Dellabona P, Lanzavecchia A, Sallusto F (2002) T cell priming by dendritic cells: thresholds for proliferation, differentiation and death and intraclonal functional diversification. Eur J Immunol 32:2046–2054

Lanzavecchia A, Sallusto F (2001a) Antigen decoding by T lymphocytes: from synapses to fate determination. Nat Immunol 2:487–492

Lanzavecchia A, Sallusto F (2001b) Regulation of T cell immunity by dendritic cells. Cell 106:263–266

Lanzavecchia A, Sallusto F (2001c) The instructive role of dendritic cells on T cell responses: lineages, plasticity and kinetics. Curr Opin Immunol 13:291–298

Leung BP, Conacher M, Hunter D, McInnes IB, Liew FY, Brewer JM (2002) A novel dendritic cell-induced model of erosive inflammatory arthritis: distinct roles for dendritic cells in T cell activation and induction of local inflammation. J Immunol 169:7071–7077

Lien E, Sellati TJ, Yoshimura A, Flo TH, Rawadi G, Finberg RW, Carroll JD, Espevik T, Ingalls RR, Radolf JD, Golenbock DT (1999) Toll-like receptor 2 functions as a pattern recognition receptor for diverse bacterial products. J Biol Chem 274:33419–33425

Liu Y, Gao X, Masuda E, Redecha PB, Blank MC, Pricop L (2006) Regulated expression of FcgammaR in human dendritic cells controls cross-presentation of antigen-antibody complexes. J Immunol 177:8440–8447

Liu Y, Masuda E, Blank MC, Kirou KA, Gao X, Park MS, Pricop L (2005) Cytokine-mediated regulation of activating and inhibitory Fc gamma receptors in human monocytes. J Leukoc Biol 77:767–776

Lotze MT, Tracey KJ (2005) High-mobility group box 1 protein (HMGB1): nuclear weapon in the immune arsenal. Nat Rev Immunol 5:331–342

Lubberts E (2007) IL-17/Th17 targeting: On the road to prevent chronic destructive arthritis? Cytokine 41:84–91

Luo X, Tarbell KV, Yang H, Pothoven K, Bailey SL, Ding R, Steinman RM, Suthanthiran M (2007) Dendritic cells with TGF-beta1 differentiate naive CD4 + CD25− T cells into islet-protective Foxp3+ regulatory T cells. Proc Natl Acad Sci USA 104:2821–2826

Luross JA, Williams NA (2001) The genetic and immunopathological processes underlying collagen-induced arthritis. Immunology 103:407–416

Mahnke K, Guo M, Lee S, Sepulveda H, Swain SL, Nussenzweig M, Steinman RM (2000) The dendritic cell receptor for endocytosis, DEC-205, can recycle and enhance antigen presentation via major histocompatibility complex class II-positive lysosomal compartments. J Cell Biol 151:673–684

Mahnke K, Qian Y, Knop J, Enk AH (2003) Induction of CD4 + /CD25+ regulatory T cells by targeting of antigens to immature dendritic cells. Blood 101:4862–4869

Marshak-Rothstein A, Busconi L, Lau CM, Tabor AS, Leadbetter EA, Akira S, Krieg AM, Lipford GB, Viglianti GA, Rifkin IR (2004) Comparison of CpG s-ODNs, chromatin immune complexes, and dsDNA fragment immune complexes in the TLR9-dependent activation of rheumatoid factor B cells. J Endotoxin Res 10:247–251

Marshak-Rothstein A, Rifkin IR (2007) Immunologically active autoantigens: the role of toll-like receptors in the development of chronic inflammatory disease. Annu Rev Immunol 25:419–441

Marshall AS, Willment JA, Lin HH, Williams DL, Gordon S, Brown GD (2004) Identification and characterization of a novel human myeloid inhibitory C-type lectin-like receptor (MICL) that is predominantly expressed on granulocytes and monocytes. J Biol Chem 279:14792–14802

Matyszak MK, Citterio S, Rescigno M, Ricciardi-Castagnoli P (2000) Differential effects of corticosteroids during different stages of dendritic cell maturation. Eur J Immunol 30:1233–1242

Matzinger P (2002) An innate sense of danger. Ann N Y Acad Sci 961:341–342

Mellman I (2005) Antigen processing and presentation by dendritic cells: cell biological mechanisms. Adv Exp Med Biol 560:63–67

Mellman I, Steinman RM (2001) Dendritic cells: specialized and regulated antigen processing machines. Cell 106:255–258

Menges M, Rossner S, Voigtlander C, Schindler H, Kukutsch NA, Bogdan C, Erb K, Schuler G, Lutz MB (2002) Repetitive injections of dendritic cells matured with tumor necrosis factor alpha induce antigen-specific protection of mice from autoimmunity. J Exp Med 195:15–21

Moghaddami M, Cleland LG, Radisic G, Mayrhofer G (2007) Recruitment of dendritic cells and macrophages during T cell-mediated synovial inflammation. Arthritis Res Ther 9:R120

Morita Y, Yang J, Gupta R, Shimizu K, Shelden EA, Endres J, Mule JJ, McDonagh KT, Fox DA (2001) Dendritic cells genetically engineered to express IL-4 inhibit murine collagen-induced arthritis. J Clin Invest 107:1275–1284

Napolitani G, Rinaldi A, Bertoni F, Sallusto F, Lanzavecchia A (2005) Selected Toll-like receptor agonist combinations synergistically trigger a T helper type 1-polarizing program in dendritic cells. Nat Immunol 6:769–776

Nimmerjahn F, Ravetch JV (2006) Fcgamma receptors: old friends and new family members. Immunity 24:19–28

Nimmerjahn F, Ravetch JV (2007) Fc-receptors as regulators of immunity. Adv Immunol 96: 179–204

O'Neill LA, Fitzgerald KA, Bowie AG (2003) The Toll-IL-1 receptor adaptor family grows to five members. Trends Immunol 24:286–290

Okamura Y, Watari M, Jerud ES, Young DW, Ishizaka ST, Rose J, Chow JC, Strauss JF, III (2001) The extra domain A of fibronectin activates Toll-like receptor 4. J Biol Chem 276:10229–10233

Page G, Lebecque S, Miossec P (2002) Anatomic localization of immature and mature dendritic cells in an ectopic lymphoid organ: correlation with selective chemokine expression in rheumatoid synovium. J Immunol 168:5333–5341

Page G, Miossec P (2004) Paired synovium and lymph nodes from rheumatoid arthritis patients differ in dendritic cell and chemokine expression. J Pathol 204:28–38

Penna G, Adorini L (2000) 1 Alpha,25-dihydroxyvitamin D3 inhibits differentiation, maturation, activation, and survival of dendritic cells leading to impaired alloreactive T cell activation. J Immunol 164:2405–2411

Pricop L, Redecha P, Teillaud JL, Frey J, Fridman WH, Sautes-Fridman C, Salmon JE (2001) Differential modulation of stimulatory and inhibitory Fc gamma receptors on human monocytes by Th1 and Th2 cytokines. J Immunol 166:531–537

Probst HC, McCoy K, Okazaki T, Honjo T, van den Broek M (2005) Resting dendritic cells induce peripheral CD8 + T cell tolerance through PD-1 and CTLA-4. Nat Immunol 6:280–286

Pulendran B, Smith JL, Caspary G, Brasel K, Pettit D, Maraskovsky E, Maliszewski CR (1999) Distinct dendritic cell subsets differentially regulate the class of immune response in vivo. Proc Natl Acad Sci USA 96: 1036–1041

Radstake TR, Blom AB, Sloetjes AW, van Gorselen EO, Pesman GJ, Engelen L, Torensma R, van den Berg WB, Figdor CG, van Lent PL, Adema GJ, Barrera P (2004a) Increased FcgammaRII expression and aberrant tumour necrosis factor alpha production by mature dendritic cells from patients with active rheumatoid arthritis. Ann Rheum Dis 63:1556–1563

Radstake TR, Roelofs MF, Jenniskens YM, Oppers-Walgreen B, van Riel PL, Barrera P, Joosten LA, van den Berg WB (2004b) Expression of toll-like receptors 2 and 4 in rheumatoid synovial tissue and regulation by proinflammatory cytokines interleukin-12 and interleukin-18 via interferon-gamma. Arthritis Rheum 50:3856–3865

Radstake TR, van Lent PL, Pesman GJ, Blom AB, Sweep FG, Ronnelid J, Adema GJ, Barrera P, van den Berg WB (2004c) High production of proinflammatory and Th1 cytokines by dendritic cells from patients with rheumatoid arthritis, and down regulation upon FcgammaR triggering. Ann Rheum Dis 63:696–702

Radstake TR, Nabbe KC, Wenink MH, Roelofs MF, Oosterlaar A, van Lieshout AW, Barrera P, van Lent PL, van den Berg WB (2005) Dendritic cells from patients with rheumatoid arthritis lack the interleukin 13 mediated increase of Fc gamma RII expression, which has clear functional consequences. Ann Rheum Dis 64:1737–1743

Radstake TR, Franke B, Wenink MH, Nabbe KC, Coenen MJ, Welsing P, Bonvini E, Koenig S, van den Berg WB, Barrera P, van Riel PL (2006) The functional variant of the inhibitory Fcgamma receptor IIb (CD32B) is associated with the rate of radiologic joint damage and dendritic cell function in rheumatoid arthritis. Arthritis Rheum 54:3828–3837

Randolph GJ, Sanchez-Schmitz G, Angeli V (2005) Factors and signals that govern the migration of dendritic cells via lymphatics: recent advances. Springer Semin Immunopathol 26:273–287

Ravetch JV, Bolland S (2001) IgG Fc receptors. Annu Rev Immunol 19:275–290

Reise Sousa C (2004a) Activation of dendritic cells: translating innate into adaptive immunity. Curr Opin Immunol 16:21–25

Reise Sousa C (2004b) Toll-like receptors and dendritic cells: for whom the bug tolls. Semin Immunol 16:27–34

Roelofs MF, Joosten LA, Abdollahi-Roodsaz S, van Lieshout AW, Sprong T, van den Hoogen FH, van den Berg WB, Radstake TR (2005) The expression of toll-like receptors 3 and 7 in rheumatoid arthritis synovium is increased and costimulation of toll-like receptors 3, 4, and 7/8 results in synergistic cytokine production by dendritic cells. Arthritis Rheum 52:2313–2322

Roelofs MF, Boelens WC, Joosten LA, Abdollahi-Roodsaz S, Geurts J, Wunderink LU, Schreurs BW, van den Berg WB, Radstake TR (2006) Identification of small heat shock protein B8 (HSP22) as a novel TLR4 ligand and potential involvement in the pathogenesis of rheumatoid arthritis. J Immunol 176:7021–7027

Roelofs MF, Abdollahi-Roodsaz S, Joosten LA, van de berg WB, Radstake T (2008) The orchestra of Toll-Like Receptors (TLRs) and their potential role in frequently occurring rheumatic conditions. Arthritis Rheum 58:338–348

Ronnblom L, Alm GV (2002) The natural interferon-alpha producing cells in systemic lupus erythematosus. Hum Immunol 63:1181–1193

Salmon JE, Pricop L (2001) Human receptors for immunoglobulin G: key elements in the pathogenesis of rheumatic disease. Arthritis Rheum 44:739–750

Seder RA, Paul WE, Davis MM, Fazekas de St Groth B (1992) The presence of interleukin 4 during in vitro priming determines the lymphokine-producing potential of CD4+ T cells from T cell receptor transgenic mice. J Exp Med 176:1091–1098

Srivastava PK, Maki RG (1991) Stress-induced proteins in immune response to cancer. Curr Top Microbiol Immunol 167:109–123

Steinbrink K, Wolfl M, Jonuleit H, Knop J, Enk AH (1997) Induction of tolerance by IL-10-treated dendritic cells. J Immunol 159:4772–4780

Steinman RM, Banchereau J (2007) Taking dendritic cells into medicine. Nature 449:419–426

Steinman RM, Cohn ZA (1973) Identification of a novel cell type in peripheral lymphoid organs of mice. I. Morphology, quantitation, tissue distribution. J Exp Med 137:1142–1162

Steinman RM, Nussenzweig MC (2002) Avoiding horror autotoxicus: the importance of dendritic cells in peripheral T cell tolerance. Proc Natl Acad Sci USA 99:351–358

Svensson L, Jirholt J, Holmdahl R, Jansson L (1998) B cell-deficient mice do not develop type II collagen-induced arthritis (CIA). Clin Exp Immunol 111:521–526

Tacken PJ, de Vries IJ, Torensma R, Figdor CG (2007) Dendritic-cell immunotherapy: from ex vivo loading to in vivo targeting. Nat Rev Immunol 7:790–802

Takeuchi O, Kawai T, Muhlradt PF, Morr M, Radolf JD, Zychlinsky A, Takeda K, Akira S (2001) Discrimination of bacterial lipoproteins by Toll-like receptor 6. Int Immunol 13:933–940

Terato K, Hasty KA, Reife RA, Cremer MA, Kang AH, Stuart JM (1992) Induction of arthritis with monoclonal antibodies to collagen. J Immunol 148:2103–2108

Termeer C, Benedix F, Sleeman J, Fieber C, Voith U, Ahrens T, Miyake K, Freudenberg M, Galanos C, Simon JC (2002) Oligosaccharides of Hyaluronan activate dendritic cells via toll-like receptor 4. J Exp Med 195:99–111

Thomas R, Lipsky PE (1996a) Dendritic cells: origin and differentiation. Stem Cells 14:196–206

Thomas R, Lipsky PE (1996b) Presentation of self peptides by dendritic cells: possible implications for the pathogenesis of rheumatoid arthritis. Arthritis Rheum 39:183–190

Thomas R, Quinn C (1996) Functional differentiation of dendritic cells in rheumatoid arthritis: role of CD86 in the synovium. J Immunol 156:3074–3086

Thomas R, Davis LS, Lipsky PE (1994) Rheumatoid synovium is enriched in mature antigen-presenting dendritic cells. J Immunol 152:2613–2623

Trombetta ES, Mellman I (2005) Cell biology of antigen processing in vitro and in vivo. Annu Rev Immunol 23:975–1028

Ueno H, Klechevsky E, Morita R, Aspord C, Cao T, Matsui T, Di Pucchio T, Connolly J, Fay JW, Pascual V, Palucka AK, Banchereau J (2007) Dendritic cell subsets in health and disease. Immunol Rev 219:118–142

Unger WW, Hauet-Broere F, Jansen W, van Berkel LA, Kraal G, Samsom JN (2003) Early events in peripheral regulatory T cell induction via the nasal mucosa. J Immunol 171:4592–4603

van der Pouw Kraan TC, Wijbrandts CA, van Baarsen LG, Voskuyl AE, Rustenburg F, Baggen JM, Ibrahim SM, Fero M, Dijkmans BA, Tak PP, Verweij CL (2007) Rheumatoid arthritis subtypes identified by genomic profiling of peripheral blood cells: assignment of a type I interferon signature in a subpopulation of patients. Ann Rheum Dis 66:1008–1014

van Duivenvoorde LM, Louis-Plence P, Apparailly F, van der Voort EI, Huizinga TW, Jorgensen C, Toes RE (2004) Antigen-specific immunomodulation of collagen-induced arthritis with tumor necrosis factor-stimulated dendritic cells. Arthritis Rheum 50:3354–3364

van Duivenvoorde LM, Han WG, Bakker AM, Louis-Plence P, Charbonnier LM, Apparailly F, van der Voort EI, Jorgensen C, Huizinga TW, Toes RE (2007) Immunomodulatory dendritic cells inhibit Th1 responses and arthritis via different mechanisms. J Immunol 179:1506–1515

van Vliet SJ, den Dunnen J, Gringhuis SI, Geijtenbeek TB, van Kooyk Y (2007) Innate signaling and regulation of Dendritic cell immunity. Curr Opin Immunol 19:435–440

Wakkach A, Fournier N, Brun V, Breittmayer JP, Cottrez F, Groux H (2003) Characterization of dendritic cells that induce tolerance and T regulatory 1 cell differentiation in vivo. Immunity 18:605–617

Waldner H, Collins M, Kuchroo VK (2004) Activation of antigen-presenting cells by microbial products breaks self tolerance and induces autoimmune disease. J Clin Invest 113:990–997

Weyand CM, Goronzy JJ (2003) Ectopic germinal center formation in rheumatoid synovitis. Ann N Y Acad Sci 987:140–149

Wilson NJ, Boniface K, Chan JR, McKenzie BS, Blumenschein WM, Mattson JD, Basham B, Smith K, Chen T, Morel F, Lecron JC, Kastelein RA, Cua DJ, McClanahan TK, Bowman EP, de Waal Malefyt R (2007) Development, cytokine profile and function of human interleukin 17-producing helper T cells. Nat Immunol 8:950–957

Zhang D, Facchinetti V, Wang X, Huang Q, Qin J, Su B (2006) Identification of MEKK2/3 serine phosphorylation site targeted by the Toll-like receptor and stress pathways. Embo J 25:97–107

Zwickey HL, Unternaehrer JJ, Mellman I (2006) Presentation of self-antigens on MHC class II molecules during dendritic cell maturation. Int Immunol 18:199–209

Lung Dendritic Cells: Targets for Therapy in Allergic Disease

Bart N. Lambrecht and Hamida Hammad

Contents

Abstract Dendritic cells (DCs) are crucial in determining the functional outcome of allergen encounter in the lung. Antigen presentation by myeloid DCs leads to Th2 sensitization typical of allergic disease, whereas antigen presentation by plasmacytoid DCs serves to dampen inflammation. It is increasingly clear that DCs have an antigen presenting function beyond sensitisation. DCs therefore constitute a novel target for the development of antiallergic therapy aimed at the origin of the inflammatory cascade. A careful study of DC biology and of the receptors expressed by lung DCs has provided a framework for the discovery of novel antiallergic compounds.

B.N. Lambrecht (✉)
Department of Pulmonary Medicine, Erasmus M.C. Dr. Molerwaterplein 50, 3015 GE. Rotterdam, The Netherlands
b.lambrecht@erasmusmc.nl

G. Lombardi, Y. Riffo-Vasquez (eds.), *Dendritic Cells,* Handbook of Experimental Pharmacology 188,

1 General Function of Dendritic Cells in the Immune System: Induction of Immunity

Dendritic cells (DCs) were originally described by their capacity to efficiently process and present antigens and to prime naïve T cells (Steinman and Cohn 1973). Over the last three decades, multiple DC subtypes have been defined, differing in phenotype, localization, and immune function (Shortman and Liu 2002). In the most general view, immature DCs are situated in the periphery at sites of antigen exposure. Here, DCs are specialized in antigen recognition and uptake. A degree of discrimination between harmless antigen and dangerous pathogens can be inferred from their expression of pathogen associated molecular pattern receptors (such as the Toll-like receptors (TLRs)). Under homeostatic conditions and particularly upon recognition of pathogens, DCs subsequently migrate to the T cell area of draining nodes, where they screen the repertoire of naïve T cells for antigen-specific T cells directed against the pathogen. Upon cognate TCR–MHC–peptide interaction, DCs subsequently form more stable interactions, and optimally induce T cell effector function by providing costimulatory molecules and T cell stimulatory and T cell survival cytokines. In homeostatic conditions, only harmless antigens or self antigens are being presented to T cells. Because these antigens fail to induce the complete maturation of DCs, these antigens induce the abortive T cell proliferation and/or lead to a T cell response, in which regulatory T cells (Tregs) are induced. This system allows for dangerous antigens to be eliminated, while avoiding overt immune-mediated damage in response to harmless environmental and self antigens.

2 Function of Lung Dendritic Cells: Induction of Tolerance in Steady State and Bridging Innate and Adaptive Immunity

Immature DCs are distributed throughout the lung and are at the focal control point determining the induction of pulmonary immunity or tolerance (Akbari et al. 2001, 2002; Lambrecht and Hammad 2003; de Heer et al. 2005). Airway DCs form a dense network in the lung ideally placed to sample inhaled antigens, by forming tight junctions with airway epithelial cells and extending their dendrites into the airway lumen, analogous to the situation in the gut. Indeed, lamina propria DCs were found to depend on the chemokine receptor CX3CR1 to form transepithelial dendrites, which enable the cells to directly sample luminal antigens. Thus, CX3CR1-dependent processes, which control host interactions of specialized DCs with commensal and pathogenic bacteria, may regulate immunological tolerance and inflammation. Whether a similar CX3CR1 dependent mechanism exists in the lung remains to be shown (Niess et al. 2005).

Following antigen uptake across the airway epithelial barrier, DCs migrate to draining mediastinal LNs to stimulate naive T cells (Vermaelen et al. 2001; Lambrecht et al. 1998). As most allergens are immunologically inert proteins, the usual outcome of their inhalation is tolerance. In true sense, this means that when the antigen is subsequently given to mice as an adjuvant setting (e.g. in combination with the Th2 adjuvant alum), it no longer induces an immunological response that leads to effector cells causing inflammation (De Heer et al. 2004; Van Hove et al. 2007; Ostroukhova et al. 2004). This is shown best for the model antigen ovalbumin (OVA). When given to the airways of naïve mice, it induces tolerance to a subsequent immunization with OVA in adjuvant, and effectively inhibits the development of airway inflammation, a feature of true immunological tolerance (De Heer et al. 2004; Ostroukhova et al. 2004). This tolerance is mediated in part by deletion of Ag reactive T cells as well as induction and/or expansion of regulatory T cells in the mediastinal nodes (Akbari et al. 2002; Van Hove et al. 2007; Ostroukhova et al. 2004; Hintzen et al. 2006), which is dominant and can be transferred to other mice by adoptive transfer.

It was therefore long enigmatic, how sensitization to natural allergens occurred. An important discovery was the fact that most clinically important allergens, such as the major Der p 1 allergen from HDM, are proteolytic enzymes that can directly activate DCs or epithelial cells to break the process of tolerance and promote Th2 responses (Hammad et al. 2001; Kheradmand et al. 2002). However, other allergens, such as the experimental allergen OVA, do not have any intrinsic activating properties. For these antigens, contaminating molecules or environmental exposures (respiratory viruses, air pollution) might pull the trigger on DC activation (Dahl et al. 2004). Eisenbarth showed that low level TLR4 agonists admixed with harmless OVA prime DCs induce a Th2 response by inducing their full maturation, yet not their production of IL-12 (Eisenbarth et al. 2004). This process has been recently described as being dependent on the activation of the adaptor molecule MyD88 in pulmonary DCs (Piggott et al. 2005). This is clinically important information as most natural allergens such as HDM, cockroach, and animal dander contain endotoxin and undoubtedly other TLR agonists (Braun-Fahrlander et al. 2002).

From the above, it seems that the decision between tolerance or immunity (in the lungs) is controlled by the degree of maturity of mDCs interacting with naïve T cells, a process driven by signals from the innate immune system (de Heer et al. 2005; Herrick and Bottomly 2003). It is often claimed that induction of tolerance is a function of "immature" DCs, meaning that these cells lack the expression of high levels of MHC, adhesion, and costimulatory molecules. It has indeed been shown that immature mDCs induce abortive T cell proliferation in responding T cells and induce regulatory T cells (Tregs) (Akbari et al. 2001; Ostroukhova et al. 2004; Brimnes et al. 2003). Another level of complexity arose, when it was shown that (respiratory) tolerance might be a function of a subset of plasmacytoid DCs (De Heer et al. 2004; Oriss et al. 2005). pDCs depletion from mice using antibodies led to a break in inhalational tolerance to OVA and to development of asthmatic inflammation (De Heer et al. 2004). For more detailed discussion on this topic, see de Heer et al. (2005) and Hammad and Lambrecht (2006). If pDCs promote tolerance and mDCs immunity, it is logical to assume that the balance between both subsets is tightly controlled. In support, the administration of Flt-3 ligand, a cytokine that induces the differentiation of pDCs, to sensitized mice reduced all the features of asthma (Edwan et al. 2004), whereas administration of GM-CSF expanded mDCs, and strongly enhanced sensitization and inflammation (Stampfli et al. 1998). Xanthou and colleagues demonstrated, by using osteopontin deficient mice and using blocking antibodies, that the secreted form of osteopontin promoted respiratory sensitization to inhaled antigen, an effect mediated by alteration of pDC to mDC balance (Xanthou et al. 2007). Along the same lines, the mucosal adjuvant cholera toxin has the capacity to break inhalational tolerance and promote Th2 sensitization to inhaled harmless antigens by promoting mDC over pDC balance (Oriss et al. 2005).

3 Dendritic Cells in Established Allergic Airway Inflammation

Not only do DCs play a role in the primary immune response to inhaled allergens, but are also crucial for the outcome of the effector phase in asthma. Indeed, the number of $CD11b^{+}$ mDCs is increased in the conducting airways and lung interstitium of sensitized and challenged mice during the acute phase of the response (van Rijt et al. 2002; Vermaelen and Pauwels 2003). Similar findings have been reported in the rat (Huh et al. 2003). The mechanisms for this enhanced recruitment are that DC-precursors, most likely at the monocyte stage of development, which are attracted from the bone marrow, via the bloodstream to the lung in a CCR2 dependent and generally CCR5 and CCR6 independent way (Robays et al. 2007). However, during the chronic phase of the pulmonary response induced by prolonged exposure to a large number of aerosols, respiratory tolerance develops through unclear mechanisms. During this regulatory phase, the number of mDCs in the lungs steadily decreased, and this was associated with a reduction of BHR. Inflammation, however, reappeared when mDCs were given (Koya et al. 2006). The role of mDCs in the secondary immune response was further supported by the fact that their depletion at the time of allergen challenge abrogated all the features of asthma, including airway inflammation, goblet cell hyperplasia, and bronchial hyperresponsiveness (Lambrecht et al. 1998; van Rijt et al. 2005). Again the defect was restored by intratracheal injection of $CD11b^{+}$ inflammatory mDCs, but not other APCs such as macrophages. The same effects were observed, when DCs were depleted in the nose of an animal model for allergic rhinitis (KleinJan et al. 2006). It therefore seems that inflammatory mDCs are both necessary and sufficient for secondary immune responses to allergen. The reasons for this could be manyfold. Costimulatory molecules expressed by DCs could play a crucial role in established asthma. Pulmonary DCs upregulate the expression of CD40, CD80, CD86, ICOS-L, PD-L1 and PD-L2 during eosinophilic airway inflammation, particularly upon contact with Th2 cells (De Heer et al. 2004; Huh et al. 2003; Van Rijt et al. 2004, 2005). Costimulatory molecules might be involved in activation of effector T cells in the tissues. In allergen challenged mice, mDCs might also be a prominent source of the chemokines CCL17 and CCL22, involved in attracting $CCR4^{+}$ Th2 cells to the airways (Kohl et al. 2006; Vermaelen et al. 2003). The production of chemokines by lung DC subsets is furthermore differentially regulated, with $CD11b^+$ inflammatory DCs being the most prominent source of proinflammatory chemokines (Beaty et al. 2007). The proallergic cytokine thymic stromal lymphopoeitin (TSLP) induces the production of large amounts of CCL17 by mDCs, thus contributing to the recruitment of a large number of Th2 cells to the airways, explaining how it may act to enhance inflammation (Zhou et al. 2005).

In humans, allergen challenge leads to an accumulation of myeloid, but not plasmacytoid DCs to the airways of asthmatics, concomitantly with a reduction in circulating $CD11c^+$ cells, showing that these cells are recruited from the bloodstream in response to allergen challenge (Upham et al. 2002; Jahnsen et al. 2001). A recent report suggests that pDCs are also recruited into the BAL fluid, but are poor APCs (Bratke et al. 2007). The exact role of plasmacytoid DCs in ongoing allergen specific responses in asthma is currently unknown. It was shown that pDCs accumulate in the nose, but not lungs, of allergen challenged atopics (Jahnsen et al. 2000). In stable asthma, the number of $CD1a^+$ DCs is increased in the airway epithelium and lamina propria, and these numbers are reduced by treatment with inhaled corticosteroids (Moller et al. 1996). Based on the above argumentation in mice studies of asthma, it is very likely that part of the efficacy of inhaled steroids might be due to their effects in dampening airway DC function.

4 Control of Lung DC Function by Regulatory T Cells

Induction of DC maturation and provision of peptide-MHC to T cells is not sufficient to generate effector cells (Sporri and Reise Sousa 2005). During generation of an efficient effector immune response, DCs have to overcome suppression by regulatory T (Treg) cells, and the dominant way by which they seem to do this is by producing the cytokine IL-6, which counteracts the suppression by naturally occurring $CD4^+CD25^+$ Tregs (Doganci et al. 2005). The lung DCs of mice with allergic inflammation produce enhanced amounts of IL-6 (Dodge et al. 2003). Established airway inflammation seems to be regulated by Tregs expressing membrane TGFβ (Ostroukhova et al. 2004) or secreting bioactive TGFβ and possibly IL-10 (Kearley et al. 2005). This is a pleiotropic cytokine with significant antiinflammatory and immunosuppressive properties in the lungs, as reduced expression of this cytokine exacerbates airway pathology in an asthma model (Ostroukhova et al. 2004). Several papers now support the concept that Tregs alter airway DC function. Mice lacking the transcription factor RunX3, involved in downstream TGFβ signalling, spontaneously develop asthma features (Fainaru et al. 2004). In the lungs of these mice, there is a strong increase in the number of alveolar myeloid DCs, displaying a mature phenotype with increased expression of MHC II, OX40-Ligand, and CCR7 (Fainaru et al. 2005) and demonstrating an increased immunostimulatory capacity. Moreover, $RunX3^{-/-}$ DCs are able to mount inflammatory responses to otherwise harmless inhaled antigens, possibly through their lack of responsiveness to locally secreted TGF-β (Fainaru et al. 2004). In mice normally resistant to HDM-induced asthma and AHR (C3H mice), Treg cell depletion similarly led to increased numbers of pulmonary myeloid DCs with elevated expression of MHCII, CD80, and CD86 and an increased capacity to stimulate T cell proliferation and Th2 cytokine production. In normally susceptible A/J mice, Tregs did not suppress inflammation and AHR. These data suggest, therefore, that resistance to allergen-driven AHR is mediated partly by $CD4^+CD25^+$ Treg cell suppression of DC activation and that the absence of this regulatory pathway contributes to susceptibility (Lewkowich et al. 2005). In the rat, it was shown that Tregs also control the level of CD86 expression on lung DCs and are responsible for the tolerance to inhaled allergen that occurs upon repeated exposure to allergens (Strickland et al. 2006). In humans with allergy, there is a reduction in the number and possibly, function of Tregs (Kuipers and Lambrecht 2004), but it is unclear at present whether this would also lead to an altered function of DCs in these patients.

5 Perpetuation of Allergic Inflammation and Remodelling: A Role for Cytokine Driven Activation of DCs?

According to current thinking, epithelial dysfunction, either intrinsic to asthma or caused by persistent inflammation, leads to epithelial release of profibrotic cytokines such as epidermal growth factor and transforming growth factor-β acting on fibroblasts and smooth muscle cells, disturbing the equilibrium between epithelial destruction and growth and repair. The exact consequences of this epithelial remodelling, myofibroblast differentiation, altered matrix distribution, and neovascularization on the functioning of the airway DCs are currently unknown.

Chronically inflamed asthmatic epithelium might release growth factors such as GM-CSF, VEGF, or TSLP that profoundly influence DC survival and/or function. TSLP is a 140 amino acid, IL-7-like four-helix-bundle cytokine that has potent DC-modulating capacities by binding its receptor complex, composed of the IL-7 receptor (IL-7R) and the TSLP receptor (TSLPR) (Liu et al. 2007; Leonard 2002). TSLP can directly activate DCs to prime naive $CD4^+$ T cells to differentiate into proinflammatory Th2 cells that secrete IL4, IL-5, IL-13 and TNFα, but not IL-10, and express the prostaglandin D_2 receptor CRTH2 (chemoattractant receptor-homologous molecule expressed on TH2 cells), a T-cell phenotype that is also found in asthmatic airways (Ito et al. 2005; Wang et al. 2006). The way by which this polarization occurs has been studied in detail (see Fig. 1). The polarization of Th2 cells induced by TSLP-matured DCs is further enhanced by IL-25, which is produced by epithelial cells, basophils, and eosinophils (Wang et al. 2007). A recent report showed that airway epithelial cells can produce IL-25 in response to an innate immune response to allergen (Angkasekwinai et al. 2007). In addition to its effects on DCs, TSLP can also activate human mast cells to produce Th2-associated effector cytokines in the absence of T cells or IgE cross linking (Allakhverdi et al. 2007). The most convincing evidence for a role for TSLP in DC-driven Th2-cell development came from studies in mice that conditionally overexpressed TSLP in the lungs. These

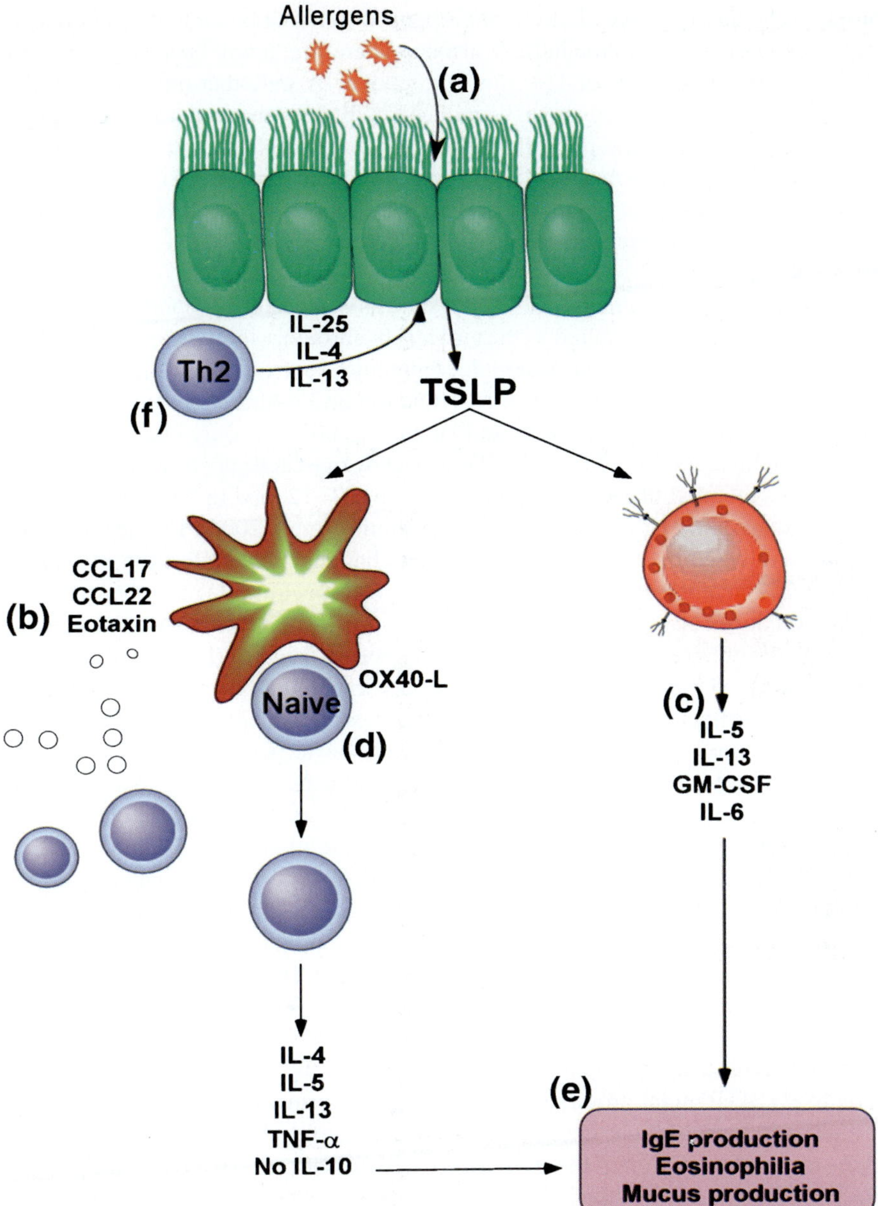

Fig. 1 TSLP takes centre stage in driving DC maturation for Th2-cell responses

mice mounted a vigorous DC-driven primary Th2-cell response in the airways. In contrast, $Tlspr^{-/-}$ mice fail to develop an antigen-specific Th2-cell inflammatory response in the airways unless supplemented with wild-type $CD4^+$ T cells (Zhou et al. 2005; Al-Shami et al. 2005). Taken together, these data suggest that TSLP produced by the lung epithelium might represent a crucial factor that can initiate allergic responses at the epithelial-cell surface. Therefore, it will be very important to study how the production of TSLP by epithelial cells and other inflammatory cells is regulated. TSLP production can be induced by ligands that activate TLR2, TLR3, TLR8, and TLR9, by the proinflammatory cytokines TNF, IL-1α and IL-1β, and by the proallergic cytokines IL-4 and IL-13 (Bogiatzi et al. 2007). In the airways of patients with asthma, the levels of TSLP are increased, but it is not yet known whether exposure to enzymatically active allergens stimulates TSLP release (Ying et al. 2005).

Finally, many inflammatory cell types such as mast cells, basophils, eosinophils, and even platelets are recruited to the airways in chronic asthma. These cells release many mediators such as cytokines, neuropeptides, enzymes, and lipid mediators that may also profoundly influence DC function and in this way might perpetuate ongoing inflammation (Lambrecht and Hammad 2003). As only one example, it is known that histamine and PGD2, both released by mast cells upon IgE cross linking, reduce the potential of DCs to produce bioactive IL-12, and in this way contribute to Th2 polarization (Idzko et al. 2002a,b; Hammad et al. 2003). Extracellular ATP might be released by platelets upon allergen challenge. Neutralization of ATP via administration of the enzyme, apyrase or the broad spectrum P2 receptor antagonist, suramin reduced all the cardinal features of asthma by interfering with DC function, although the precise receptor involved has not been elucidated (Idzko et al. 2007a,b). How exactly ATP promotes DC-driven airway inflammation and how its blockade suppresses asthma is insufficiently known at present. Strikingly, the levels of the major eosinophil (CCL11, CCL24) and Th2 lymphocyte (CCL17, CCL22) selective chemokines were not reduced upon apyrase treatment, suggesting that ATP more likely controls responsiveness of inflammatory cells to chemokine gradients, as recently suggested by in vitro studies using apyrase to reduce neutrophil chemotaxis (Chen et al. 2006). In vitro experiments suggested that purinergic signalling has potent chemotactic effects on immature DCs in humans (Idzko et al. 2002a,b) and mice (Idzko et al. 2007a,b). In support, ATP administration induced a marked increase in the DC chemokine CCL20, a predominant chemokine attracting immature DCs into the mucosa. The subsequent enhanced migration of ATP exposed lung DCs to the mediastinal LN was explained by the upregulation of the CCR7 chemokine receptor, involved in directing the interest of maturing DCs to the T cell area of the node. Alternatively, ATP might promote Th2 responses by formation of the inflammasome, a multimeric intracellular complex of signalling molecules that lead to caspase-1 activation and activation of the IL-1 family of cytokines (IL-1β, IL-18, and possibly IL-33). The formation of the inflammasome has been shown to occur following triggering of the P2X7 receptor by ATP, widely expressed on murine and human DCs, in conjunction with TLR triggering (Mariathasan et al. 2006; Ogura et al. 2006; Ferrari et al. 2006). Clearly, blockade of ATP might also affect other inflammatory cells. Nucleotides cause the release of inflammatory mediators such as eosinophil cationic protein (ECP), radical oxygen intermediates (ROIs), and interleukin-8 (IL-8) from human eosinophils (Ferrari et al. 2006; Idzko et al. 2003).

6 Dendritic Cells as Drug Targets in Allergic Diseases

If DCs are so crucial in mounting immune responses during ongoing inflammation in the lung, nose and skin, then interfering with their function could constitute a novel form of treatment for allergic diseases. Additionally, pharmacological modification of DCs might fundamentally reset the balance of the allergic immune response in favour of regulatory T cells and thus lead to a more long lasting effect on the natural course of allergic disease. Steroids are currently the cornerstone of antiinflammatory treatment in allergic disease. Inhaled steroids reduce the number of lung and nose DCs in patients with allergic asthma and allergic rhinitis (Hammad and Lambrecht 2006). Steroids might also interfere with a GITRL driven induction of the enzyme indoleamine 2,3-dioxygenase (IDO) in plasmacytoid DCs, thus broadly suppressing inflammation (Grohmann et al. 2007). Inhaled steroids reduce the number of lung and nose DCs in patients with AA and AD, whereas local application of steroids to the skin of AD patients reduces the influx of DCs (Moller et al. 1996; Holm et al. 1995). The immunosuppressant drug tacrolimus is currently in use for topical treatment for AD. It suppresses the expression of MHCII and costimulatory molecules and Fc RI on LC from AD patients in vitro and reduces the number of IDECs in lesional skin.

Recently, several other new molecules have surfaced that may alter DC function in allergic inflammation and thus treat disease. Many of these compounds were first discovered by their potential to interfere with DC driven Th2 sensitization. The sphingosine-1-P analogue FTY720 is currently used in clinical trials for multiple sclerosis and transplant rejection. When given locally to the lungs of mice with established inflammation, it strongly reduced inflammation by suppressing the T cell stimulatory capacity and migratory behaviour of lung DCs, without the commonly observed lymphopenia, when the drug is given orally (Idzko et al. 2006). FTY720 inhibited the potential of DCs to form stable synapses with naive Ag specific T cells as well as Th2 effector cells, possibly explaining how these drugs might work to inhibit allergic inflammation.

Selective agonists of particular prostaglandin series receptors might suppress DC function. Prostaglandin D_2 has pleiotropic effects in the immune system, due to its activity on the DP1 and DP2 (also known as CRTH2) receptor, widely expressed on immune cells. The airways of chimeric $DP1^{-/-}$ deficient mice have more mature DCs, pointing to a suppressing role of endogenously released PGD_2 on DC function (Idzko et al. 2007a, b). The DP1 agonist BW245C, strongly suppressed the spontaneous migration of lung DCs to the mediastinal LN (Hammad et al. 2003). More importantly, BW245C suppressed airway inflammation and bronchial hyperreactivity, when given to allergic mice by inhibiting the maturation of lung DCs. In the presence of BW245C, DCs induced the formation of $Foxp3^+$ induced Tregs from $Foxp3^-$ antigen specific T cells (Hammad et al. 2007). A very similar mechanism was described for inhaled iloprost, a prostacyclin analogue acting on the IP receptor expressed by lung DCs (Idzko et al. 2007a,b; Zhou et al. 2007).

As the number and activation status of lung $CD11b^+$ DCs during secondary challenge seems critical for controlling allergic inflammation, studying the factors that control recruitment, survival, or egress from the lung during allergic inflammation will be important, as this might reveal therapeutic targets. In an elegant study using mixed bone marrow chimeras, in which half the hematopoietic cells were $CCR2^{-/-}$ and half were $CCR2^{+/+}$, it was shown by Robays et al. that CCR2 (and not CCR5 or CCR6) is crucial for releasing DC precursors from the bone marrow and attracting them into allergically inflamed lung. This was unexpected, as CCR6 is generally seen as the chemokine receptor attracting immature DCs into peripheral tissues (Robays et al. 2007). Lung mDCs use CCR7 ligands and CCR8 for emigration to the draining lymph node, but not the leukotriene C4 transporter multidrug-related protein-1 as they do in the skin (Jakubzick et al. 2006). Unexpectedly, disruption of CCR7 selective chemokines in paucity of lymphocyte T cell (plt) mutant mice, deficient in CCL21 and CCL19, airway inflammation, and Th2 activity were enhanced (Grinnan et al. 2006). Still, increased numbers of mDCs could be found in the draining lymph node of these mice. So, other factors than CCR7 ligands are involved in the migration of DCs to the draining LN, including other chemokine receptors (Jakubzick et al. 2006). Eicosanoid lipid mediators, like prostaglandins and leukotrienes can also influence the migration of lung DCs (Hammad et al. 2007). Leukotriene LTB4 promoted the migration of immature and mature skin DCs, but these effects seem to be indirect (Del Prete et al. 2007). It will be important to study, if well known inducers of LTB4 in the lungs, such as the environmental biopolymer chitin, derived from fungi, helminthes, and insects, also induces DC migration (Reese et al. 2007).

Some novel drugs are emerging, which effect DC function without a clear mechanism of action. A specific small molecular compound (VAF347) that blocks the function of B cells and DCs was shown to be effective in suppressing allergic airway inflammation in a mouse model of asthma (Ettmayer et al. 2006). Finally, specific inhibitors of *syk* kinase were shown to suppress DC function and cure established inflammation (Matsubara et al. 2006). More detailed information on the interactions between DCs, other inflammatory cells, and epithelial cells will undoubtedly lead to the discovery of more potentially interesting drugs. In this regard, blocking the interaction of TSLP and GMCSF with its respective receptor through small molecule inhibitor or blocking antibodies might prove very useful. Ideally, novel drugs for asthma should also try to restore epithelial barrier function, as this might reduce the threshold for allergen recognition.

7 Conclusion

Dendritic cells are crucial in determining the functional outcome of allergen encounter in the lung, nose and skin and antigen presentation by myeloid DCs leads to Th2 sensitization typical of allergic disease. It is increasingly clear that DCs have an antigen presenting function beyond sensitisation. DCs therefore constitute a novel target for the development of antiallergic therapy aimed at the origin of the inflammatory cascade.

Allergens as well as effector T helper 2 (Th2)-cell-associated cytokines and loss of epithelium barrier function can trigger the production of TSLP by airway epithelial cells. Allergen triggering of protease-activated receptor 2 (PAR2) or by contaminating endotoxin acting on TLRs triggers the activation of *Tslp* gene transcription (a) TSLP induces immediate innate immune functions in DCs leading to chemokine-driven recruitment of Th2 cells and eosinophils to the airways, possibly providing a source for polarizing Th2-cell-associated cytokines. (b) In mast cells, there is immediate release of the Th2 effector cytokines that can attract and activate eosinophils in a T-cell independent way. (c) Following innate immune induction, TSLP triggers the maturation of DCs so that they migrate to the mediastinal lymph nodes and induce the polarization of inflammatory Th2 cells in an OX40L-dependent fashion. In contrast to most other triggers that induce DC maturation, TSLP-induced maturation is not accompanied by the production of interleukin-12 (IL-12), thereby explaining Th2-cell polarization. (d) The effector cytokines produced by adaptive Th2 cells and mast cells trigger the salient features of asthma. (e) Effector cytokines can also perpetuate TSLP-driven inflammation by further triggering the release of TSLP by airway epithelial cells. This process is enhanced by epithelial production of the proallergenic cytokine IL-25.

Acknowledgements The author is supported by an Odysseus grant of the FWO Vlaanderen and by a VIDI grant of the Dutch Organization for Scientific Research.

References

Akbari O, DeKruyff RH, Umetsu DT (2001) Pulmonary dendritic cells producing IL-10 mediate tolerance induced by respiratory exposure to antigen. Nat Immunol 2:725–731

Akbari O, Freeman GJ, Meyer EH, Greenfield EA, Chang TT, Sharpe AH, Berry G, DeKruyff RH, Umetsu DT (2002) Antigen-specific regulatory T cells develop via the ICOS-ICOS-ligand pathway and inhibit allergen-induced airway hyperreactivity. Nat Med 8:1024–1032

Allakhverdi Z, Comeau MR, Jessup HK, Yoon BR, Brewer A, Chartier S, Paquette N, Ziegler SF, Sarfati M, Delespesse G (2007) Thymic stromal lymphopoietin is released by human epithelial cells in response to microbes, trauma, or inflammation and potently activates mast cells. J Exp Med 204:253–258

Al-Shami A, Spolski R, Kelly J, Keane-Myers A, Leonard WJ (2005) A role for TSLP in the development of inflammation in an asthma model. J Exp Med 202:829–839

Angkasekwinai P, Park H, Wang YH, Wang YH, Chang SH, Corry DB, Liu YJ, Zhu Z, Dong C (2007) Interleukin 25 promotes the initiation of proallergic type 2 responses. J Exp Med 204:1509–1517

Beaty SR, Rose CE, Jr., Sung SS (2007) Diverse and potent chemokine production by lung CD11bhi dendritic cells in homeostasis and in allergic lung inflammation. J Immunol 178:1882–1895

Bogiatzi SI, Fernandez I, Bichet JC, Marloie-Provost MA, Volpe E, Sastre X, Soumelis V (2007) Cutting edge: Proinflammatory and Th2 cytokines synergize to induce thymic stromal lymphopoietin production by human skin keratinocytes. J Immunol 178:3373–3377

Bratke K, Lommatzsch M, Julius P, Kuepper M, Kleine HD, Luttmann W, Christian Virchow J (2007) Dendritic cell subsets in human bronchoalveolar lavage fluid after segmental allergen challenge. Thorax 62:168–175

Braun-Fahrlander C, Riedler J, Herz U, Eder W, Waser M, Grize L, Maisch S, Carr D, Gerlach F, Bufe A, Lauener RP, Schierl R, Renz H, Nowak D, von Mutius E (2002) Environmental exposure to endotoxin and its relation to asthma in school-age children. N Engl J Med 347: 869–877

Brimnes MK, Bonifaz L, Steinman RM, Moran TM (2003) Influenza virus-induced dendritic cell maturation is associated with the induction of strong T cell immunity to a coadministered, mormally nonimmunogenic protein. J Exp Med 198:133–144

Chen Y, Corriden R, Inoue Y, Yip L, Hashiguchi N, Zinkernagel A, Nizet V, Insel PA, Junger WG (2006) ATP release guides neutrophil chemotaxis via P2Y2 and A3 receptors. Science 314:1792–1795

Dahl ME, Dabbagh K, Liggitt D, Kim S, Lewis DB (2004) Viral-induced T helper type 1 responses enhance allergic disease by effects on lung dendritic cells. Nat Immunol 5:337–343

De Heer HJ, Hammad H, Soullie T, Hijdra D, Vos N, Willart MA, Hoogsteden HC, Lambrecht BN (2004) Essential role of lung plasmacytoid dendritic cells in preventing asthmatic reactions to harmless inhaled antigen. J Exp Med 200:89–98

de Heer HJ, Hammad H, Kool M, Lambrecht BN (2005) Dendritic cell subsets and immune regulation in the lung. Semin Immunol 17:295–303

Del Prete A, Shao WH, Mitola S, Santoro G, Sozzani S, Haribabu B (2007) Regulation of dendritic cell migration and adaptive immune response by leukotriene B4 receptors: a role for LTB4 in up-regulation of CCR7 expression and function. Blood 109:626–631

Dodge IL, Carr MW, Cernadas M, Brenner MB (2003) IL-6 production by pulmonary dendritic cells impedes Th1 immune responses. J Immunol 170:4457–4464

Doganci A, Eigenbrod T, Krug N, De Sanctis GT, Hausding M, Erpenbeck VJ, Haddad el B, Lehr HA, Schmitt E, Bopp T, Kallen KJ, Herz U, Schmitt S, Luft C, Hecht O, Hohlfeld JM, Ito H, Nishimoto N, Yoshizaki K, Kishimoto T, Rose-John S, Renz H, Neurath MF, Galle PR, Finotto S (2005) The IL-6R alpha chain controls lung CD4 + CD25+ Treg development and function during allergic airway inflammation in vivo. J Clin Invest 115:313–325

Edwan JH, Perry G, Talmadge JE, Agrawal DK (2004) Flt-3 ligand reverses late allergic response and airway hyper-responsiveness in a mouse model of allergic inflammation. J Immunol 172:5016–5023

Eisenbarth SC, Zhadkevich A, Ranney P, Herrick CA, Bottomly K (2004) IL-4-dependent Th2 collateral priming to inhaled antigens independent of toll-like receptor 4 and myeloid differentiation factor 88. J Immunol 172:4527–4534

Ettmayer P, Mayer P, Kalthoff F, Neruda W, Harrer N, Hartmann G, Epstein MM, Brinkmann V, Heusser C, Woisetschlager M (2006) A novel low molecular weight inhibitor of dendritic cells and B cells blocks allergic inflammation. Am J Respir Crit Care Med 173:599–606

Fainaru O, Woolf E, Lotem J, Yarmus M, Brenner O, Goldenberg D, Negreanu V, Bernstein Y, Levanon D, Jung S, Groner Y (2004) Runx3 regulates mouse TGF-beta-mediated dendritic cell function and its absence results in airway inflammation. Embo J 23:969–979

Fainaru O, Shseyov D, Hantisteanu S, Groner Y (2005) Accelerated chemokine receptor 7-mediated dendritic cell migration in Runx3 knockout mice and the spontaneous development of asthma-like disease. Proc Natl Acad Sci U S A 102:10598–10603

Ferrari D, Pizzirani C, Adinolfi E, Lemoli RM, Curti A, Idzko M, Panther E, Di Virgilio F (2006) The P2X7 receptor: a key player in IL-1 processing and release. J Immunol 176:3877–3883

Grinnan D, Sung SS, Dougherty JA, Knowles AR, Allen MB, Rose CE, 3rd, Nakano H, Gunn MD, Fu SM, Rose CE, Jr (2006) Enhanced allergen-induced airway inflammation in paucity of lymph node T cell (plt) mutant mice. J Allergy Clin Immunol 118:1234–1241

Grohmann U, Volpi C, Fallarino F, Bozza S, Bianchi R, Vacca C, Orabona C, Belladonna ML, Ayroldi E, Nocentini G, Boon L, Bistoni F, Fioretti MC, Romani L, Riccardi C, Puccetti P (2007) Reverse signaling through GITR ligand enables dexamethasone to activate IDO in allergy. Nat Med 13:579–586

Hammad H, Lambrecht BN (2006) Recent progress in the biology of airway dendritic cells and implications for understanding the regulation of asthmatic inflammation. J Allergy Clin Immunol 118:331–336

Hammad H, Charbonnier AS, Duez C, Jacquet A, Stewart GA, Tonnel AB, Pestel J (2001) Th2 polarization by Der p 1–pulsed monocyte-derived dendritic cells is due to the allergic status of the donors. Blood 98:1135–1141

Hammad H, de Heer HJ, Souillie T, Hoogsteden HC, Trottein F, Lambrecht BN (2003) Prostaglandin D2 modifies airway dendritic cell migration and function in steady state conditions by selective activation of the DP-receptor. J Immunol 171:3936–3940

Hammad H, Kool M, Soullie T, Narumiya S, Trottein F, Hoogsteden HC, Lambrecht BN (2007) Activation of the D prostanoid 1 receptor suppresses asthma by modulation of lung dendritic cell function and induction of regulatory T cells. J Exp Med 204:357–367

Herrick CA, Bottomly K (2003) To respond or not to respond: T cells in allergic asthma. Nat Rev Immunol 3:405–412

Hintzen G, Ohl L, del Rio ML, Rodriguez-Barbosa JI, Pabst O, Kocks JR, Krege J, Hardtke S, Forster R (2006) Induction of tolerance to innocuous inhaled antigen relies on a CCR7-dependent dendritic cell-mediated antigen transport to the bronchial lymph node. J Immunol 177:7346–7354

Holm AF, Fokkens WJ, Godthelp T, Mulder PG, Vroom TM, Rijntjes E (1995) Effect of 3 months' nasal steroid therapy on nasal T cells and Langerhans cells in patients suffering from allergic rhinitis. Allergy 50:204–209

Huh JC, Strickland DH, Jahnsen FL, Turner DJ, Thomas JA, Napoli S, Tobagus I, Stumbles PA, Sly PD, Holt PG (2003) Bidirectional interactions between antigen-bearing respiratory tract dendritic cells (DCs) and T cells precede the late phase reaction in experimental asthma: DC activation occurs in the airway mucosa but not in the lung parenchyma. J Exp Med 198:19–30

Idzko M, Dichmann S, Ferrari D, Di Virgilio F, la Sala A, Girolomoni G, Panther E, Norgauer J (2002a) Nucleotides induce chemotaxis and actin polymerization in immature but not mature human dendritic cells via activation of pertussis toxin-sensitive P2y receptors. Blood 100: 925–932

Idzko M, la Sala A, Ferrari D, Panther E, Herouy Y, Dichmann S, Mockenhaupt M, Di Virgilio F, Girolomoni G, Norgauer J (2002b) Expression and function of histamine receptors in human monocyte-derived dendritic cells. J Allergy Clin Immunol 109:839–846

Idzko M, Panther E, Bremer HC, Sorichter S, Luttmann W, Virchow CJ, Jr., Di Virgilio F, Herouy Y, Norgauer J, Ferrari D (2003) Stimulation of P2 purinergic receptors induces the release of eosinophil cationic protein and interleukin-8 from human eosinophils. Br J Pharmacol 138:1244–1250

Idzko M, Hammad H, van Nimwegen M, Kool M, Muller T, Soullie T, Willart MA, Hijdra D, Hoogsteden HC, Lambrecht BN (2006) Local application of FTY720 to the lung abrogates experimental asthma by altering dendritic cell function. J Clin Invest 116:2935–2944

Idzko M, Hammad H, van Nimwegen M, Kool M, Vos N, Hoogsteden HC, Lambrecht BN (2007a) Inhaled iloprost suppresses the cardinal features of asthma via inhibition of airway dendritic cell function. J Clin Invest 117:464–472

Idzko M, Hammad H, van Nimwegen M, Kool M, Willart MA, Muskens F, Hoogsteden HC, Luttmann W, Ferrari D, Di Virgilio F, Virchow JC, Jr., Lambrecht BN (2007b) Extracellular ATP triggers and maintains asthmatic airway inflammation by activating dendritic cells. Nat Med 13:913–919

Ito T, Wang YH, Duramad O, Hori T, Delespesse GJ, Watanabe N, Qin FX, Yao Z, Cao W, Liu YJ (2005) TSLP-activated dendritic cells induce an inflammatory T helper type 2 cell response through OX40 ligand. J Exp Med 202:1213–1223

Jahnsen FL, Lund-Johansen F, Dunne JF, Farkas L, Haye R, Brandtzaeg P (2000) Experimentally induced recruitment of plasmacytoid (CD123high) dendritic cells in human nasal allergy. J Immunol 165:4062–4068

Jahnsen FL, Moloney ED, Hogan T, Upham JW, Burke CM, Holt PG (2001) Rapid dendritic cell recruitment to the bronchial mucosa of patients with atopic asthma in response to local allergen challenge. Thorax 56:823–826

Jakubzick C, Tacke F, Llodra J, van Rooijen N, Randolph GJ (2006) Modulation of dendritic cell trafficking to and from the airways. J Immunol 176:3578–3584

Kearley J, Barker JE, Robinson DS, Lloyd CM (2005) Resolution of airway inflammation and hyperreactivity after in vivo transfer of CD4 + CD25+ regulatory T cells is interleukin 10 dependent. J Exp Med 202:1539–1547

Kheradmand F, Kiss A, Xu J, Lee SH, Kolattukudy PE, Corry DB (2002) A protease-activated pathway underlying Th cell type 2 activation and allergic lung disease. J Immunol 169:5904–5911

KleinJan A, Willart M, van Rijt LS, Braunstahl GJ, Leman K, Jung S, Hoogsteden HC, Lambrecht BN (2006) An essential role for dendritic cells in human and experimental allergic rhinitis. J Allergy Clin Immunol 118:1117–1125

Kohl J, Baelder R, Lewkowich IP, Pandey MK, Hawlisch H, Wang L, Best J, Herman NS, Sproles AA, Zwirner J, Whitsett JA, Gerard C, Sfyroera G, Lambris JD, Wills-Karp M (2006) A regulatory role for the C5a anaphylatoxin in type 2 immunity in asthma. J Clin Invest 116: 783–796

Koya T, Kodama T, Takeda K, Miyahara N, Yang ES, Taube C, Joetham A, Park JW, Dakhama A, Gelfand EW (2006) Importance of myeloid dendritic cells in persistent airway disease after repeated allergen exposure. Am J Respir Crit Care Med 173:42–55

Kuipers H, Lambrecht BN (2004) The interplay of dendritic cells, Th2 cells and regulatory T cells in asthma. Curr Opin Immunol 16:702–708

Lambrecht BN, Hammad H (2003) Taking our breath away: dendritic cells in the pathogenesis of asthma. Nat Rev Immunol 3:994–1003

Lambrecht BN, Salomon B, Klatzmann D, Pauwels RA (1998) Dendritic cells are required for the development of chronic eosinophilic airway inflammation in response to inhaled antigen in sensitized mice. J Immunol 160:4090–4097

Leonard WJ (2002) TSLP: finally in the limelight. Nat Immunol 3:605–607

Lewkowich IP, Herman NS, Schleifer KW, Dance MP, Chen BL, Dienger KM, Sproles AA, Shah JS, Kohl J, Belkaid Y, Wills-Karp M (2005) CD4 + CD25+ T cells protect against experimentally induced asthma and alter pulmonary dendritic cell phenotype and function. J Exp Med 202:1549–1561

Liu YJ, Soumelis V, Watanabe N, Ito T, Wang YH, Malefyt Rde W, Omori M, Zhou B, Ziegler SF (2007) TSLP: an epithelial cell cytokine that regulates T cell differentiation by conditioning dendritic cell maturation. Annu Rev Immunol 25:193–219

Mariathasan S, Weiss DS, Newton K, McBride J, O'Rourke K, Roose-Girma M, Lee WP, Weinrauch Y, Monack DM, Dixit VM (2006) Cryopyrin activates the inflammasome in response to toxins and ATP. Nature 440:228–232

Matsubara S, Koya T, Takeda K, Joetham A, Miyahara N, Pine P, Masuda ES, Swasey CH, Gelfand EW (2006) Syk activation in dendritic cells is essential for airway hyperresponsiveness and inflammation. Am J Respir Cell Mol Biol 34:426–433

Moller GM, Overbeek SE, Van Helden-Meeuwsen CG, Van Haarst JM, Prens EP, Mulder PG, Postma DS, Hoogsteden HC (1996) Increased numbers of dendritic cells in the bronchial mucosa of atopic asthmatic patients: downregulation by inhaled corticosteroids. Clin Exp Allergy 26:517–524

Niess JH, Brand S, Gu X, Landsman L, Jung S, McCormick BA, Vyas JM, Boes M, Ploegh HL, Fox JG, Littman DR, Reinecker HC (2005) CX3CR1-mediated dendritic cell access to the intestinal lumen and bacterial clearance. Science 307:254–258

Ogura Y, Sutterwala FS, Flavell RA (2006) The inflammasome: first line of the immune response to cell stress. Cell 126:659–662

Oriss TB, Ostroukhova M, Seguin-Devaux C, Dixon-McCarthy B, Stolz DB, Watkins SC, Pillemer B, Ray P, Ray A (2005) Dynamics of dendritic cell phenotype and interactions with CD4+ T cells in airway inflammation and tolerance. J Immunol 174:854–863

Ostroukhova M, Seguin-Devaux C, Oriss TB, Dixon-McCarthy B, Yang L, Ameredes BT, Corcoran TE, Ray A (2004) Tolerance induced by inhaled antigen involves CD4(+) T cells expressing membrane-bound TGF-beta and FOXP3. J Clin Invest 114:28–38

Piggott DA, Eisenbarth SC, Xu L, Constant SL, Huleatt JW, Herrick CA, Bottomly K (2005) MyD88-dependent induction of allergic Th2 responses to intranasal antigen. J Clin Invest 115:459–467

Reese TA, Liang HE, Tager AM, Luster AD, Van Rooijen N, Voehringer D, Locksley RM (2007) Chitin induces accumulation in tissue of innate immune cells associated with allergy. Nature 447:92–96

Robays LJ, Maes T, Lebecque S, Lira SA, Kuziel WA, Brusselle GG, Joos GF, Vermaelen KV (2007) Chemokine receptor CCR2 but not CCR5 or CCR6 mediates the increase in pulmonary dendritic cells during allergic airway inflammation. J Immunol 178:5305–5311

Shortman K, Liu YJ (2002) Mouse and human dendritic cell subtypes. Nat Rev Immunol 2: 151–161

Sporri R, Reise Sousa C (2005) Inflammatory mediators are insufficient for full dendritic cell activation and promote expansion of CD4+ T cell populations lacking helper function. Nat Immunol 6:163–170

Stampfli MR, Wiley RE, Scott Neigh G, Gajewska BU, Lei XF, Snider DP, Xing Z, Jordana M (1998) GM-CSF transgene expression in the airway allows aerosolized ovalbumin to induce allergic sensitization in mice. J Clin Invest 102:1704–1714

Steinman RM, Cohn ZA (1973) Identification of a novel cell type in peripheral lymphoid organs of mice.I. Morphology, quantitation, tissue distribution. J Exp Med 137:1142–1162

Strickland DH, Stumbles PA, Zosky GR, Subrata LS, Thomas JA, Turner DJ, Sly PD, Holt PG (2006) Reversal of airway hyperresponsiveness by induction of airway mucosal CD4+CD25+ regulatory T cells. J Exp Med 203:2649–2660

Upham JW, Denburg JA, O'Byrne PM (2002) Rapid response of circulating myeloid dendritic cells to inhaled allergen in asthmatic subjects. Clin Exp Allergy 32:818–823

Van Hove CL, Maes T, Joos GF, Tournoy KG (2007) Prolonged inhaled allergen exposure can induce persistent tolerance. Am J Respir Cell Mol Biol 36:573–584

van Rijt LS, Prins JB, deVries VC, Leenen PJ, Thielemans K, Hoogsteden HC, Lambrecht BN (2002) Allergen-induced accumulation of airway dendritic cells is supported by an increase in $CD31^{hi}$ $Ly\text{-}6C^{neg}$ hematopoietic precursors. Blood 100:3663–3671

Van Rijt LS, Vos N, Willart M, Kleinjan A, Coyle AJ, Hoogsteden HC, Lambrecht BN (2004) Essential role of dendritic cell CD80/CD86 costimulation in the induction, but not reactivation, of TH2 effector responses in a mouse model of asthma. J Allergy Clin Immunol 114:166–173

van Rijt LS, Jung S, Kleinjan A, Vos N, Willart M, Duez C, Hoogsteden HC, Lambrecht BN (2005) In vivo depletion of lung CD11c+ dendritic cells during allergen challenge abrogates the characteristic features of asthma. J Exp Med 201:981–991

Vermaelen K, Pauwels R (2003) Accelerated airway dendritic cell maturation, trafficking, and elimination in a mouse model of asthma. Am J Respir Cell Mol Biol 29:405–409

Vermaelen K, Cataldo D, Tournoy KG, Maes T, Dhulst A, Louis R, Foidart J-M, Noel A, Pauwels RA (2003) Matrix metalloproteinse-9-mediated dendritic cell recruitment into the airways is a critical step in mouse model of asthma. J Immunol 171:1016–1022

Vermaelen KY, Carro-Muino I, Lambrecht BN, Pauwels RA (2001) Specific migratory dendritic cells rapidly transport antigen from the airways to the thoracic lymph nodes. J Exp Med 193: 51–60

Wang YH, Ito T, Wang YH, Homey B, Watanabe N, Martin R, Barnes CJ, McIntyre BW, Gilliet M, Kumar R, Yao Z, Liu YJ (2006) Maintenance and polarization of human TH2 central memory T cells by thymic stromal lymphopoietin-activated dendritic cells. Immunity 24:827–838

Wang YH, Angkasekwinai P, Lu N, Voo KS, Arima K, Hanabuchi S, Hippe A, Corrigan CJ, Dong C, Homey B, Yao Z, Ying S, Huston DP, Liu YJ (2007) IL-25 augments type 2 immune responses by enhancing the expansion and functions of TSLP-DC-activated Th2 memory cells. J Exp Med 204:1837–1847

Xanthou G, Alissafi T, Semitekolou M, Simoes DC, Economidou E, Gaga M, Lambrecht BN, Lloyd CM, Panoutsakopoulou V (2007) Osteopontin has a crucial role in allergic airway disease through regulation of dendritic cell subsets. Nat Med 13:570–578

Ying S, O'Connor B, Ratoff J, Meng Q, Mallett K, Cousins D, Robinson D, Zhang G, Zhao J, Lee TH, Corrigan C (2005) Thymic stromal lymphopoietin expression is increased in asthmatic airways and correlates with expression of Th2-attracting chemokines and disease severity. J Immunol 174:8183–8190

Zhou B, Comeau MR, De Smedt T, Liggitt HD, Dahl ME, Lewis DB, Gyarmati D, Aye T, Campbell DJ, Ziegler SF (2005) Thymic stromal lymphopoietin as a key initiator of allergic airway inflammation in mice. Nat Immunol 6:1047–1053

Zhou W, Hashimoto K, Goleniewska K, O'Neal JF, Ji S, Blackwell TS, Fitzgerald GA, Egan KM, Geraci MW, Peebles RS (2007) Prostaglandin I2 analogs inhibit proinflammatory cytokine production and T cell stimulatroy function of dendritic cells. J Immunol 178:702–710

Dendritic Cells in Rhinitis

Alex KleinJan and Bart N. Lambrecht

Contents

A. KleinJan (✉)
Department of Pulmonary Medicine, Erasmus MC, Room Ee2257b, Dr. Molewaterplein 50, 3015 GE. Rotterdam, The Netherlands
a.kleinjan@erasmusmc.nl

G. Lombardi, Y. Riffo-Vasquez (eds.), *Dendritic Cells,* Handbook of Experimental Pharmacology 188,

Abstract Dendritic cells (DCs) play an important role in all kind of rhinitis and sinusitis. One of the most important upper airway diseases is allergic rhinitis. DCs are the professional antigen presenting cells that have the capacity to present antigen to naive–T cells and T-effector cells. In the context of a broad spectrum of rhinitis, from allergic rhinitis via upper respiratory tract virus infection to chronic sinusitis, DCs have an important role in the immunological outcome of the disease. Studies in humans and animal models that have highlighted the role of DC were evaluated. This article reviews recent information on the involvement of DC in rhinitis, and the mechanisms by which DC could be employed as targets for therapeutic intervention.

1 Introduction

The nose is the part of the human body with mucosal tissue that gets in contact with inhaled air. It functions like an air conditioner, which filters and humidifies air that is inhaled. Because of these functions, the nose is continuously exposed to pathogens and, when dry air is inhaled, mucosa becoming over-dry is also a possibility. These dangers need to be prevented by good defense mechanisms that protect against pathogens and dried mucosa.

The mucosa is covered with a thin layer of mucous (fluid), the epithelial lining fluid. This has the function of preventing dehydration of the mucosa, humidifying the inspired air and also trapping pathogens. The lining fluid contains enzymes, chemicals, anti-microbial peptides, etc. that prevent the growth of pathogens. The fluid has a continuous flow in the direction of the nasopharynx, due to the movement of the cilia from epithelial cells.

Between the epithelial cells are goblet cells, situated for the production of the epithelial lining fluid. If pathogens survive in the epithelial lining fluid, then the epithelium can dispose of these by the flow of the epithelial lining fluid. In the case that this is insufficient, there is another defense mechanism, which is caused by immune cells. These immune cells stay in the epithelium until they have been activated by a stimulus that is recognized by that particular cell. The most important immune competent cells in the epithelium are the dendritic cells (DCs), in steady state condition a few of these professional antigen presenting cells (APC) are present. These DCs formed an intensive network of cells in between the epithelial cells (Jahnsen et al. 2002; Kleinjan et al. 2006; Takano et al. 2005). DCs have the possibility to open the tight junctions enabling dendrite sprouting beyond the epithelium. The DC can sample the lumen in the lower airway as observed by Hammad et al (unpublished observation). When the DCs are triggered, they get activated and change from an immature DC into a mature DC phenotype. The sentinel function of DCs is very important for inducing an immune response.

2 Passive and Active Antigen Migration

2.1 Migration of Antigens in the Upper Airways

The deposition of the airways depends on the method of administration antigens. Mice and other rodents are obligate nose breathers. When Evans blue dye is applied to the nose of an anesthetized mouse, 25% of the dye can found back in the nose, 13% in the esophagus and stomach and 31% can found back in the trachea and lower airways, as described in a model for asthma (Tomaki et al. 2000). If the antigen is introduced only locally in the nose for models of AR then the dye should affect only the upper airways and not the lower airways. For this reason, it is important to confirm that there is no involvement of the lower airways or significant overspill of the antigen in the lower airways. The exposure of antigen to only the upper airways is confirmed by several authors. Saito et al and McCusker et al describe the distribution of an intranasal application in non-anesthetized mice including nasal mucosa, oral mucosa, pharynx, larynx, subglottic region, and gastrointestinal tract; however, from below the tracheal region to the lower airways or spleen as a control method, no significant dye uptake was observed (McCusker et al. 2002; Saito et al. 2001; Wang and McCusker 2005). Studying the deposition of airborne particles indicated that 83% of the particles were indeed trapped in the nasal mucosa and 13% in the lower airway (Hellings and Ceuppens 2004). Airborne particle studies illustrate that size, weight, and the manner of inhalation influence the deposition of the particles in the airways (Barry and O'Callaghan 1996), which suggests that different models of applying antigen in solution or aerosol damp or airborne particles give different deposition of the antigens. An important question is how do antigens appear in the draining lymph node, just by passive transport via the lymph conduits or by cellular uptake and transport?

2.2 DC Migration from Peripheral Tissue to the Draining LN

Once DCs have been activated, they expressed receptors and react to chemokines signaling. Then DCs start to migrate in the direction of a lymph node (LN). Data strongly suggests that these activated maturated DCs migrate via the lymphatic vessel and appear in the draining lymph node. Once they have arrived in the draining LN, they present antigen to antigen specific T-cells and decide in which of them the immune response should occur. This process is generally the same for all immune responses. This migration pattern is made clear by the skin. Experiments performed with skin painting showed the migration of DC/Langerhans Cells (LC) from the epidermis to the draining LN. The question is: "Does this migration occur in the nasal mucosa as well?"

In a human migration study of the respiratory tract, it is indicated that tumor-specific pulsed dendritic cells that are introduced by injection in the nasal inferior lysate turbinates can be traced back to the injection side of the nose and the regional lymph nodes (Horiguchi et al. 2007). Tumor specific T-cell reaction was detected in the ipsilaterals but not in the contra lateral LN (Horiguchi et al. 2007). Although DCs used in this study were monocyte derived DCs, they still clearly show a localized draining and migration pattern. Moreover, introduction of CFSE labeled murine DCs in the nasal mucosa in droplet form resulted in detectable CFSE labeled DCs in the nasal mucosa in the nasal associated lymphoid tissue (NALT) and in the cervical LN, which drains the nose. No CFSE labeled cells could be detected either in the mediastinal LN or in the lung (KleinJan et al unpublished observations). An earlier study showed the presence and function of migratory cells, which transport the antigen from the nasal epithelial side to other sides. Administration of a fluorescent dye (DiY) dissolved in glycerine, in the nasal cavity of mice was followed by a time curve of harvesting the nasal mucosa containing the nasal associated lymphoid tissue and the cervical LN, the mediastinal LN. These DiY experiments indicate that DiY positive cells appear in the NALT within 2 h and in the cervical LN within 6 h and last for up to 48 h. No DiY could be observed in the mediastinal LN nor in mesenteric LN suggesting that the nasal mucosa side is drained by NALT and CLN and that there is no uptake of the antigen in places other than the nasal mucosa as indicated by the absence of DiY in the draining LN of the lung or intestinal mucosa (Vinke and Fokken 1999).

Recent studies with confocal microscopy indicate that soluble antigen-immune complex reach the draining lymph node very fast within 15 min just by passive transport due to the lymph flow (Phan et al. 2007).

3 DCs in the Nasal Mucosa

3.1 DCs and DC Related Cytokine Predict the Immunological Outcome in Infants

Once captured and transported, antigens by DCs into the lymph node are followed by a T-cell response. The initial hallmark of DC function is that, it is a potent stimulator of T-cell response. Not only DCs play an important role in the induction of a T cell response in an allergic sensitization contexts but also in all kinds of infections.

The percentage of IL-10 positive cells in nasal epithelium is high in infants suggesting a pro Th2 milieu. In infants, a nasal Th1 immune response is induced during rhinovirus or RSV-induced upper respiratory tract infections, which show an increase in the response of TNF-α and a reduction in the regulatory cytokine response of IL10. In the epithelium of the nasal mucosa of children, DCs are present as measured by nasal brushes. The nasal brush harvests the upper part of the epithelium (van Benten et al. 2005). Although in nasal mucosal biopsies, DCs are present in quite large numbers in children (age 4–12 years) 293 cells mm^2, median value with a range of 32–683 cells mm^2 in the epithelium and 25 (0–90) cells mm^2 in the lamina propira suggest an active presence of these cells in the epithelium (Vinke et al. 1999). A cohort study showed that infants are born with a high natural expression of IL-10 in their nasal epithelial cells. During respiratory viral infection down regulation of IL-10 occurs, TNF-α as a marker of pro-inflammator cytokine is elevated during infection. About 2 years after birth, the high baseline levels of IL-10 positive epithelial cells reduce (van Benten et al. 2005). Children with an RSV infection showed no enhancement of Th2 related cytokine but rather an increased pro-inflammatory Th1 related response as measured by IL-18 (van Benten et al. 2003) as a strong inducer of IFN-γ as an important Th1 representative. IL-18 synergizes with IL-12 in the induction of IFN-γ production of NK-cells and T-cells. Also, in skin it is observed that IL-18 is capable of initiating LC/DC migration from an epidermal site with subsequent accumulation of mature DC in draining LN (Antonopoulos et al. 2008). This suggests that the minimal amount of DCs observed during upper respiratory tract infection and the high levels of IL-18 that a similar process of DC migration could have taken place in the nasal mucosa, as observed in the skin during URTI.

DC related cytokine, IL-10 production of DCs has a proTh2 direction, suggests that infants have a proTh2 milieu in the nasal mucosa tissue although this could also be considered as a regulatory or anti-inflammatory cytokine. IL-10 may also directly act on immature resting DCs, resulting in DCs that stimulate T-cells to become unresponsive.

When DCs produce low amounts of IL-12, the outcome of the T-cell response is proTh2 as measured by the cytokines produced by T-cells. When DCs produce IL-12, the T-cell response is proTh1. The IL-12 production of DCs is mainly dependent on the presence of bacterial product like LPS (Martin et al. 2003; Trinchieri 2003).

The induction of IL-12 by microbial patterns is not only a marker of Th1 bias, but also it seems to inhibit the sensitization (Kuipers et al. 2004). The exposure to microbial products in early life is inversely correlated with the development of atopic sensitization (Braun-Fahrlander 2003). This observation is in agreement with the high level of IL-10 in nasal epithelial cells as observed in infants, which can alter in pro Th1 by IL-12 or IL-18, the IL-12 production is induced by the exposure to viruses and LPS.

3.2 DCs in the Local Micro Environment

The local microenvironments of the nasal mucosa have a pro-maturating feature on DCs (Faith et al. 2005). An important cell is the epithelial cell, which can influence DCs and vice versa. From the epithelial cells itself, it is suggested that these have also some antigen presenting capacities, although (Takizawa et al. 2007) no comparable data was available regarding the strength of these capacities in a DC context and this should be regarded with caution. Moreover, epithelial cells are structural cells and are unable to migrate to the draining LN, which is an unique feature for DCs as being sentinels. That epithelial cells indeed have an enormous

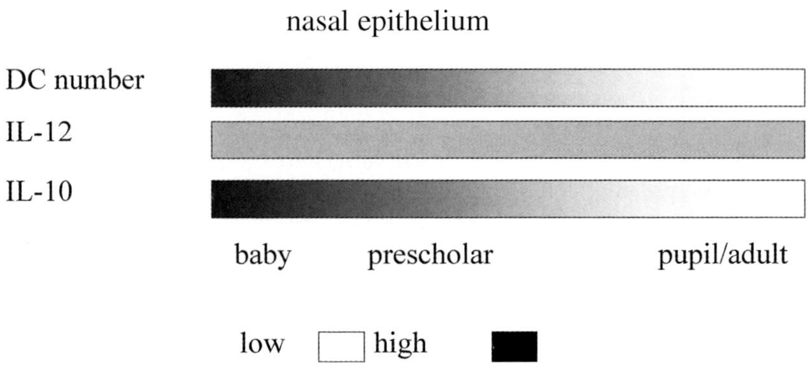

Fig. 1 The nasal epithelial cell produced cytokines. Studies in infants and children showed that the immune system of infants mature during childhood in an adult immune system. Impressing are the observations that nasal mucosa epithelial cells produce large amount of IL-10. After several upper airway infections the epithelial cells seem to change and produce less IL-10. Children at prescholar age showed no significant levels of IL-10 in nasal epithelial cells. The IL-12 production is very low. Regarding the numbers of DCs they are at the age 2 years still present and slightly seem to decline, when they become adults DC were present only in limited numbers

influence on DCs is clear. Epithelial cells form an important barrier against invading pathogens. Within the epithelium, DCs form a dense network, the dendrites can open or even can be a part of the tight junctions barrier function and penetrate beyond well-developed epithelial tight junctions in human nasal mucosa of allergic rhinitis. (Kleinjan et al. 2006; Takano et al. 2005). DCs express CD103 (alpha E-beta7 the ligand for E-cadherin) Fc receptors; langerin and tight junction proteins (Sung et al. 2006). Epithelial cells can produce an enormous amount of cytokines (Salib et al. 2005), which influence DCs and support the recruitment of DCs and other inflammatory cells like eosinophils mast cells and T-cells. Moreover, specific chemokine attracting DCs are produced in epithelial cells for the recruitment of DCs (Marcet et al. 2007). These clarify the elevated DC numbers in the epithelial side of the nasal mucosa in symptomatic allergic rhinitis patients (Fig. 1).

DCs present in the epithelium can be stimulated and matured after being triggered by their TLR's. Matured DCs migrate from the epithelium by down regulation of their so called anchor molecules like E-cadherin, CD103, etc. followed by the migration towards the lamina propria for stimulation of T-cells or by migrating to the draining LN. In skin, down regulation of E-cadherin is associated with DC maturation (Jiang et al. 2007). As well as in pre-neoplastic cervic HPV associated abnormalities, loss of E-cadherin has been observed together with the lack of DCs in the epithelium (Hubert et al. 2005).

3.3 DCs Act in General as Sentinels, Which Take up Antigens

The presence of DCs in quite large numbers in children in the epithelium and lamina propira, suggests an active presence of these cells (Vinke et al. 1999). In adults, these number were less (Braunstahl et al. 2003). In samples taken from virus infected children, almost no DCs could be detected in cells from nasopharyngeal washes, although there are significant numbers of monocytes 4.4% (0–15.6) around (Brandenburg et al. 2000). Nasal brushes obtained from children during an infection showed minimal numbers of DCs varying from complete absence in samples of more than 50,000 cells up to 25 per 50,000 cells. Analysis of inflammatory cells' nasal mucosa brushes showed the presence of only minimal DCs, during viral infection almost below the detection levels. Moreover, $CD14^+$ cells can always detected at high levels during viral infection in the nasal mucosa (Brandenburg et al. 2000; van Benten et al. 2001). This means that the number of DCs is very small in these samples, and that there are only limited numbers of DCs after the first 2 days of infection. In vivo influenza infections in mice show that there is an almost complete absence of DCs in tracheal whole mounts at fourth day post infection (Geurts van Kessel manuscript in preparation).

The dynamics of DCs in this study strongly suggest that after DCs have been taken up antigens, they migrate to the draining lymph node. These observations in mice are in agreement with the human data in which DCs seem to be absent in the nasal mucosa during infection in children as well as in adults. We have observed only limited numbers of DCs in natural occurring upper respiratory tract virus infections (van Benten et al. 2001). The number of monocytes and macrophages increase significantly during the acute phase of the infection. In general, the numbers of DCs in healthy or asymptomatic allergic rhinitis patients are very limited. We report only a few DCs at baseline level in the nasal mucosa of healthy controls and allergic rhinitis patients with or without asthma (Braunstahl et al. 2003). The numbers of other subtypes of DCs like langerin (CD207) positive cells and DC-LAMP (CD208) positive cells were too few for reliable analysis in this studied population (unpublished observations).

4 DC Characterization

4.1 Phenotype of Nasal Mucosal DCs

Faith et al. studied the role of nasal mucosa dendritic cells (NMDC) and compare their function with peripheral blood DCs. The phenotype of NMDCs obtained from non-atopic chronic rhinitis patients or healthy nasal mucosa showed cells positive for CD1a, HLA-DR, CD11c, CD116, CD1c, TLR4, CD40, CD80, CD86, CCR6 and lack the expression of CCR7, which is important for the migration to the draining LN (Faith et al. 2005). The absence of CCR7 could be due to the fact that patients with chronic rhinitis have also abnormalities in blood granulocytes polarization that can be restored by G-CSF (Kalkman et al. 2002). In the nasal mucosa, CD86 can easily be identified by immunohistochemical stainings. At baseline level, the expression of CD86 is higher in the nasal mucosa of perennial allergic rhinitis patients compared to healthy controls (Hattori et al. 2001). Moreover, CD86 is induced in perennial HDM sensitive allergic rhinitis and the percentage DCs expressing CD86 is higher in HDM allergic patients than in healthy controls in the nasal mucosa (Kleinjan et al. 2006). More cells express CD86 and CD80 after allergen provocation in the nasal mucosa in allergic rhinitis patients (Hattori et al. 2001). The expression of costimulatory molecules were weakly expressed compared to blood DCs in which expression could be increased by GM-CSF into a more mature phenotype (Faith et al. 2005). Flow cytometric data indicates the lack of CD86 on DCs from the epithelium of nasal turbinates of healthy controls (Hartmann et al. 2006).

4.2 Subtypes of DCs

In the airways of humans, there are currently several different DC subtypes characterized as resident DCs (CD1a^{+} or langerin CD207^{+} cells), Inflammatory DCs (CD11c^{+} MHC II^{+} cells), and pDCs (CD123^{+} or BDCA2^{+} or BDCA 4^{+}). Animal studies prove differences in DC subtypes in the capacity of antigen presentation and cross presentation (del Rio et al. 2007).

Inflammatory DCs (in mice characterized as CD103^{-}CD11b^{+}CD11^{+}DC) particularly under conditions of inflammation, for priming and restimulating effector CD4 cells (Hintzen et al. 2006), can easily be grown from bone marrow cells in the presence of GM-CSF that closely resemble human in vitro monocyte-derived DCs. When an adoptive transfer of inflammatory DCs is given intra nasally in AR animals, the features of AR exacerbates, indicates the important role of inflammatory DCs in the ongoing inflammation and disease (Kleinjan et al. 2006).

Resident DCs (characterized as CD103^{+}CD11b^{-}CD11c^{+}DC) seem to have an important function in sampling the luminal side of the airways. These cells express junctional antigens, which keep the epithelial barrier intact, and are thought to play an important role in taking up antigens and migration to the draining LN in a CCR7 dependent manner (del Rio et al. 2007; Sung et al. 2006) and by the expression of CD103 they could be a mouse counterpart of the human langerhans cells. Similar histological data was observed in allergic rhinitis patients. Takano et al. showed that HLA-DR- and CD11c-positive DCs expressed claudin-1 and penetrated beyond occludin in the epithelium of the nasal mucosa with, but not without, allergic rhinitis (Takano et al. 2005). Moreover, the epithelial barrier function measured by a dye tracer was well maintained in occludin-positive tight junctions in the epithelium of the nasal mucosa (Takano et al. 2005. The CD11c positive DCs almost completely overlap with the population of CD1a (Kleinjan et al. 2006) suggesting that the nasal mucosa langerhans cells have the same properties.

Functional studies in human nasal mucosal DCs were only limited to describing the costimulator molecules and comparison between markers with flow cytometry. Allan et al. showed that 40% of the CD1a positive DCs were CD207 (langerin) positive, suggesting that this part were the Langerhans Cells (Allam et al. 2006). Almost 80% of the CD1a positive cells expressed CD11b as a marker of inflammatory DCs (Allam et al. 2006). This result suggested that at least a part of the LC has a more in-

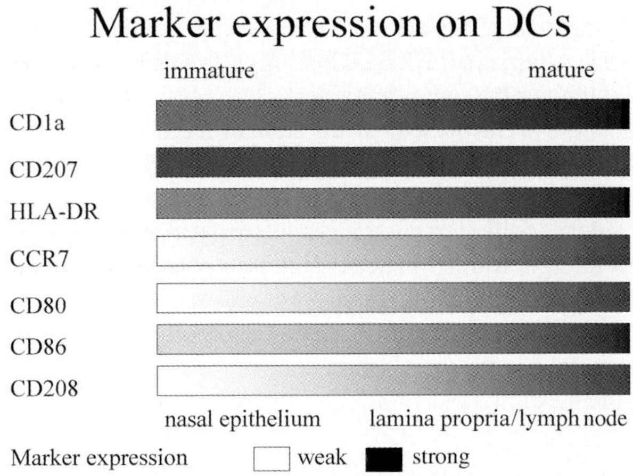

Fig. 2 Marker expression in the nasal mucosa of DCs. DCs express several markers reflecting their maturation stage. DCs are immature if they are found in the epithelium. After DCs picked up antigens they activate and express maturation markers. Costimulatoir molecule expression increases as measured by CD80 and CD86 when DCs move from the epithelium in the lamina propria in which they have a higher expression of these costimulatoir molecules. The expression of MHC-II as measured by HLA-DR in humans or I-A in mouse increase along maturation. The CCR7 chemokine receptor is highly expressed when DCs are ready for migration to the draining lymph node. It is not clear so far when DCs migrate to the lamina propria if they are underway to the draining lymph node or that they get specific signals for staying in the lamina propria to stimulate T-effector cells. The expression of marker CD208 increases during maturation

flammatory phenotype, while the absence of CD11b suggests a resident phenotype and that DCs in human tend to show similar phenotypic characteristics as in mouse (Fig. 2).

4.3 Role of Plasmacytoid DCs in Rhinitis

Since Jahnsen et al. 2002 first described the plamacytoid DCs in the nasal mucosa, several other authors confirm this observation (Hartmann et al. 2006; Jahnsen et al. 2002; Kleinjan et al. 2006). The dynamics of pDCs follow almost the same trend as mDCs do in the nasal mucosa of seasonal allergic rhinitis (Jahnsen et al.), although symptomatic perennial house dust mite allergic rhinitis patients do not differ from healthy controls (Kleinjan et al. 2006). Flowcytometric analysis suggests a lower percentage of pDCs in allergics than healthy controls (Hartmann et al. 2006). Although, these observations should refer to a standard cell, which is not different between tissues from patients and healthy controls and therefore these data are difficult to interpret. Calculating the mDCs: pDCs ratio data shows that there is a higher proportion in favor of mDCs in case of Th2 disease and in favor of pDCs in case of infections. The mDC:pDC ratio in healthy is nearly one (Hartmann et al. 2006).

The oral mucosa lacks pDCs and the DCs present in the oral mucosa have an epidermal phenotype (Allam et al. 2006). This suggests a difference between respirator epithelium and the mucosa from other sides.

Plasmacytoid DCs were present in the human nasal mucosa as well as in animals. No initial differences in pDCs were observed in mild–moderate symptomatic HDM allergic rhinitis patients compared to healthy controls (Kleinjan et al. 2006). Although after relevant allergen challenges, increase of pDCs were observed in the nasal mucosa of allergic rhinitis patients (Jahnsen et al. 2000). In an animal model for asthma, more severe asthma features were observed when pDCs were depleted (de Heer et al. 2004). No effect of pDC depletion could be observed when this was performed in a model for allergic rhinitis in mice. Moreover, hardly any pDC could be observed in the nasal mucosa of allergic rhinitis mouse (Kleinjan et al. 2006).

4.4 The Role of Costimulatory Molecules on DCs

Functional in vivo studies indicate a blockade of CD80 at the induction phase significantly inhibits the manifestation of AR as measured by tissue eosinophilia and the production of IL-4 and IL-5 by nasal lymphocytes (Okano et al. 2001). There is no effect on the blockade of CD86 at the induction phase. Blockade of CD80 and CD86 prevents and inhibits the development of allergic rhinitis features as measured by levels of serum IgE and IgG1 and tissue eosiophilia (Okano et al. 2001). There was no abrogation of rhinitis features observed when CD80 or CD86 was blocked. The important role of these costimulatoir molecules were confirmed with CD80/86 knockout bone marrow derived DCs, which were used to immunize mice. The lack of asthma features in these mice and the presence of it in wild type BMDC immunized mice, support the important role of these costimulatory molecules in allergic inflammation (van Rijt et al. 2004). CD40 is also very important in the development of allergic rhinitis, mDCs obtained from the nasal mucosa have a higher expression of CD40 in atopic individual compared with non-atopics (Allam et al. 2006). Animals studies with tg CD40 knockout mice showed the importance of CD40. The lack of CD40 prevents the development of the cardinal features of AR like tissue eosinophilia and the production of (specific) IgE and other features of AR (Hattori et al. 2006).

4.5 Cytokine Production of Nasal Mucosa DCs

Nasal mucosa DCs lack the production of IL12p70 on CD40L stimulation and produce TNF-α, IL-6, IL-8 and IL-10 (Faith et al. 2005). In allo MLR, nasal mucosa (NM) DCs as well as peripheral blood (PB) DC can induce Th1 and Th2 cytokines only for IFN-γ PBDCs seem to be more potent. In response on the DC maturating cytokine GM-CSF, NMDC were more potent in the allo MLR supporting higher levels of Th2 cytokins IL4, IL5 and IL-13 than PBDC that support the Th1 cytokine IFN-γ (Faith et al. 2005). Functional studies in a murine model of AR in which bone marrow derived myeloid DCs support the characteristics of AR as measured with tissue eosinophilia and elevated levels of Th2 cytokines produced in Cervical LN (Kleinjan et al. 2006).

5 LC/DC Paradigm

The characterization of nasal mucosa DCs being langerhans cells by Fokkens et al. was a big step forward in DC phenotyping (Fokkens et al. 1991). Resident DCs in skin are mainly langerhans cells, containing rod/tennis racket–shaped intracellular organelles (birbeck granulas), which was confirmed with electron microscopy (Mizumoto and Takashima 2004). Characterization of DCs in the nasal mucosa was performed in relation to allergies. In allergen provoked allergic rhinitis patients, the increase of DCs (CD1a positive cells) was up to 10 times more when compared to basal numbers (Godthelp et al. 1996). Also, about 30% of DCs characterized by CD1a bear (specific) IgE (Godthelp et al. 1996) (Kleinjan et al. 1997). Only DCs containing birbeck granules were marked as langerhans cells. Birbeck granula positive DCs were only found in the nasal mucosa of allergic rhinitis patients and not in healthy controls (Fokkens et al. 1991). Due to the use of the marker Langerin (CD207), as a marker for langerhans cells, numbers of LCs (langerin positive cells) were much more easily identified. DCs characterized as langerin positive, being the resident DCs and DCs negative for langerin, being the inflammatory DCs seem to have distinct functions (Sung et al. 2006). The expression of FcεRI and the level of membrane bound IgE and the expression of langerin CD207 were higher in atopics than in non-atopics (Allam et al. 2006).

Geismann suggested that LC with an immature phenotype can migrate to the draining lymph node in the context of a chronically inflamed skin (Geissmann et al. 2002). Each DC subset had a different immunological preference and have a significant impact on the outcome of the immune response. Comparison of nasal and oral mucosa was performed to get a better insight into the mechanism behind hyposensitisation immunotherapy as given by sublingual therapy. The phenotype of oral mucosa DCs was compared with the phenotype of nasal mucosa DCs. Oral mucosa DCs were characterized as having a more Langerhans cell phenotypes.

6 An Important Role for DCs in Nasal Tolerance

A recent important outcome of epidemiological studies by Braun-Farlander et al. was that children who have grown up on farms have less allergic reactions. The underlying mechanism could be that mother and child are exposed to environmental/house dust antigens, which contain significant amounts of LPS on farms. These differ from citizen environmental house dust antigens that contain low amounts of LPS. The exposure of the nasal mucosa with antigens in the presence of a bacterial component biases the immune response in such a way that tolerance is induced (Braun-Fahrlander 2003). From animal studies, it is known that when animals are immunized with DCs in the presence of LPS, they switch to be more pro Th1 and induce tolerance, which is mainly caused by the induction of IL-12 production of DCs (Kuipers et al. 2004).

Recent findings postulate a role in nasal tolerance for a secretory leukoprotease inhibitor (SLPI) (Samsom et al. 2007). This inhibitor is produced by DCs and influences DC activation. In SLPI −/− animals, DCs expressed higher levels of costimulator molecules like CD40, CD86 and MHC II. Lymph node cells from SLPI −/− animals produce higher amounts of IL-12p70, MCP and IL-6 after OVA treatment (Samsom et al. 2007). SLPI controls DC activation in response to antigens in the context of LPS in the mucosal environment. Another important enzyme is IDO (Indoleamine 2,3-Dioxygenase), which is thought to play an important role in induction of tolerance due to the induction of apoptose of T cells by the production of kynurenine by IDO as a result of the tryptophan metabolisation. IDO is expressed in plasmacytoid DCs and down regulates the immune response (Fallarino et al. 2002). Observation in the nose draining lymphnode strongly suggests that IDO is a key regulator in nasal tolerance (van der Marel et al. 2007). The pro-immunotolerance environment in the upper airway draining, LN should keep in mind in the context of immunotherapy and the immunogenicity of allergen immunotherapy (Lund et al. 2007) and allergen vaccine development.

Not only do the upper airways have this pro-immunotolerance environment, also in the lower airways is a micro environment of immune suppression. The alveolar macrophages that produce large amount of IL-10 to suppress the immunoresponse, also leading to immunotolerance and downregulation of the immune response.

7 Chemokines

7.1 Role of Chemokines

Mice deficient in CCL19 (MIB3β)/CCL21 (SLC), the plt mice (paucity of lymph node T cells) shows more severe nasal inflammation and severe cytokine production in nasal mucosa NALT, CLN, and spleen. Also, Takamura et al. showed higher number of mDC and less T regs and DC in plt AR mice than in WT mice. Targeting CCL19 with plasmids that encode CCL19 in PLT–mice lowers the nasal symptoms and (antigen specific) IgE in serum. Although treated WT animals, only improve in nasal symptoms and higher number of T regs in spleen and CLN. Extracting this data suggests that CCL19 and CCL21 could play a role in the induction of T-regs and simultaneously relieves the pathological function of m-DCs in allergic rhinitis animals (Takamura et al. 2007). Data obtained from peripheral blood DCs revealed that CCL22 (MDC) production was higher in AR than in healthy controls (Yanai et al. 2007). Moreover, they support these data that T-cells obtained from patients migrate in response on birch pollen extract pulsing. The reacting T-cells that migrate expressed CCR4, the receptor of CCL22. This response could be abrogated by anti CCL22 (Yanai et al. 2007). This in vitro data is nicely supported by in vivo immunohistochemical data showing the presence of CCL22 in nasal mucosa tissue of AR and the absence of CCL22 in the nasal mucosal tissue of healthy controls (Yanai et al. 2007).

7.2 TSLP in Mucosa Context

Thymic stromal lymphopoietin (TSLP) -activated DCs, primed naive T (H) cells to produce the pro-allergic cytokines (Soumelis et al. 2002). TSLP is initially described in the context of allergy being produced in keratinocytes and plays an important role in atopic dermatitis (Soumelis et al. 2002). Overexpression of TSLP in lower airway epithelial cells induces asthma features in these animals (Zhou et al. 2005). Human studies so far only describe the presence of RNA with in situ hybridization (Ying et al. 2005). In contrast, immunoreactive TSLP is only detected in squamuous nasal mucosa epithelium, which is absent in respirator epithelium (Scheel et al. 2006). Squamuous epithelium is found on that particular sides, where skin can be transferred to mucosa and have some features of skin and some of mucosa. We also detected TSLP in very low quantities in bronchial biopsies with QPCR and antibodies, although there was no difference between healthy controls and mild asthmatics. The definitive proof of TSLP production in respirator epithelial cells as having a significant impact on airway DCs has to be done for the human upper and lower airways. The presence of TSLP in skin and its absence in mucosa could be a significant difference between these organs in humans.

8 DCs in Rhinitis Models

8.1 Human Studies

An important tool in studying DCs in allergic rhinitis is allergen provocation studies. With this method, the dynamics of inflammatory cells can easily be discovered and sampling methods of nasal mucosa are easy to perform by nasal washes, nasal mucosa brushes, and nasal mucosa biopsies, although this last sampling method is a more invasive than the others. Godthelp et al. showed the increase in DCs as measured with CD1a in the epithelium and in the lamina propria of the nasal mucosa of allergic rhinitis patients during prolonged allergen provocation (Godthelp et al. 1996). In this study, we created a small grass pollen season in the winter, which enabled us to study the cellular dynamics of isolated grass pollen allergic rhinitis patients. The numbers reach a maximum during several days of allergen challenge and remain stable at that high level for a few weeks (Godthelp et al. 1996). Other studies confirm this observation that DCs increase in number after allergen provocation (Jahnsen et al. 2000). A definitive prove of the important role of DCs in nasal allergy has been performed by the use of transgenic and wild type mouse enabling us to reach this goal.

8.2 Animal Studies

In essence, if one wants to prove that DCs are functionally important in AR, the DCs should be present in higher numbers in diseased tissues, administration of DCs should exacerbate disease, and depleting DCs from diseased tissue should cure disease (Lambrecht and Hammad 2003). We prove these points in a mouse model of AR (Kleinjan et al. 2006). In mice, AR has been modeled using OVA as a model allergen, but most models are accompanied by lung inflammation (Hellings and Ceuppens 2004; McCusker 2004; Saito et al. 2001). We first sensitized mice to OVA and subsequently challenged intranasal by application of small volume of OVA solution in the nose of awake mice for a period of three weeks. Awake mouse was use to avoid aspiration of the antigen in the lungs because they can swallow. This procedure of sensitization and challenge indeed led to tissue eosinophilia and localized Th2 responses in the nose, and to systemic levels of OVA-specific IgE, while leaving the lungs unaffected. In accordance with the human data, we again found an increase in myeloid DCs in the nose of mice with artificially induced AR and these DCs formed clusters with $CD4^+$ T cells (Kleinjan et al. 2006).

When OVA-pulsed myeloid DCs were next administered intranasally to OVA sensitized mice, they boosted the production of Th2 cytokines in the nasal local draining cervical lymph nodes, which also led to stronger eosinophilic tissue inflammation. This increase did not occur in the lungs, suggesting that the DCs acted locally to enhance inflammation (Kleinjan et al. 2006). The boosting of allergic inflammation by adoptive transfer of DCs directly to the trachea has previously been shown to enhance asthmatic inflammation in the lungs of mice and humanized SCID mice. This suggests that DCs can enhance localized Th2 responses depending on the site of administration (Hammad et al. 2002; Lambrecht and Hammad 2003; van Rijt et al. 2005).

To definitively prove that endogenous DCs are important for ongoing nasal inflammation, we made use of a conditional DC depletion model, employing mice in which the monkey diphteria toxin receptor is expressed only in CD11c positive cells, including DCs, alveolar macrophages, and intraepithelial CD8 cells (Jung et al. 2002; van Rijt et al. 2004; Zammit et al. 2005). Systemic administration of DT in the CD11c-DTR Tg mice leads to a rapid decline in $CD11c^+$ cells in all organs including the spleen, lymph nodes, and lungs leading to a defect in $CD8^+$ T cell priming, as well as CD4 and CD8 effector cell generation (Jung et al. 2002;

van Rijt et al. 2004; Zammit et al. 2005). In these mice, DCs were depleted using DT administration in the middle of a period of ongoing allergen exposure. When DCs were depleted, all the cardinal features of AR disappeared (Kleinjan et al. 2006). Strikingly, Th2 cytokine production was totally reduced. There was almost complete absence of nasal eosinophilia dependent on IL-5, and serum IgE levels dependent on IL-4 were abolished or returned to control or unimmunized levels (Kleinjan et al. 2006). These findings, therefore, strongly suggest that DCs are necessary for generating effector CD4 function in primed Th cells during ongoing inflammation in already sensitized mice. This data also suggests that DCs are crucial for ongoing IgE synthesis by B cells. Dendritic cells can boost IgE responses by enhancing Th2 effector function, leading to enhanced IL-4 production critical for IgE synthesis. Alternatively, DCs can also directly interact with B cells, thus inducing class switching and plasma cell formation (Dubois et al. 1997). Although it is possible that DC depletion interference with localized production of IgE in the nose, as previously shown to occur in AR patients (Durham et al. 1997; Kleinjan et al. 2000b), another possibility would be the synthesis of IgE in the cervical lymph nodes, as previously shown in rats (McMenamin et al. 1992).

In a murine model of allergic rhinitis, Stat-1 seems to be involved in the induction of allergy; a lacking of Stat-1 completely prevents the appearance of AR (Hattori et al. 2007). No attention was paid to the role of DCs in the development of AR, although Stat-1 signaling seem to be very important in DC production of IFN's (Remoli et al. 2002).

Allergic inflammation in a murine model of rhinitis seems to be affected by different bacterial ligands with the involvement of mast cells and DCs. Peptidoglycan (PGN) exposure increased the OVA induced specific IL-4 response and exacerbated the nasal allergic symptoms and eosinophilia, whereas CpG exposure decreased the OVA induced IL-4 response and suppressed nasal allergic symptoms (Yamamoto et al. 2006). In vitro work supports these observations and suggests that mast cells are responsible for PGN induced response and the DCs seem to be responsible for the CpG induced effects (Yamamoto et al. 2006). Moreover, nasal symptoms induced by the allergen OVA were induced via the mast cell dependent route, while the DC dependent route suppresses allergic symptoms (Yamamoto et al. 2006).

9 Follicle and Germinal Center Formation

DCs play an important role in the secondary immune response in stimulation of the circulating Th2 effector cells and vice versa. DCs matured locally due to the production of cytokines by Th2 cells. One consistent finding was that CD11c^{+} DCs formed intense clusters with CD3^{+} T cells in inflamed tissues, suggesting a functional interaction between DCs and T cells, necessary for generating effector function in these T cells (Kleinjan et al. 2006). It is known that CD4^{+} T cells produce Th2 cytokines locally in the nose of AR patients (Durham et al. 1992; Humbert et al. 1997, 1999; Kleinjan et al. 1999; Masuyama et al. 1998). This supports the idea of local interactions between DCs and effector T cells. These DCs present their antigens to T-cells and T-cell can interact with B-cells in the periphery tissue like the nasal mucosa. DCs can act as a platform on which T-cell interaction and B-cell interaction can take place (Takahashi et al. 2006). DCs together with T-cells and B-cells were often found in clusters of at least 20 or more cells. These clusters suggest at least the presence of local, peripheral antigen presentation from DCs with T-cells. Studying the cognate interaction between T-B-cells shows that in allergic rhinitis patients more clusters were observed than in healthy controls (Gevaert et al. 2005; Gould et al. 2006; Kleinjan et al. 2000). An important confirmation of the T-B-cell interaction in peripheral tissue is the observation of the local IgE isotype switch of B-cells in allergic rhinitis patients (Cameron et al. 2000; Coker et al. 2003; Gould et al. 2006; Smurthwaite et al. 2001) leading to the production of allergen specific IgE in the nasal mucosa (Kleinjan et al. 2000). Besides these physical observations, there are more reasons to expect that this localized immune response is ongoing. Germinal centre formation goes hand in hand with the development of plasma cell formation. It is also thought that DCs can play an important role in these germinal centre formations. Taking this into account, DCs have a function in the B-cell immunoglobulin production. Depletion of DCs in our rhinitis model also abrogate the production of IgE (Kleinjan et al. 2006). This observation strongly supports the indirect influence of DCs on immunoglobulin production and could play a role in the local production of IgE in allergic context (Gould et al. 2006).

10 Intervention

10.1 Altering the Balance in Disease

New therapies have tried to change the balance of pro Th2 in a pro T reg and also to induce IL-10 or TGF-beta as tried with *Lactobacillus*. Some of these treatments seem to improve daily nasal symptoms and reduce the use of additional medicines (Cross and Gill 2001; Ishida et al. 2005). Sublingual hyposensitization is also an important tool to cure allergics from their disease. The lack of TLR4, associated with the LPS receptor (CD14) prevents oral mucosa DCs to react against bacterial antigens, which were frequently found in oral mucosa. Due to the use of TLR4 agonist as an adjuvant for sublingual immunotherapy, this is an effective alternative for subcutaneous immunotherapy (Allam et al. 2008).

10.2 Pharmacological Targeting DCs

In nasal allergy, one of the first therapeutics is topical steroids. Use of topical steroids reduces the number of DCs dramatically in the nasal mucosa (Fokkens et al.

1997, 1998; Holm et al. 2001; Till et al. 2001). Although, almost any inflammatory cell and cytokine is affected by steroids (Holm et al. 2001; Kleinjan et al. 2000).

In other nasal mucosa related diseases like sinusitis, treatment with G-CSF gives improvement, which can clarified also by the improvement of cell function in which DCs could play a role although G-CSF mainly act on granulocytes and restore their function (Kalkman et al. 2002). Moreover, topical antifungal therapy in patients with chronic sinusitis seem to be less effective (Weschta et al. 2004) and suggest that this is not the effective treatment. TLR2 on DCs can recognize fungal pathogens (Funderburg et al. 2007; Goodridge and Underhill 2008). By the use of an adjuvant, which additionally triggers DCs in a inflammatory context, DCs should be able to recognize these pathogens and induce a T-cell response.

In general, newly developed drugs that are under investigation in lower airway allergy pathology can be used for the treatment of the upper airways as well. Recently,

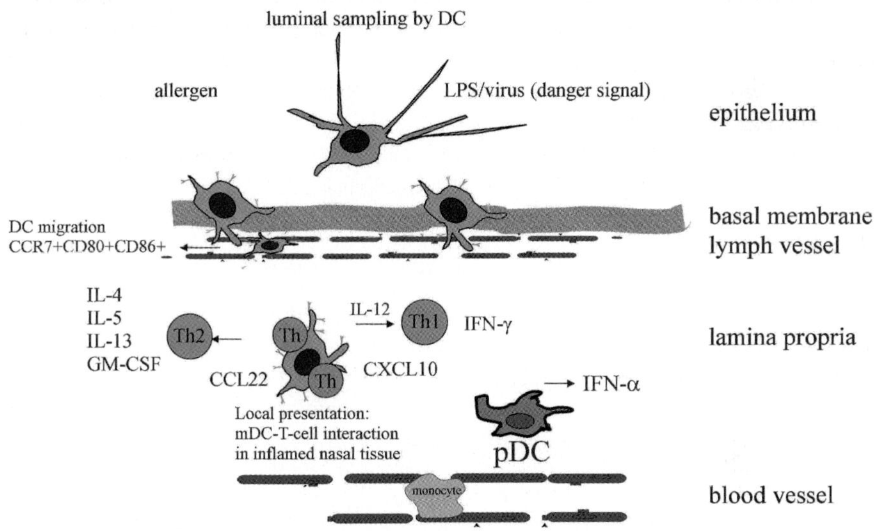

Fig. 3 DCs in rhinitis. The most important immune competent cells in the epithelium are the dendritic cells (DCs), in steady state condition a few of these professional antigen presenting are present. DCs formed an intensive network of cells in between the epithelial cells. They have the possibility to open the tight junctions enabling dendrite sprouting beyond the epithelium to sample the lumen. After been triggered by environmental pathogens and antigens they got activated and express chemokine receptors and migrate into lymph vessels or in the lamina propria of the nasal mucosa. Nasal mucosa DCs appearing in the draining lymph node interact with T-cells. Nasal mucosa DCs who migrated into the lamina propria interact with effector T-cells, upon this interaction T-cells produce cytokines and chemokines for the recruitment of new inflammatory cells. Plasmacytoid DCs are present in the nasal mucosa, it is unclear what the precise function is of these DCs. In the lower airways they play an important role in the production of Type I IFN, this could be an important function although this need confirmation. Myeloid DCs in the nose formed clusters with $CD4^+$ T cells. It is known that $CD4^+$ T cells produce Th2 cytokines locally in the nose of AR patients. This supports the idea of local interactions between DCs and effector T cells. Follicle formation occurs in the inflamed nasal mucosa suggesting that the nasal mucosa itself can act as a kind of lymphoid tissue during chronic inflammation

it was described that compound VAF347, a low molecular weight inhibitor is an effective drug in targeting DCs and B-cells (Ettmayer et al. 2006) and could have benefits in treatment. There are more target genes and compounds influencing the immune system like BW245c, a DP1 agonist which strongly suppressed the lower airway inflammation (Hammad et al. 2007). New therapies should be developed in the context of inducing a tollerogenic environment by local application of secretory leukoprotease inhibitor (SLPI) (Samsom et al. 2007) or by the induction of IDO (van der Marel et al. 2007).

New employment of already established therapies in other diseases like in virus mediated diseases of imiquimod as a TLR7 agonist. An important recent observation was that topical application of imiquimod could cure HPV associated VIN III, a premalign based vulva disease (van Seters et al. 2008). It is suggested to use imiquimod in common cold to induce the production of type I IFN as a topical effective drug in the treatment of common colds (Clejan et al. 2005).

In chronic sinusitis, it could be of benefit to make use of ex vivo generated monocyte derived DCs, which can be loaded with a mixture of sonificated bacteria that cause the sinusitis to support the immune system. DC vaccination therapies already seem to be successful in the treatment of cancers and mesothelioma (Hegmans et al. 2005; Worgall et al. 2001; Yu et al. 2004) (Fig. 3).

11 Conclusion

The current understanding of the DC biology of the upper airways is increasing. Therapies targeting DCs lead to an improvement in symptoms, although underlying disease were not always completely cured. The important role of DCs in established disease is stressed and new therapies should influence DC function and therefore manipulate the T-cell response in particular cases.

References

Allam JP et al (2006) Comparative analysis of nasal and oral mucosa dendritic cells. Allergy 61:166–172

Allam JP et al (2008) Toll-like receptor 4 ligation enforces tolerogenic properties of oral mucosal Langerhans cells. J Allergy Clin Immunol 121:368–374

Antonopoulos C et al (2008) IL-18 is a key proximal mediator of contact hypersensitivity and allergen-induced Langerhans cell migration in murine epidermis. J Leukoc Biol 83:361–367

Barry PW, O'Callaghan C (1996) Inhalational drug delivery from seven different spacer devices. Thorax 51:835–840

Brandenburg AH et al (2000) Type 1-like immune response is found in children with respiratory syncytial virus infection regardless of clinical severity. J Med Virol 62:267–277

Braun-Fahrlander C (2003) Environmental exposure to endotoxin and other microbial products and the decreased risk of childhood atopy: evaluating developments since April 2002. Curr Opin Allergy Clin Immunol 3:325–329

Braunstahl GJ et al (2003) Mucosal and systemic inflammatory changes in allergic rhinitis and asthma: a comparison between upper and lower airways. Clin Exp Allergy 33:579–587

Cameron L et al (2000) Local synthesis of epsilon germline gene transcripts, IL-4, and IL-13 in allergic nasal mucosa after ex vivo allergen exposure. J Allergy Clin Immunol 106:46–52

Clejan S et al (2005) Immune responses induced by intranasal imiquimod and implications for therapeutics in rhinovirus infections. J Cell Mol Med 9:457–461

Coker HA, Durham SR, Gould HJ (2003) Local somatic hypermutation and class switch recombination in the nasal mucosa of allergic rhinitis patients. J Immunol 171:5602–5610

Cross ML, Gill HS (2001) Can immunoregulatory lactic acid bacteria be used as dietary supplements to limit allergies? Int Arch Allergy Immunol 125:112–119

de Heer HJ et al (2004) Essential role of lung plasmacytoid dendritic cells in preventing asthmatic reactions to harmless inhaled antigen. J Exp Med 200:89–98

del Rio ML et al (2007) CD103- and CD103$^+$ bronchial lymph node dendritic cells are specialized in presenting and cross-presenting innocuous antigen to CD4$^+$ and CD8$^+$ T cells. J Immunol 178:6861–6866

Dubois B et al (1997) Dendritic cells enhance growth and differentiation of CD40-activated B lymphocytes. J Exp Med 185:941–951

Durham SR et al (1992) Cytokine messenger RNA expression for IL-3, IL-4, IL-5, and granulocyte/macrophage-colony-stimulating factor in the nasal mucosa after local allergen provocation: relationship to tissue eosinophilia. J Immunol 148:2390–2394

Durham SR et al (1997) Expression of epsilon germ-line gene transcripts and mRNA for the epsilon heavy chain of IgE in nasal B cells and the effects of topical corticosteroid. Eur J Immunol 27:2899–2906

Ettmayer P et al (2006) A novel low molecular weight inhibitor of dendritic cells and B cells blocks allergic inflammation. Am J Respir Crit Care Med 173:599–606

Faith A et al (2005) Functional plasticity of human respiratory tract dendritic cells: GM-CSF enhances T(H)2 development. J Allergy Clin Immunol 116:1136–1143

Fallarino F et al (2002) T cell apoptosis by tryptophan catabolism. Cell Death Differ 9:1069–1077

Fokkens WJ et al (1991) Langerhans cells in nasal mucosa of patients with grass pollen allergy. Immunobiology 182:135–142

Fokkens WJ et al (1997) Allergic rhinitis and inflammation: the effect of nasal corticosteroid therapy. Allergy 52:29–32

Fokkens WJ et al (1998) Local corticosteroid treatment: the effect on cells and cytokines in nasal allergic inflammation. Am J Rhinol 12:21–26

Funderburg N et al (2007) Human -defensin-3 activates professional antigen-presenting cells via Toll-like receptors 1 and 2. Proc Natl Acad Sci U S A 104:18631–18635

Geissmann F et al (2002) Accumulation of immature Langerhans cells in human lymph nodes draining chronically inflamed skin. J Exp Med 196:417–430

Gevaert P et al (2005) Organization of secondary lymphoid tissue and local IgE formation to Staphylococcus aureus enterotoxins in nasal polyp tissue. Allergy 60:71–79

Godthelp T et al (1996) Antigen presenting cells in the nasal mucosa of patients with allergic rhinitis during allergen provocation. Clin Exp Allergy 26:677–688

Goodridge HS, Underhill DM (2008) Fungal Recognition by TLR2 and Dectin-1. Handb Exp Pharmacol 87–109

Gould HJ et al (2006) Germinal-centre reactions in allergic inflammation. Trends Immunol 27:446–452

Hammad H et al (2002) Monocyte-derived dendritic cells induce a house dust mite-specific Th2 allergic inflammation in the lung of humanized SCID mice: involvement of CCR7. J Immunol 169:1524–1534

Hammad H et al (2007) Activation of the D prostanoid 1 receptor suppresses asthma by modulation of lung dendritic cell function and induction of regulatory T cells. J Exp Med 204:357–367

Hartmann E et al (2006) Analysis of plasmacytoid and myeloid dendritic cells in nasal epithelium. Clin Vaccine Immunol 13:1278–1286

Hattori H et al (2001) Expression of costimulatory CD80/CD86-CD28/CD152 molecules in nasal mucosa of patients with perennial allergic rhinitis. Clin Exp Allergy 31:1242–1249
Hattori H et al (2006) Signals through CD40 play a critical role in the pathophysiology of Schistosoma mansoni egg antigen–induced allergic rhinitis in mice. Am J Rhinol 20:165–169
Hattori H et al (2007) STAT1 is involved in the pathogenesis of murine allergic rhinitis. Am J Rhinol 21:241–247
Hegmans JP et al (2005) Immunotherapy of murine malignant mesothelioma using tumor lysate-pulsed dendritic cells. Am J Respir Crit Care Med 171:1168–1177
Hellings PW, Ceuppens JL (2004) Mouse models of global airway allergy: what have we learned and what should we do next? Allergy 59:914–919
Hintzen G et al (2006) Induction of tolerance to innocuous inhaled antigen relies on a CCR7-dependent dendritic cell-mediated antigen transport to the bronchial lymph node. J Immunol 177:7346–7354
Holm A et al (2001) Fluticasone propionate aqueous nasal spray reduces inflammatory cells in unchallenged allergic nasal mucosa: effects of single allergen challenge. J Allergy Clin Immunol 107:627–633
Horiguchi S et al (2007) Migration of tumor antigen-pulsed dendritic cells after mucosal administration in the human upper respiratory tract. J Clin Immunol 27:598–604
Hubert P et al (2005) E-cadherin-dependent adhesion of dendritic and Langerhans cells to keratinocytes is defective in cervical human papillomavirus-associated (pre)neoplastic lesions. J Pathol 206:346–355
Humbert M et al (1997) Relationship between IL-4 and IL-5 mRNA expression and disease severity in atopic asthma. Am J Respir Crit Care Med 156:704–708
Humbert M et al (1999) The immunopathology of extrinsic (atopic) and intrinsic (non-atopic) asthma: more similarities than differences. Immunol Today 20:528–533
Ishida Y et al (2005) Clinical effects of Lactobacillus acidophilus strain L-92 on perennial allergic rhinitis: a double-blind, placebo-controlled study. J Dairy Sci 88:527–533
Jahnsen FL et al (2000) Experimentally induced recruitment of plasmacytoid (CD123high) dendritic cells in human nasal allergy. J Immunol 165:4062–4068
Jahnsen FL et al (2002) Involvement of plasmacytoid dendritic cells in human diseases. Hum Immunol 63:1201–1205
Jiang A et al (2007) Disruption of E-cadherin-mediated adhesion induces a functionally distinct pathway of dendritic cell maturation. Immunity 27:610–624
Jung S et al (2002) In vivo depletion of CD11c(+) dendritic cells abrogates priming of CD8(+) T cells by exogenous cell-associated antigens. Immunity 17:211–220
Kalkman PM et al (2002) A hampered chemoattractant-induced cytoskeletal rearrangement in granulocytes of patients with unexplained severe chronic and relapsing infections of the upper and lower airways. In vitro restoration by G-CSF exposure. Clin Exp Immunol 127:115–122
Kleinjan A et al (1997) Allergen binding to specific IgE in the nasal mucosa of allergic patients. J Allergy Clin Immunol 99:515–521
Kleinjan A et al (1999) Increase in IL-8, IL-10, IL-13, and RANTES mRNA levels (in situ hybridization) in the nasal mucosa after nasal allergen provocation. J Allergy Clin Immunol 103:441–450
Kleinjan A et al (2000a) Preventive treatment of intranasal fluticasone propionate reduces cytokine mRNA expressing cells before and during a single nasal allergen provocation. Clin Exp Allergy 30:1476–1485
Kleinjan A et al (2000b) Local production and detection of (specific) IgE in nasal B-cells and plasma cells of allergic rhinitis patients. Eur Respir J 15:491–497
Kleinjan A et al (2006) An essential role for dendritic cells in human and experimental allergic rhinitis. J Allergy Clin Immunol 118:1117–1125
Kuipers H et al (2004) Dendritic cells retrovirally overexpressing IL-12 induce strong Th1 responses to inhaled antigen in the lung but fail to revert established Th2 sensitization. J Leukoc Biol 76:1028–1038

Lambrecht BN, Hammad H (2003) Taking our breath away: dendritic cells in the pathogenesis of asthma. Nat Rev Immunol 3:994–1003

Lund L et al (2007) Comparison of allergenicity and immunogenicity of an intact allergen vaccine and commercially available allergoid products for birch pollen immunotherapy. Clin Exp Allergy 37:564–571

Marcet B et al (2007) Extracellular nucleotides regulate CCL20 release from human primary airway epithelial cells, monocytes and monocyte-derived dendritic cells. J Cell Physiol 211: 716–727

Martin E et al (2003) The combination of plasmid interleukin-12 with a single DNA vaccine is more effective than Mycobacterium bovis (bacille Calmette-Guerin) in protecting against systemic Mycobacterim avium infection. Immunology 109:308–314

Masuyama K et al (1998) Nasal eosinophilia and IL-5 mRNA expression in seasonal allergic rhinitis induced by natural allergen exposure: effect of topical corticosteroids. J Allergy Clin Immunol 102:610–617

McCusker C et al (2002) Site-specific sensitization in a murine model of allergic rhinitis: role of the upper airway in lower airways disease. J Allergy Clin Immunol 110:891–898

McCusker CT (2004) Use of mouse models of allergic rhinitis to study the upper and lower airway link. Curr Opin Allergy Clin Immunol 4:11–16

McMenamin C, Girn B, Holt PG (1992) The distribution of IgE plasma cells in lymphoid and non-lymphoid tissues of high-IgE responder rats: differential localization of antigen-specific and 'bystander' components of the IgE response to inhaled antigen. Immunology 77:592–596

Mizumoto N, Takashima A (2004) CD1a and langerin: acting as more than Langerhans cell markers. J Clin Invest 113:658–660

Okano M et al (2001) Differential role of CD80 and CD86 molecules in the induction and the effector phases of allergic rhinitis in mice. Am J Respir Crit Care Med 164:1501–1507

Phan TG et al (2007) Subcapsular encounter and complement-dependent transport of immune complexes by lymph node B cells. Nat Immunol 8:992–1000

Remoli ME et al (2002) Selective expression of type I IFN genes in human dendritic cells infected with Mycobacterium tuberculosis. J Immunol 169:366–374

Saito H et al (2001) Allergen-induced murine upper airway inflammation: local and systemic changes in murine experimental allergic rhinitis. Immunology 104:226–234

Salib RJ, Lau LC, Howarth PH (2005) The novel use of the human nasal epithelial cell line RPMI 2650 as an in vitro model to study the influence of allergens and cytokines on transforming growth factor-beta gene expression and protein release. Clin Exp Allergy 35:811–819

Samsom JN et al (2007) Secretory leukoprotease inhibitor in mucosal lymph node dendritic cells regulates the threshold for mucosal tolerance. J Immunol 179:6588–6595

Scheel C et al (2006) CD1c^{+} myeloid dendritic cells and TSLP are involved in human nasal allergy. Abstracth 9th International Conference Dendritic Cells. Edinburg, 16–20 September 2006 No.123

Smurthwaite L et al (2001) Persistent IgE synthesis in the nasal mucosa of hay fever patients. Eur J Immunol 31:3422–3431

Soumelis V et al (2002) Human epithelial cells trigger dendritic cell mediated allergic inflammation by producing TSLP. Nat Immunol 3:673–680

Sung SS et al (2006) A major lung CD103 (alphaE)-beta7 integrin-positive epithelial dendritic cell population expressing Langerin and tight junction proteins. J Immunol 176:2161–2172

Takahashi K et al (2006) Dendritic cells interacting mainly with B cells in the lymphoepithelial symbiosis of the human palatine tonsil. Virchows Arch 448:623–629

Takamura K et al (2007) Regulatory role of lymphoid chemokine CCL19 and CCL21 in the control of allergic rhinitis. J Immunol 179:5897–5906

Takano K et al (2005) HLA-DR- and CD11c-positive dendritic cells penetrate beyond well-developed epithelial tight junctions in human nasal mucosa of allergic rhinitis. J Histochem Cytochem 53:611–619

Takizawa R et al (2007) Increased expression of HLA-DR and CD86 in nasal epithelial cells in allergic rhinitics: antigen presentation to T cells and up-regulation by diesel exhaust particles. Clin Exp Allergy 37:420–433

Till SJ et al (2001) Recruitment of CD1a^{+} Langerhans cells to the nasal mucosa in seasonal allergic rhinitis and effects of topical corticosteroid therapy. Allergy 56:126–131

Tomaki M et al (2000) Eosinophilopoiesis in a murine model of allergic airway eosinophilia: involvement of bone marrow IL-5 and IL-5 receptor alpha. J Immunol 165:4040–4050

Trinchieri G (2003) Interleukin-12 and the regulation of innate resistance and adaptive immunity. Nat Rev Immunol 3:133–146

van Benten IJ et al (2001) Prolonged nasal eosinophilia in allergic patients after common cold. Allergy 56:949–956

van Benten IJ et al (2003) RSV-induced bronchiolitis but not upper respiratory tract infection is accompanied by an increased nasal IL-18 response. J Med Virol 71:290–297

van Benten IJ et al (2005) Reduced nasal IL-10 and enhanced TNFalpha responses during rhinovirus and RSV-induced upper respiratory tract infection in atopic and non-atopic infants. J Med Virol 75:348–357

van der Marel AP et al (2007) Blockade of IDO inhibits nasal tolerance induction. J Immunol 179:894–900

van Rijt LS et al (2004) Essential role of dendritic cell CD80/CD86 costimulation in the induction, but not reactivation, of TH2 effector responses in a mouse model of asthma. J Allergy Clin Immunol 114:166–173

van Rijt LS et al (2005) In vivo depletion of lung CD11c^{+} dendritic cells during allergen challenge abrogates the characteristic features of asthma. J Exp Med 201:981–991

van Seters M et al (2008) Treatment of Vulvar Intraepithelial Neoplasia with Topical Imiquimod. N Engl J Med 358:1465–1473

Vinke JG, Fokken WJ (1999) The role of the adenoid in allergic sensitisation. Int J Pediatr Otorhinolaryngol 49(Suppl 1):S145–S149

Vinke JG et al (1999) Differences in nasal cellular infiltrates between allergic children and age-matched controls. Eur Respir J 13:797–803

Wang Y, McCusker CT (2005) Interleukin-13-dependent bronchial hyper-responsiveness following isolated upper-airway allergen challenge in a murine model of allergic rhinitis and asthma. Clin Exp Allergy 35:1104–1111

Weschta M et al (2004) Topical antifungal treatment of chronic rhinosinusitis with nasal polyps: a randomized, double-blind clinical trial. J Allergy Clin Immunol 113:1122–1128

Worgall S et al (2001) Protection against pulmonary infection with Pseudomonas aeruginosa following immunization with P. aeruginosa-pulsed dendritic cells. Infect Immun 69:4521–4527

Yamamoto K et al (2006) Modification of allergic inflammation in murine model of rhinitis by different bacterial ligands: involvement of mast cells and dendritic cells. Clin Exp Allergy 36:760–769

Yanai M et al (2007) The role of CCL22/macrophage-derived chemokine in allergic rhinitis. Clin Immunol 125:291–298

Ying S et al (2005) Thymic stromal lymphopoietin expression is increased in asthmatic airways and correlates with expression of Th2-attracting chemokines and disease severity. J Immunol 174:8183–8190

Yu JS et al (2004) Vaccination with tumor lysate-pulsed dendritic cells elicits antigen-specific, cytotoxic T-cells in patients with malignant glioma. Cancer Res 64:4973–4979

Zammit DJ et al (2005) Dendritic cells maximize the memory CD8 T cell response to infection. Immunity 22:561–570

Zhou B et al (2005) Thymic stromal lymphopoietin as a key initiator of allergic airway inflammation in mice. Nat Immunol 6:1047–1053

Role of Epidermal Dendritic Cells in Drug-Induced Cutaneous Adverse Reactions

Maria Dolores Ramírez-González, Miguel Herrera-Enríquez, Luisa Geraldine Villanueva-Rodríguez, and Andrés Eliu Castell-Rodríguez

Contents

Abstract Drug-induced adverse reactions (ADR) include any undesirable pharmacological effect that occurs following drug administration at therapeutic doses. The appearance of ADR significantly limits the use of drugs in as much as their clinical symptoms may range from very mild discomfort such as cutaneous rash, up to very severe, or even fatal tissue necrolysis such as the Stevens Johnson syndrome.

One of the most frequently involved organ during ADR is the skin. Drug-induced cutaneous reactions (CDR) incidence is variable but they may appear in 2–3% of ambulatory patients, and it may increase to 10–15% when patients are hospitalized, or even be as high as 60% when co morbidity includes the presence of virus, bacteria, or parasites.

Due to the fact that skin is one of the organs most frequently involved in ADR, in this work we analyze and propose a mechanism by which epidermal dendritic cells

M.D. Ramírez-González (✉)
Department of Pharmacology, School of Medicine, National Autonomous University of Mexico, Mexico
mdrg@servidor.unam.mx

G. Lombardi, Y. Riffo-Vasquez (eds.), *Dendritic Cells,* Handbook of Experimental Pharmacology 188,

operating as the sentinels of the skin neuro-immune-endocrine system may contribute to CDR via either immunogenic or tolerogenic immune responses towards drugs, whenever they are administered topic or systemically.

1 Drug-Induced Adverse and Cutaneous Drug Reactions

World Health Organization's definition of adverse drug reaction (ADR) refers to a noxious and unintended response that occurs at doses used in humans for prophylaxis, diagnosis, or therapy of disease, or for the modification of any physiologic function. This definition excludes therapeutic failure, overdose, drug abuse, noncompliance, and medication errors (WHO 2007).

Due to the fact that ADR recognition depends on both their clinical recognition and their medical report to pharmacovigilance programs, the magnitude of the problem is difficult to quantify. In the United States, it is estimated that 5–15% of therapeutic drug courses are complicated by ADR with over 100,000 annual deaths due to severe ADR; 3–6% of hospital admissions are related to ADR and 6–15% of hospitalized patients can experience a serious ADR (Riedl and Casillas 2003). ADR may include hematologic, CNS, dermatologic, allergic, metabolic, cardiovascular, gastrointestinal, renal, genitourinary, respiratory and/or sensory reactions, with 3–90% chance of becoming life-threatening ADR (Mockenhaupt 2005, French 2006). Cutaneous drug reactions (CDR) of varying severity (Table 1) may occur in 3–60% of patients receiving drugs. In addition to this, incidence rapidly increases when dealing with immune compromised patients. For example, toxic epidermal necrolysis (TEN) in adults occurs in 2.6 per 100,000 exposures but in HIV patients this rate increases to 8.4 cases per 100,000 exposures (Luther and Glesby 2007; Knowles and Shear 2007); and it further worsens when comorbidity aggregates, for example, thiacetazone induces ADR in 20–29% of HIV-infected patients with tuberculosis, but only in 1–7% of HIV negative tuberculosis patients (Flacher et al. 2007).

1.1 Criteria to Define ADR and CDR

ADR can be classified according to their onset as acute, if appearing within 60 mins, subacute when observed between 1–24 h and latent when they appear two or more days after treatment. Another criteria relates to the severity of symptoms, hence ADR can be mild which is bothersome for the patient, but requires no change in therapy; moderate, when requires change in therapy, the use of additional forms of treatment, or even when hospitalization of the patient needs to be done. Severe ADR are those disabling or life-threatening. And according to the Food and Drug Administration (FDA 2004), serious ADR include those that require intervention to prevent permanent injury, are life threatening, require prolonged hospitalization and may result in death, cause disability or can cause congenital anomalies.

Table 1 Drug Induced Cutaneous Reactions (CDR)

Morbiliform reactions. Most common within 2 weeks of drug use. Confluent fine pink macules and papules on trunk and pressure-bearing areas, may progress to large body areas. Dermis and dermal–epidermal junction edema. Dermal eosinophilia and cytotoxic CD4+ Tcells perforin + and granzyme B+. Increased IFNγ, TNFα, IL-5, and eotaxin/CCL-11
Drugs: Allopurinol, amphotericin B, barbiturates, benzodiazepines, captopril, carbamazepine, gold, lithium, NSAIDS, penicillin and derivatives, phenothiazines, phenytoin, quinidine, sulfonamides (clotrimazol), oral antifungals, thiazides, proton pump inhibitors, H2 receptor antagonists
Urticaria. The second most common. Pink skin wheals with pruritus, and subcutaneous angioedema. Clinically undistinguishable from non-drug urticaria. Single lesions last less than 24 h, but new lesions may continue to arise. Swelling of the lips or eyes may last for several days. Most reactions are related to an IgE
Drugs: Aminoglycosides, angiotensin converting enzyme inhiitors, antiretrovirals, hydralazine, narcotic analgesics, penicillin and derivatives, phenytoin, protamine, quinidine, sulfonamides, systemic azole antifungals, tetracyclines. Non steroidal antiinflammatory drugs (NSAIDS) and acetysalicylic acid can exacerbate or trigger chronic urticaria
Fixed drug eruption (FDE). Skin lesion(s) within hours that recur at the same anatomic site(s). Dusky erythematous macule, usually on the lips and genitalia with a burning sensation, that may progress to central vesicles and bullae. Fever, malaise, nausea, and vomiting are common. Dermal epidermal junction mixed inflammatory infiltrate of lymphocytes, neutrophils (NE), eosinophils (EO), melanin containing Mφ. Epidermal necrotic keratinocytes (KE) and CD4+ Tcells producing IL-10. Chronic epidermal acanthosis, hypergranulosis, and hyperkeratosis. For disseminated or bullous FDE, differential diagnosis should consider EM, SJS, and TEN. FDE may resolve without scarring
Drugs: Allopurinol, barbiturates, dapsone, NSAIDS, oral contraceptives, metronidazole, pseudoephedrine, sulfonamides, tetracycline
Toxic pustuloderma. Rare widespread macular erythemathous rash with fever and blood leucocytosis. Intraepidermal pustules surrounded by CD4+ and CD8+ Tcells, and KE producing high levels of IL-8. Systemic drugs can produce acute generalized exanthematous pustulosis in more than 90% of the cases
Drugs: Aminopenicillins, cephalosporins, macrolides.
Erythema Multiform (EM)/Stevens Johnson Syndrome (SJS)/Toxic Epidermal Necrolysis (TEN). Most severe forms of CDR. EM lesions are targetoid dusky erythematous patches mainly on the extremities. In SJS, bullae form on an erythematous base with confluent areas of skin detachment on face and trunk with a burning sensation or pain. TEN is the most severe form with large areas of skin sloughing affecting over 30% of the total body surface area. Fever preceds mucocutaneous eruption by 1–3 days and SJS and TEN progress within hours. Incidences of SJS or TEN range from 1.2 to 6 per million per year, and 0.4 to 1.2 per million per year, respectively; but SJS is fatal in about 5% and TEN in 30% of cases. In EM there is a dense dermal inflammatory cell infiltrate and necrotic KE. In TEN there is complete epidermal necrosis and a sparse mononuclear cell infiltrate
Drugs: Sulfonamide may provoke immediate as well as delayed reactions occurring 7–14 days after the initiation of therapy, and patients may quickly progress from a multiorgan syndrome to SJS or TEN. Other: .allopurinol, amoxicillin, amoxicillin-clavulanate, ampicillin, antiretorvirals, barbiturates, carbamazepine, cefaclor, diclofenac, NSAIDS, nevirapine, nitrofurantoin, phenobarbital, phenytoin, piroxicam
Beltraminelli et al. (2005); Bronnimann and Yawalkar (2005); Demirkan et al. (2006); Hertl-Yazdi and Hertl (2005); Knowles and Shear (2007); Mockenhaupt (2005); Nikkels et al. (2006); Rojeau (2006); Roychowdhury and Svensson (2005); Segal et al. (2007); Tan and Grattan (2004); Yawalkar (2005)

From a clinical point of view, ADR can be grouped in five types: A or augmented, which represents an extension of primary or secondary pharmacologic effect; these are often predictable and dose dependent, their appearance may be related to genetic factors that determine susceptibility. Type B or idiosyncratic, also known as bizarre or immune related reactions, they are typically unpredictable. Type C includes ADR associated with long-term use of drugs and may involve dose accumulation. In some cases this type of ADR can be predicted from the chemical structure of drug metabolites. Type D or delayed are dose independent ADR that can cause carcinogenicity or teratogenicity. And Type E or of the end of dose, that include withdrawal reactions that follow discontinuation of the drug. Up to two-thirds of observed ADR are considered of type A in as much as they disappear when the drug is withdrawn or the dose decreased (WHO 2007; FDA 2004).

In pharmacology texts, ADR fall within the scope of toxicology and include undesirable effects that lead to toxic pharmacological, pathological, or genotoxic effects following acute or chronic exposure to drugs. The endogenous production of toxic metabolites or reactive oxygen species may be related to ADR such as in phototoxic and photoallergic reactions. While idiosyncratic reactions may take the form of extreme sensitivity to low doses or extreme insensitivity to high doses of chemicals; while chemical allergy is referred to as an ADR that results from previous sensitization to a particular chemical or to one that is structurally similar (Brunton et al. 2006).

From an immunology point of view, allergic reactions to drugs are classified in four types according to the extent and type of tissue damage produced. Type I, immediate or anaphylactic, result of IgE binding to the surface of mast cells (mastocytes, MA) or basophils (BA) with consequent degranulation and release of histamine and other mediators or inflammation. Type II allergic reactions are those where cytotoxic antigenic determinants on cell surfaces are the target of IgG or IgM, leading to cell and tissue damage by activation of complement or cytotoxic killing cells, by binding through Fcε receptors. Type III or serum sickness reactions are those where circulating immune complexes are deposited in vascular beds or on tissue surfaces and activate complement and attract neutrophils (NE). In the case of Type IV, or delayed hypersensitivity, effector T lymphocytes are activated after recognition of the antigen for which they are specific; the antigen is presented as peptide(s) in the groove of major histocompatibility molecules (MHC): CD4+ T cells are activated via MHC II and CD8+ T cells via MHC I molecules; and T cells can act as cytotoxic causing tissue damage (Descotes and Choquet-Kastylevsky 2001).

However, the terminology for ADR that are believed to be immune-mediated is an area of debate. The term allergy implies "a disease mediated by the immune system to an otherwise innocuous agent", a definition that properly includes foodstuffs and environmental allergens, but this term excludes drugs since they are not innocuous. For clinical allergology, an allergic reaction occurs only when an immunological mechanism can be demonstrated, but this drug allergy falls within the unpredictable Type B of hypersensitivity reactions, that also includes non immune hypersensitivity reactions and those reactions related to genetic susceptibilities or undefined mechanisms, either idiosyncratic or intolerance reactions (Demoly and Hillaire-Buys 2004). This controversy has led some authors to the use of "idiosyncratic drug reactions" interchangeably with "drug hypersensitivity". However, idiosyncratic refers to events encountered "infrequently" in the population, which it is not the case for ADR such as nausea or diarrhea caused in 30–40% of patients taking varenicline or misoprostol (Romano and Demoly 2007; Zaccara et al. 2007).

CDR can also pose a challenging problem since they can mimic a large variety of skin diseases, and causality assessment is limited by the ethical constraints of re-challenging patients with a drug that may evoke a life-threatening or seriously disabling reaction. In addition to this, CDR not requiring hospitalization are usually underreported and/or non diagnosed (Roychowdhury and Svensson 2005; Rodríguez-Velasco et al. 2006).

For the purposes of this paper we considered ADR as unexpected reactions to drugs that occur with three potential causes: immunological processes, genetic factors that may influence drug metabolism, and/or due to the production of toxic drug metabolites.

Consideration of ADR's pathogenic mechanism as a multifactorial phenomena may help to understand better the reasons determining that only a small fraction of patients who receive a drug will experience ADR; why these reactions are exacerbated when the drug is administered at a later date; and how microbial infections modify their incidence and severity.

Unraveling the underlying mechanisms of CDR and ADR may have a significant impact on the health care system, particularly considering that 5–9% of hospital costs are related to them (Riedl and Casillas 2003; Mockenhaupt 2005), in addition to the improvement of patient compliance, and entailment of otherwise effective drugs (Roychowdhury and Svensson 2005; Zaccara et al. 2007).

2 Skin as a Target for Drug Action and Reaction

2.1 Skin Structure, Function, and Development

Skin is the largest organ of the human body accounting up to 6% of body weight and containing about 30% of the total blood volume. Histologically, it comprises two different layers. The external corresponds to a keratinized stratified squamous epithelium called epidermis, and the inner layer called dermis, which corresponds to a loose connective tissue where sweat and sebaceous glands as well as hair follicles are immersed.

Human skin has a pH gradient from deep dermis (pH 7.2) towards corneum stratum (pH 5.5) as a result of sweat evaporation, sebaceous secretion, and carbon dioxide diffusion. From the granulosum stratum, are also released enzymes like glucocerebrosidases, acid lipases, and phospholipases; which are involved on ceramides production, liberation of lamellar bodies of spinosum stratum keratinotcytes (KE), and polymerization of keratin. The epidermal pH gradient and the epicutaneous physical chemical layer contribute significantly to the barrier function of normal skin (Schmid-Wendtner and Korting 2006).

Normal human skin contain, as resident cells populations, KE, Merckel cells (MK), melanocytes (ME) and Langerhans cells (LC) in the epidermis, while in the dermis are normally observed fibroblasts, macrophages (Mϕ), mast cells (MA), adipocytes, lymphocytes, and dermal dendritic cells (DDC). However, in the presence of physical, chemical, or biological agents these cells populations may be mobilized along with the arrival of specialized cell types. These transient cell populations may include LC and lymphocytes in the epidermis; and DDC, LC, Mϕ, lymphocytes, neutrophils (NE), eosinophils (EO) and basophilis (BA) in the dermis. Among these different skin cells' populations, LC are the only skin cell type that can migrate from the epidermis into the dermis, on route towards the cutaneous draining lymph nodes (CDLN), by changing their morphology, immune phenotype and genotype.

Skin development occurs into three histological defined time periods: embryonic or specification stage (0–60 days), early fetal or morphogenesis stage (2–5 months) and late fetal or differentiation stage (5–9 months). Shortly after gastrulation during the embryonic period, ectoderm subdivides into neuroectoderm and presumptive epidermis. Neural ectoderm separates from epithelial ectoderm during the 3rd–5th week of gestation occurring simultaneously with the formation and closure of the neural tube. When incomplete fusion of the neural tube occurs, known as dysraphism, this may lead to the presence of cutaneous lesions in the offspring. During morphogenesis, epidermis begins its stratification by the occurrence of periderm at the end of 8th gestational week, and keratinization of the epidermal surface, as a differentiation step, begins after 15 weeks' gestation (Chu et al. 2003).

LC are the first immigrant cell population arriving into the epidermis at 40th day of embryonic gestational age (EGA), followed by ME at 50th day EGA, and MK first detectable in the volarpads epidermis of the 11–12 week EGA human fetus. In contrast, the reticular dermis begins to take on its characteristic fibrillar appearance by 12–15 weeks EGA. Blood and lymph vasculogenesis of the dermis occurs by 45–50 days EGA, but blood vessels at the dermal – hypodermal junction are seen at 9 weeks EGA. By the end of the differentiation stage, epidermis growth as a non vascularized tissue with an intraepithelial innervation consisting of free nerve terminations of thin unmyelinated fibers, which are somatic receptors and axonic projections of sympathetic autonomic fibers (Chu et al. 2003).

Along lifetime, skin features change from hypo-developed, in early years of life, into hypo-functional when entering the fourth decade, due to both chrono-ageing and/or photo-ageing, when the clear age-related skin immune suppression appears to be associated with higher risk for suffering, annoying, and hazardous skin reactions and epidermal deterioration (Kobayashi and Flavell 2004; Sullivan and Shear 2002). How these effects are associated with the age- and gender-related changes in the density of LC epidermal population on different body regions is not well documented (Ayala-García et al. 2005); but a gender effect results in 35% higher incidence of skin reactions in adult women than in men (Rodríguez-Velasco et al. 2006).

Skin and the epithelial lining of respiratory, gastrointestinal, and genitourinary tracts serve to protect the human body depending on its integrity as a physical barrier and on its ability to display immunologic responses, of innate and adaptive types, in response to the presence of either external or internal offending agents whose earliest detection rely on epithelial dendritic cells (DC) (Roosterman et al. 2006; Schmid-Wendtner and Korting 2006).

Skin symptoms and lesions used to be considered a health problem restricted to underdeveloped countries, most of the times related to poor hygiene. However, an uprising trend is beginning to appear in developed countries apparently due to the exaggerated use of cleansing treatments, which tend to remove skin natural defenses. Allergic topic disorders such as rhinitis, asthma, and atopic dermatitis appear to be the result of systemic inflammatory reactions triggered by enhanced type 2 T helper (Th2) and attenuated T regulatory (Treg) cells mediated immune responses against "innocuous" antigens (allergens) of complex genetic and environmental origin (Schmid-Wendtner and Korting 2006).

2.2 Skin as a Main Target of CDR

Skin pathology is one of the most aggressive and complex human conditions to treat due to the medical, psychological, and social impacts on the affected patient. The list of drugs reported to produce CDR include many useful treatments such as nonsteroidal anti-inflammatory drugs (NSAIDS) and aminopenicillins. Most CDR observed following antipsychotics or antidepressants use are benign (exanthematous eruptions, skin pigmentation changes, photosensitivity, urticaria, and pruritus), but their appearance impacts patient's compliance (Knowles and Shear 2007).

Mild CDR usually occur 9 ± 5 days after initiation of treatment; most severe reactions like Stevens-Johnson syndrome (SJS) or toxic epidermal necrolysis (TEN) begin by 14 ± 7 days; whereas "drug hypersensitivity syndrome", also called drug reaction with eosinophilia and systemic symptoms are observable by 28 ± 14 days. Some eruptions may occur within minutes to hours like urticaria and anaphylaxia, and others may take from one to three days, like acute generalized pustulosis or fixed drug eruption (FDE). One of the most striking features of CDR is that exacerbated recurrences usually occur after re-challenge with the offending drug beginning within two days (Knowles and Shear 2007; Litt 2007; Rojeau 2006).

The most frequent CDR include morbilliform reactions, urticaria, FDE; and the most severe and feared include erythema multiforme (EM), SJS, and TEN (Table 1), which may be observed in 1 per 1000 hospitalized persons (Rojeua 2006; Valeyrie-Allanore et al. 2007).

When a severe CDR is suspected, immediate withdrawal of all potential offending agents is the most effective mode of therapy. Patients with extensive involvement should be cared for as a "burn patient" with fluid resuscitation, infection control measures, and nutritional support in a hospital burn-unit setting.

NSAIDS are the leading agents for causing CDR with as high as 27% of all ADR reported. Most CDR are moderate (aspirin, sulindac, naproxen, nabumetone, and ketoprofen) but in few cases CDR can be severe and account for up to 37% of TEN (oxicams). NSAIDS can also produce lichenoid eruption, photosensitivity, pruritus, and pseudoporphyria. Children are particularly sensitive to these drugs (Segal et al. 2007).

Antimicrobial drugs can also induce CDR in about 1.1% of patients, with higher frequencies (7.3%) in ambulatory pediatric population receiving penicillins, sulfonamides, or cephalosporins. The percentage of children receiving cefaclor, sulfonamides, penicillins, or other cephalosporins who exhibited a rash was 12.3, 8.5, 7.4, and 2.6%, respectively. The odds ratio of development of a rash was higher in children less than 3 years of age than other groups (Segal et al. 2007). Exfoliative dermatitis, pruritus ani, serum sickness-like reaction and vulvovaginitis can occur following cephalosporins; and clinical data suggest that there is cross reactivity with penicillins for evoking CDR (Rodriguez-Peña et al. 2006). In addition, aminopenicillins may also provoke drug-induced pemphigus, localized pustular eruption, and serum sickness-like reaction (Lopez et al. 2007).

With antiretrovirals, overall SJS and TEN are 100–1,000 times more likely for a given drug exposure in HIV patients; but other CDR induced include acne, lipodystrophy, pigmentation, pruritis, and vasculitis (Luther and Glesby 2007).

Calcium channel blockers can induce CDR with frequencies as high as 48%; the most common are ankle or pedal edema (30%), gingival hyperplasia (21%) and flushing (10%); less common are facial or truncal telangiectasia, photosensitivity reactions, exacerbation of/or new-onset psoriasis, purpuric exanthems, pemphigoid manifestations, subacute cutaneous lupus and oral ulcers, among others (Ioulios et al. 2003).

Chemotherapeutic and molecularly targeted drugs are associated with a wide array of benign to severe CDR. Interestingly, dermatologic toxicity of agents such as epidermal growth factor receptor inhibitors, multikinase inhibitors, proteosome inhibitors, BCR-ABL tyrosine kinase inhibitors, and immunomodulatory drugs appears to correlate with antitumor activity (Hammond-Thelin 2008; Sanborn and Sauer 2008); an observation that may serve as an indicator of the relevance of skin immune system in body homeosthasis.

To these lists of drugs, should also be added many of the drugs commonly recommended in dermatology texts for the treatment and care of skin diseases. Dermatologist's arsenal includes at least 132 drugs of 15 different groups; but it is of the utmost importance that some of these therapeutic agents can also provoke CDR and some life-threatening complications (Orion et al. 2005). Topical corticosteroids may produce striae, rosacea, perioral dermatitis, acne, atrophy, and purpura, as well as systemic reactions such as hyperglycemia, glaucoma, and adrenal insufficiency (Hengge et al. 2006).

CDR are also observed with well known skin contact sensitins and immunologic ernhancers. In the first group are included plants like the poison ivy and European primrose; perfumes; and chemical compounds like benzocaine, epoxy resins, mercaptans, picric acid derivatives, chlorinated hydrocarbons, ethylendiamine, paraphenylenediamine, thimerosal, neomycin, dinitrochlorobenzene, dinitrofluorobenzene; and minerals like beryllium, nickel, cadmium, chromates, silver, zirconium, and cutting oils. Immunologic enhancers include adjuvants, mineral oil, bacterial muramyl dipeptides, bacterial cell wall peptidoglycans, lipopolysacharides, bestatin, thymosin, tuftsin, liposomes, polyadenylate, levamisole, methisoprinol, IFNα. Whereas, examples of immunesuppresants include those procedures that may induce tolerance, like the desensitization schemes used for penicillin; those that exploit natural immune balance, like RhoGam that effectively suppresses the antiRh response; and immunesuppressant drugs like corticosteroids, muromonab-CD3, azathioprine, methotrexate, cyclophosphamide, cyclosporine A, tacrolimus, sirolimus, mycophenolate mofetil, FTY720, daclizumab, and basiliximab (Burrel et al. 1992; Brunton et al. 2006).

3 Role of the Immune System and Dendritic Cells in CDR

The immunesurveillance function of skin is finely tuned and tailored to the needs of the host. It guarantees the rapid recognition of and response to danger signals, like pathogen associated molecular patterns (PAMPs); and it also prevents the occurrence of such a reaction towards harmless and innocuous substances, in a tolerogenic fashion. Immune system mediation in CDR can occur within minutes, as in immediate reactions; or as a delayed response within hours, days, or even years. In either case, drugs may undergo bioactivation and haptenization or act directly on skin cells of the immune system such as DC leading to alternative forms of immune-modulation, like immunopotentiation or immunosupression (Roosterman et al. 2006).

Innate immune response of the skin immune system (SIS) is a critical first line of defense; it is rapid allowing the earliest detection of offending agents or microbial pathogens. The best studied examples of PAMP's receptors are the mannan-binding lectin, the mannose receptor, and the Toll-like receptors (TLR). After receptor ligation these cells produce both the cytokines and chemokines needed for innate response and cells immigration. These receptors do not depend on immunologic memory because they are germ-line encoded. TLR are expressed in all lymphoid tissue and highly in peripheral blood leukocytes. They are also present in monocytes, B cells, T cells, granulocytes, and DC. Monocyte-derived DC produce IL-12 but not the anti-inflammatory IL-10. Ligation of TLR on DC, triggers their maturation in terms of expression of CD83, MHC class II, CD11c, CD40, and the co-stimulatory molecules CD80 and CD86. Activation of DC via the TLR, enhances their capability to present antigens as well as an increased production of cytokines, like IL-12, TNF-β, and IFN-γ, which are critical for cell-mediated immunity, i.e., innate immune response lead to instruct the nature of adaptive T cell response (Roosterman et al. 2006; Flacher et al. 2006; Peiser et al. 2008).

In contrast, the adaptive immune response onset is delayed, is characterized by highly specific receptors that are distributed clonally on subsets of particular T or B cells, and involves immunologic memory. The innate and adaptive immune responses complement and modulate each other and, additionally, they are interactive in that the innate immune response influences the type of adaptive response; and, in turn, the adaptive immune response influences the function of innate cells (Henri et al. 2007; Randolph et al. 2008).

Evidence supporting a role of the immune system and of DC in CDR include four lines of evidence in as much as drugs can produce immediate-type immune mediated reactions; activation of T cells clones; and drugs can produce photosensitivity reactions (PS) as well as autoimmune diseases.

3.1 Drugs Induce Immediate-Type Immune-Mediated Reactions

Immediate type immune-mediated reactions develop in two phases. The immediate phase, or sensitization, can occur within seconds of drug exposure and may be associated with disseminated MA activation and degranulation. Inflammatory and cytotoxic mediators such as histamine, heparin, IL-3, IL-4, IL-5, TNFα, leukotrienes C4 and D4, platelet-activating factor, and enzymes like trypase, chymase, cathepsin G, and carboxypeptidases, are quickly released resulting in increased vascular permeability, epiglottal swelling, constriction of airways, and vascular collapse. This syndrome is known as anaphylactic shock, which is a life-threatening phenomenon that may result in death within minutes; in its mildest form, systemic drug administration results in a disseminated urticaria reaction (or hives). When precipitated by local intradermal injection, i.e., during allergy testing or an insect sting, the result is a classic wheal-and-flare reaction. A late-phase reaction, or elicitation, that generally follows is mediated by the expression of cytokines and chemokines, resulting in recruitment of a variety of inflammatory cells, including EO. This recruitment causes a more widespread edematous reaction, hence persistence of antigen can result in a chronic inflammatory condition.

Most hypersensitivity reactions produced by neuromuscular blocking agents are of immunologic origin, i.e., IgE mediated, or are related to direct stimulation of histamine release. The incidence of IgE mediated hypersensitivity or anaphylaxis is estimated between one in 10,000 and one in 20,000 anesthesias (Mertes and Laxenaire 2004). Anaphylaxis due to penicillin occurs in one per 10,000 courses of treatment and leads to death in one to five per 100,000 intramuscular courses. The mainstay treatment for anaphylaxis consists of epinephrine (adrenaline) and supportive measures to control breathing and cardiovascular functions (Dermirkan et al. 2006).

The signals initiating MA degranulation may require that drugs undergo a process of hapten-protein conjugate formation before antigenic recognition by a surface or soluble IgE and the formation of antigen-IgE complexes (Pichler et al. 2006). Then MA's high affinity Fcε receptors cross-link the complex and trigger the release of primary and secondary inflammatory mediators. Sera from subjects who have experienced an immediate-type reaction to penicillin exhibit heterogeneity in the IgE antibody response to antigenic determinants. In the case of penicillins, conjugation often occurs via amide linkage to the side chain -amino group on lysine or tyrosine residues and this may explain differences in antigenicity among penicillin derivatives; although antigenic recognition of the beta-lactam ring or thiazolidine rings will lead to a high degree of cross-reactivity among the various penicillin derivatives.

LC appears to contribute to MA degranulation because both cell types have Fcε receptors and RANK proteins (Ali et al. 2007).

3.2 Drugs Induce T Cell Mediated CDR

The clinical course of many CDR may evolve as a hypersensitivity delayed type reactions with either a variable time frame (Type II), or in a delayed form lasting over 24 h (Types IVA or IVB). These CDR types usually involve a majority of drug specific CD4+, CD8+, and some TCR$\alpha\beta$ and TCR$\gamma\delta$ T cells clones, which have been identified in the peripheral blood of patients with a history of CDR to penicillin G, amoxicillin, cephalosporins, carbamazepine, lidocaine, phenytoin, or sulfamethoxazole, phenobarbital (Roychowdhury and Svensson 2005; Rojeau 2006; Naisbitt et al. 2007).

T-cells possess clonally distributed receptors (TCR) that recognize antigen on the cell surface, when those are presented by antigen presenting cells (APC) in the context of MHC molecules, and so this cell surface-dependent recognition is referred to as MHC-restricted antigen recognition. CD4+ T cells recognize antigens presented in the context of MHC class II; while those antigens presented in the context of MHC class I are recognized by CD8+ T cells. Drug-induced TEN appears associated with an increased cutaneous infiltration CD4+ and sparse CD8+ T cells, and these drug immunocompetent T cells also show CLA+ and are capable to secrete IFN-γ (Naisbitt et al. 2007).

Considering that in drug-induced hypersensitivity reactions, small chemical compounds (SMW of $<1,000$ Da) can elicit a strong systemic T cell mediated immune response. Pichler and others (Pichler et al. 2006; Uetrecht 2008) proposed that the original compound or a drug metabolite may bind in a covalent and non covalent form with MHC, but it additionally may interact simultaneously with TCR, much like a superantigen even though requiring idiotypic residues in the TCR. DC and T cells recruitment occurs after exposure to allergens or bacterial superantigens and induces atopic skin inflammation (Pivarsci et al. 2004). Divalent nickel ions are the best studied example of such reversible coordination complexes (Martin 2004), but drugs like sulfamethoxazole, lidocaine, mepivacaine, celecoxib, carbamazepine, lamotrgine, ciproxin, and p-phneylendiamine may also trigger this mechanism (Pichler et al. 2006).

Examples of drugs that undergo bioactivation reactions before binding covalently with proteins, in a haptenization reaction, include penicillins, sulfonamides, phenytoin, carbamazepine, and dapsone; which are among the highest CDR producing drugs. Hepatic and/or cutaneous bioactivation via cytochrome P450 in DC may produce cytotoxic metabolites in the skin. The individual capability of LC and other skin cells to cope with the detoxification of these reactive metabolites may be an important predisposing factor that could account for the variable CDR observed with these drugs (Rojeau 2006; Roychowdhury and Svensson 2005; Saeki et al. 2002; Uetrecht 2005).

The importance of the possible bypassing of the innate immune system by noncovalent binding and direct interaction of drugs with T cells, relates to the shorter time necessary to activate a secondary memory response, where memory T cells would have a lower threshold of reactivity when compared with naïve T cells; features that would explain the higher incidence of drug hypersensitivity reactions during microbial infections or autoimmune diseases (Knowles and Shear 2007; Luther and Glesby 2007; Mohamadzadeh et al. 2007). For example, sulfamethoxazole allergy rises from 2–4 to 50% in HIV positive patients, or the change of 4–5% hypersensitivity to amoxicillin raising up to 90% in patients with acute infectious mononucleosis (Pichler et al. 2006). Viral infection of LC uncouples the activation and maturation from the migration processes (Flacher et al. 2006), an effect very likely to modify both innate and acquired immune responses to drugs (Mohamadzadeh et al. 2007). Whether this occurs as a result of changes in drug metabolism and antigenic presentation and/or altered immune response (immune dysregulation) caused by the presence of the microbe, their toxins and/or debris, it is an issue that remains to be elucidated.

3.3 Drugs can Produce Photosensitivity Reactions (Phototoxicity and Photoallergy)

Photosensitivity (PS) describes an increased incidence of erythema upon patient exposure to ultraviolet radiation or electromagnetic radiation, and as such it is considered a form of delayed type immune mediated CDR. Drugs like sulfonamide, tetracyclines, fluoroquinilones (sparfloxacin), NSAIDS (oxicams, naproxen), diuretics, and calcium channel blockers can provoke PS. Drug-induced PS can be phototoxic, where drug or drug's metabolites cause direct cellular damage by a mechanism that appears to be related to the production of free radicals highly reactive towards lipids and proteins (Stein and Scheinfeld 2007).

Drug-induced photoallergy, an alternative form of PS, only develops in sensitized individuals and appears to be a T cell mediated response. Allergic contact photosensitizing agent like TCSA (3,3,4,5-tetrachlorosalicylanilide) undergoes haptenization in epidermal strata but fluoroquinolones, like fleroxacin given systemically can also produce epidermal adducts when the skin is exposed to UVA; an effect that appears related to a photomodification of LC (Schwarz et al. 2005).

3.4 Drugs can Induce Autoimmune Diseases

Data from the literature indicated that LC and DC may have a pathogenic role in autoimmune diseases like pemphigus (PE), linear IgA bullous dermatosis (IgAD) and lupus like syndrome (LLS) (Ayala-García et al. 2005). PE as an ADR is induced by cephalosporins, penicillins, penicillamine, enalapril, and captopril; amiodarone, captopril, diclofenac, phenytoin, and vancomycin can trigger IgAD; while LLS can be observed following treatment with procainamide, hydralazine, chlorpromazine, isoniazide, and minocycline even years after initiation of treatment (Jones et al. 2004; Knowles et al. 2003; Roychowdhury and Svensson 2005). However, experimental evidence is lacking to document the direct effect of these drugs on LC.

In conclusion, LC have a large number of functional receptors for hormones, neuropeptides, and neurotransmitters (Roosterman et al. 2006); but only for activation of β adrenergic receptors there are reports indicative of a autocrine and paracrine adrenergic regulation of LC antigen presentation capability (Maestroni 2004). This observation could explain the mechanism by which adrenaline can control anaphylaxis symptoms, well beyond its effects on the cardiovascular system. It also opens the venue for further research on adrenergic regulation of LC functions considering that adrenaline is the only drug of this type available to treat anaphylactic shock (Dermiken et al. 2006), and for looking into the effect of other drugs on LC.

4 LC are Highly Mobile Professional Skin APC with Immunephenotype and Genotype Plasticity

The cellular basis of the immune response relies on the concerted operation of cell types including lymphocytes of B, T and natural killer (NK) lineages, and APC within the main organs of the immune system, i.e., thymus, spleen, lymphatics, lymph nodes, and lymphoid folicles. The supportive tissues in which lymphoid and myeloid elements mature and function are of prime importance, as it is often in these locations that drugs may induce ADR or CDR.

In the epidermis, LC are the primary cells responsible for the recognition, uptake, processing, and presentation of antigens and haptens to sensitized T lymphocytes. Due to this, LC have been implicated in the pathogenic mechanisms underlying allergic contact dermatitis, cutaneous leishmaniasis, and human immunedeficiency virus infection. LC are reduced in epidermis of patients with skin disorders such as psoriasis, sarcoidiosis, contact dermatitis, and neoplasic lesion; they are impaired by UV radiation; and they are significantly increased in LC Histiocytosis (Ayala-García et al. 2005; Senechal et al. 2007).

LC were originally described by Paul Langerhans in 1868 as dendritically shaped cells in the suprabasal regions of the epidermis; but it was until 1975 when Silberberg pointed to their possible immunological role during elicitation of contact allergic reactions. Over the time, one of the most intriguing recognized features of LC is the rapid morphologic and immunologic changes that LC undergo when the epidermal microenvironment is modified. As illustrated in Table 2, even the key markers of LC, langerin (Lang) and the Birbeck granules (BG) disappear during skin inflammation. The underlying mechanisms for the transitions listed in Table 2 are not yet fully understood but they certainly highlight the enormous biochemical and immune phenotype plasticity of LC.

In 1991, Steinman proposed that immature DC patrol peripheral tissues upon encounter with microbial products or other danger signals undergo maturation as they migrate to lymphoid tissue where they present antigen and activate naive T cells. Shortly after it was reported that human CD34+ hematopoietic progenitor cells can generate two subsets of myeloid DC after being cultured in vitro with GM-CSF and TNFα. One of these monocyte subsets corresponds to the immunephenotype of LC including BG; while the other subset has characteristics of interstitial dermal DC, i.e., express CD14 and factor XIIIa (Caux et al. 1992).

Later on, data in vivo indicated that Gr-1hi monocytes that express the inflammatory chemokine receptor CCR2 are the direct precursors of LC in the epidermis, and these two markers are lost after LC maturation. In the report by Ginoux et al., it is also demonstrated that the receptor for colony-stimulating factor 1 (CSF-1) is a specific requirement of LC to reconstitute following inflammation in situ (Ginhoux 2006). The proposal of specific subsets of monocytes as immediate precursors of LC is consistent with the observation that some subtypes of monocytes can cross endothelial barriers back and forth in an in vitro system, a property reminiscent of extravasation into tissue and entry to lymphatics (Randolph et al. 2008). Ginhoux's work also pointed out to the specific requirement of CSF-1 for epidermal repopulation, while the CCR2- mediated signaling is relevant for bone marrow egress but not for entry into tissues such as spleen, lung, or liver (Serbina and Pamer 2006). Thus, migration of LC precursors into skin seems to be regulated differently from the migration of precursors of other DC into spleen and other tissues. The relevance of these observations rely upon the potential use of CCR2 receptor as a target to modulate skin LC and DC repopulation.

LC as a member of DC professional APC system in other squamous epithelia (oral cavity, oesophagus, and vagina) are capable of migrating continuously to lymphoid organs such as the cutaneous draining lymph nodes (CDLN) even under steady state, i.e., in the absence of skin damage (Steinman and Bancherau 2007). As illustrated in Table 2, their differentiation can be followed by the expression of cell surface molecules like cutaneous lymphocyte antigen (CLA+), E-cadherin, $\alpha 6$ $\alpha 4$ integrin, very-late activation antigens (VLA), CD44, integrins of the CD11/CD18 class, as well as intercellular adhesion molecules (ICAM1, ICAM3, and LFA3). These markers serve a role in LC trafficking and cell adhesion (Randolph et al. 2008).

LC in the quiescent skin are characterized by the presence of heterogeneous expression of MHC II and low levels of expression of CD40, CD80, and CD86 (see Table 2); a phenotype that also corresponds to the blood borne lymph node resident DC populations. BG are more abundant in human epidermis, but few of them can still be observed in migrating LC in lymph nodes and vessels with their main molecular constituent Lang; which is a C-type lectin that accumulates where BG conform subdomains of the endosomal recycling compartment, following a process apparently controlled by the Rab GTPases Rab-11A (Uzan-Gafsou et al. 2007). Lang can be observed in endosomal recycling organelles and in BG, but it is present also on

Table 2 Surface molecules expressed on human LC[a]

Marker	Normal skin	Inflamed skin	Isolated fresh	Isolated and cultured	Cultured and cytokine-activated
Phenotype					
LAG (CD207)[b]	++	n.d.	++	n.d./+	
Langerin[b]	+++	n.d.	++	n.d./+	
ATPase[b]	+++	+	++	n.d./+	
Antigenic immunophenotype					
Antigen uptake/processing	+++	++	+++	+++	+++
Antigen presenting	+/−	+++	+	+	+++
MHC class I	+	+++	++	+++	++
MHC class II (DR, DP, DQ)[b]	+	+++	++	+++	+++
CD1a (T6 49 kD)	+++	+/++	++	n.d./+	+
CD1b	n.d.	+/++	?	?	n.d.
CD1c (T6, 43 kD)	+++	+/n.d.	+	n.d./+	n.d.
CD4	+				
CD8	n.d.				+/n.d.
CD11a (LFA-1)	n.d.	++	n.d.	n.d.	
CD11b (C3biR)	n.d./±	+++	+	n.d.	
CD11c (gp 150/95)	+	+++	+	n.d.	
CD18 (ß chain of CD11)			+	n.d.	
CD45 RB			n.d.	+	
CD45 RO	+		+	n.d./+	
FcεRI	+++	n.d.	+	n.d.	
FcεRII (CD23)	n.d./+	n.d./++	n.d.	±	
FcγRI (CD64)	n.d.	++			n.d.
FcγRII (CD32)	++	n.d.	+	n.d.	n.d.
FcγRIII (CD16)	n.d.	n.d./+			n.d.
Adhesion molecules					
β1 Integrins	++	α4 ↑ /α6 ↓			
CD44 v4–v6, v9	+	+++			
CD50 (ICAM-3)	++		++	++	
CD54 (ICAM-1)	+/n.d.	++	+/n.d.	++	
CD58 (LFA-3)	+/n.d.	++	+/n.d.	++	
E-cadherin	+				
CLA	+				
Costimulatory molecules/Activation markers					
CD24			n.d.	+	++
CD40	+/n.d.	++	+		+
CD80 (B7-1)	n.d./±	+	n.d.	++	+
CD86 (B7-2)	n.d./±	+	n.d.	++	++
Activation markers					
CD83	n.d.	++			+
CD25 (IL-2R)	n.d.	++	n.d.	+	++
CD69	+	n.d.	+	n.d./+	n.d.
VLA4α	+	+/++			
ICAM-1 (CD54)			+/n.d.	++	
ICAM-3			++	++	

(continued)

Table 2 *Continued*

Marker	Normal skin	Inflamed skin	Isolated fresh	Isolated and cultured	Cultured and cytokine-activated
LFA-3 (CD58)			+/n.d.	++	
RFD1 (DQ-like)			+	+++	
Cytokine/chemokine receptors					
GM-CSFRα (CD116)	++	+++			
GM-CSFRβ (CD131)	+/n.d.	++			
M-CSFR (CD115)	n.d.				n.d.
TNFR II (75 kD) (CD120b)	+++	+			
IL-1RI (CD121a)	+	++			
IL-1RII (CD121b)	+	++			
IFNγ-R (CD119)	+	+			
IL-6R (CD126)	n.d.	+			
Gp-130 (CD130)	n.d.	+			
C5aR (CD88)	+/n.d.	+++			+
CCR1	+	n.d.			
CCR2	−/+				n.d.
CCR3	n.d.				n.d.
CCR4	+	+			
CCR5	+	n.d.			
CCR6	++	n.d.			
CCR7	n.d.	++			
CXCR4/Fusin	+	+			
Platelet activating factor	+	+			
Cytokine/chemokine secretion					
IL-1β	+	+			
IL-6	n.d.	+			
IL-12	+/n.d.	++			
IL-15	+	++			
IL-18	+/n.d.	++			
TNF-α	n.d.	n.d.			
IFN-γ	+	++			
SCF	+	n.d.			
MIP-1α	+	n.d.			
MIP-2	+	+			

[a]Semiquantitative data adapted from Wollenberg and Bieber 2002; Lotze and Thomson (2001)
[b]Indicates the most reliable markers of LC. Non-detectable: n.d

the surface of different DC (Cheong et al. 2007). Lang is actively involved in antigen binding, uptake, and transfer to BG for processing, and although recent reports indicate that neither Lang nor BG appear to be essential for antigen presentation (Kissenpfennig et al. 2005; Verdijk et al. 2005), these observations do not exclude the role of other DDC in antigen presentation to T cells in the CDLN.

In contrast, a mature phenotype is characterized by: (1) neo-synthesis and peptide loading of MHCII molecules followed by the transport of stable peptide-MCH complexes to and prolonged display at the surface; (2) by down regulation of antigen uptake moieties (eg. FcεR1, BG); and, (3) by a massive upregulation of stimulatory molecules of T cell activation, like CD24, CD40, CD54, CD80, CD83, CD86, etc;

and certain cytokines such as IL-1â, IL-6, IL-12, IL-15, IL-18, and CCR7 (see Table 2). As a consequence, LC acquire the capacity of stimulating naive T cells for helper function both Th1 and Th2, as well as to prime naive cytotoxic T cells (Randolph et al. 2008). Upon LC stimulation in vitro with antigens, maturation occurs along with an up regulation of co-stimulatory markers of immature cell populations isolated from lymph nodes with no major effect on already mature DC or LC (see Table 2).

Full functional maturation of LC occurs after uptake of antigens and when TLR are cross linked by some damage signal like PAMP's. LC take up intact protein antigens or protein-coupled low molecular weight haptens, which enter the endocytic pathway and are cleaved inside the cell by limited digestion into small peptides. These peptides are loaded as a rule onto MHCII or into a MHCI, by cross presentation processes, before antigen presentation to TCD4+ or TCD8+ cells; in contrast lipidic bacterial antigens are usually presented in the context of CD1 molecules (Stoitzner et al. 2006). Bacterial recognition by LC depends on TLR2, TLR4, and TLR5; and selective activation of TLR2 stimulates LC antigenic presentation to CD4+ T cells (Peiser et al. 2008).

LC can also take up fluids by engulfment of extracellular space by the plasma membrane and subsequent translocation of the created endosomes into the endocytic pathway of the cell; but it may also occur via a mannose receptor or a high affinity receptor for IgE, i.e., FcεRI (Ali et al. 2007).

Following antigen uptake, LC migrate towards CDLN in a process tightly regulated by cytokines (TNFα, IL-1β, IL-18), chemokines (CCL19, CCL21), cell surface metalloproteinases, prostaglandins, E-cadherin, integrins, nuclear hormone receptors, etc. (Randolph et al. 2008). At a given time point, several dendritic cells CD11c+ populations can be observed in the CDLN; these can be subclassified by immune characterization in three groups depending on whether they come from the blood (CD8α+), dermis (DC) or from epidermis (LC). Noteworthy all CDLN derived DC populations can endocyte subcutaneous or intradermal lipopolysacharide antigens and present them to CD4+ T cells, with the larger capacity of the mature populations; i.e., all LN DC subtypes are able to induce cytotoxic CD8+ T cells with the participation of Ag-specific CD4+ T cells (Henri et al. 2007).

Schoeters et al. 2007 studied the contribution of human LC to allergen-induced contact dermatitis using blood derived CD34+ progenitors matured in vitro with human recombinant GMC-SF, TNFα, and IL-4. The mature phenotype criteria were the presence of CD1a+, HLA-DR, CD86, CD83, and CD14. Immature dendritic cells observed by these authors were consistently 50–60% CD1a positive, 75–90% HLA-DR positive, 5–25% CD86 positive, 1–5% CD83 positive and <5% CD14 positive as compared to isotype-stained control cells. When these in vitro matured LC were exposed to the allergens eugenol, oxazolone, nickel sufate or dinitrochlorobenzene, these authors observed that 119 genes were altered when compared with control cultures. 17 of the final 25 genes selected were considered by the authors as relevant for its relation to the immune response: PIP3E, TNFAIP6, PLAT, CD36, F13A1, NINJ1, CTSC, RGS1, CCR7 (a specific DC maturation marker), FGL2, PBEF1, SLC7A5, CCR2, SAT, PHLDA1, CREM, ABCA6, SLC2A3, and

CALCRL. As well as with signal transduction and metabolism: RGS1, CALCRL, RAB32, TNFAIP6, CREM, SLC2A3, SLC7A5, CD36, PIP3E, CTSC, PLAT and F13A1 (Schoeters et al. 2007).

The experimental approach used by Schoeters et al. (2007) is one the most advanced individualized diagnostic assays to assess the contribution of LC to contact allergic reactions in humans. An expansion of this type of studies could prove to be very useful in patients with multiple allergies and could lead to the development of reverse deoxyribonucleotides to block specific functions of the immune response targeting specific genes or gene products. It would also be very interesting to know how LC immune phenotype would be presented if LC progenitors were cultured in media containing only GMC-SF, or GMC-SF, IL-4, and IL-10 instead of TNFα; combinations proposed to lead to tolerogenic profiles of professional APC (Uszynski and Hertl 2001).

In normal skin, or steady state, the number of epidermal LC appears to depend on the division of LC or epidermal LC precursors, so they represent a long lived cell population as shown by the persistence of LC for over 4 years in human skin grafts (Kanitakis et al. 2004). However, when chronic skin inflammation occurs, immature LC will accumulate in human CDLN and epidermal replenishment must occur with arrival of either bone marrow progenitors (Hacker et al. 2003) or from monocytes (Ginhoux et al. 2006). The remaining unsettled issue is whether all the immune phenotype and genotype changes, illustrated in Table 2 and in the work by Schoeters et al. (2007), that need to undergo LC actually prepare them to die or to transform for entering in a dermal and/or epidermal recycling; a hypothetical scenario that could well contribute for antigen transfer among dendritic cells (Allan et al. 2006).

In conclusion, quiescent LC can be considered as a mature cell population from the histological and embryological point of views, in as much as they reach the epidermis as a differentiated cell population well ahead before structural organization of the skin. However, as stated above, from an immunological point of view quiescent LC are regarded as an immature cell population that reaches maturity when they function as professional APC in lymphoid organs. This is an issue not settled yet in the literature, but it should be kept in mind when interpreting controversial data on the possible role of LC in contact hypersensitivity (Kaplan et al. 2005; Kissenpfennig et al. 2005; Verdijk et al. 2005) because this discrepancy certainly challenges the role of LC as a dynamically changing unique cell population which can expand across very different tissue layers.

5 Proposed Mechanism by Which LC May Contribute to CDR

As illustrated in Fig. 1, the afferent arm of the SIS mediated skin responses may be initiated by exposure of skin cells to foreign substances after topical application, when skin is injured, or when epicutaneous environment and defense mechanisms are overflow. Most drugs are small molecular weight compounds (SMW) that may reach the epidermis by simple diffusion (SD), or flowing by SD into epidermis and

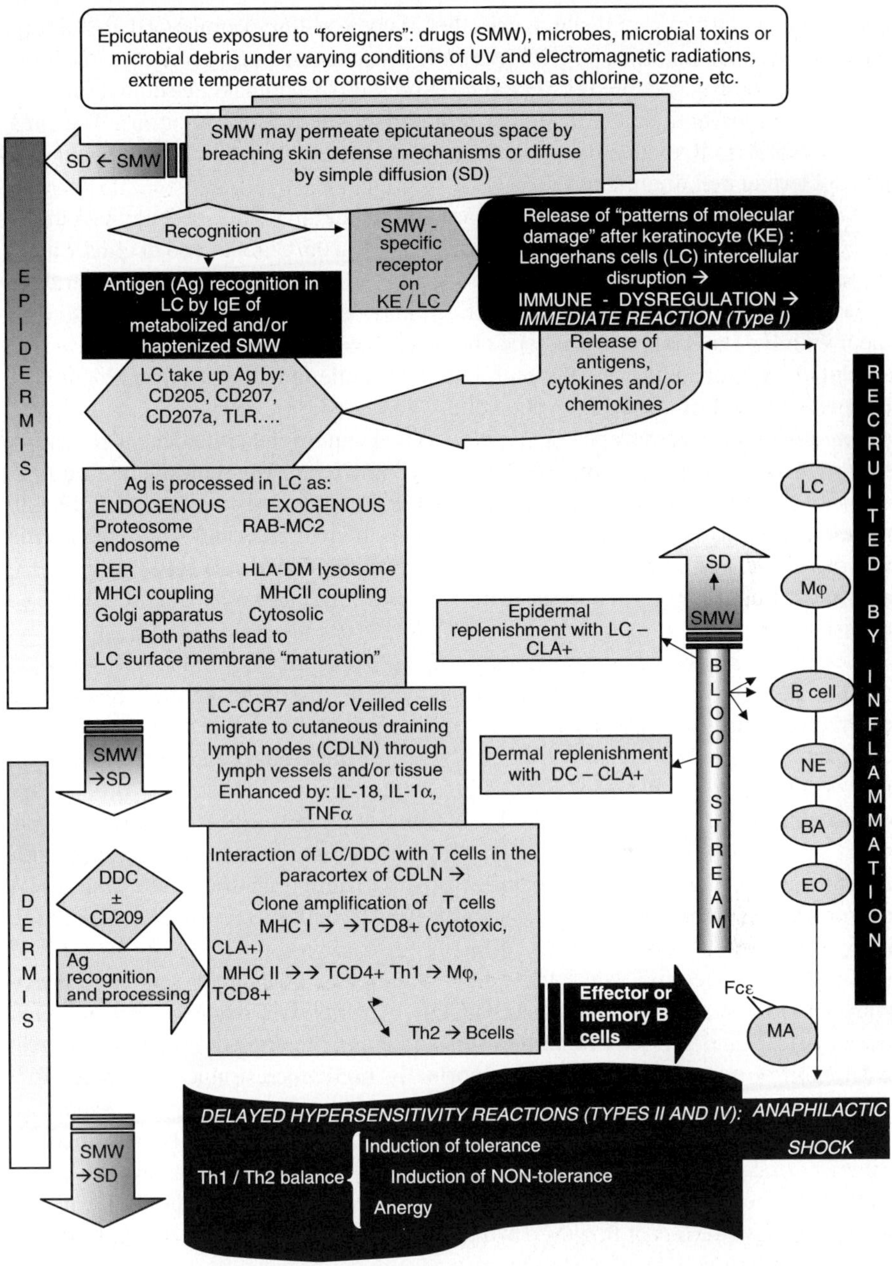

Fig. 1 Immunesurveillance function of the skin neuro-immune-endrocrine system is carried out by epidermal Langerhans cells (LC) in collaboration with dermal dendritic cells (DDC). Changes in the epicutaneous environment and/or epithelial tissues launches LC-DDC mediated innate and acquired immune responses with tolerogenic or immunogenic profiles as the underlying mechanisms of drug induced adverse systemic and cutaneous reactions. For more details see text under "Proposed Mechanism by Which LC May Contribute to CDR"

dermis when exiting from the high endothelial postcapillary venules (HEPV). Drugs may interact with pharmacological receptors on skin cells, i.e., adrenergic receptors on LC or with drug specific IgE (FcRIgE) expressed by spontaneous clonal selection due to previous antigenic encounters (epidermal immune-modulation). The presence of SMW may induce the expression of numerous costimulatory molecules on any epidermal cell, including LC.

For detecting SMW or antigens LC may use specific uptake receptors of the C-type lectin family including langerin/CD207, DEC-205/CD205, and dectins 1 and 2 (Flacher et al. 2006) or TLR (Peiser et al. 2008). The direct action on skin dendritic cells could explain how microbial infections may be priming the cutaneous environment with IL-1 or TNF-α and induce either a decrease of antioxidant defenses, such as glutathione, or induce the upregulation of proinflammatory mechanisms related to prostaglandins synthesis (Roychowdhury and Svensson 2005).

LC are the only epidermal cell population that can migrate into deeper skin strata towards CDLN, as veiled cells (VC), when KE down regulate their expression of E-cadherin (Randolph et al. 2008). Epidermal chemokines and cytokines (CCR/CCL) release that follows LC unattachment, promote their migration towards the dermis and recruitment of a multicell cascade which may involve Mϕ, B cells, NE, BA, EO and, most importantly, MA which will cause skin inflammation due to the release of histamine (Ali et al. 2007).

Severe and/or persisting inflammation along with spreading of PAMP's throughout the skin will occur depending on the type of offending stimuli, SMW concentration, duration of exposure, and the baseline state of skin and epicutaneous environment. These processes will quickly recruit the arrival of LC from bone marrow progenitors, via Id2 and TGFα signalling; effector and memory B cells, and degranulating MA. Arrival of LC-CLA+ from myeloid sources and dermal monocyte derived DC-CLA+ may occur as compensatory mechanisms for restoring skin immune barrier function. In a parallel process, offending foreigners like SMW and/or their metabolites, produced locally by LC or KE, may undergo antigenic recognition.

The time frame with which these intercellular processes may occur will differentiate the most severe forms of ADR/CDR. Anaphylaxia occurs within minutes, whereas TEN and SJS require longer time and appear restricted to those body areas where initial baseline LC density is normally high: face, trunk, and extremities (Thomas et al. 1984).

Antigen uptake and processing may occur in the epidermis only with the contribution of LC before induction of clonal expression of drug specific T cells in CDLN. To the immune response launched by immunologically matured LC, migrating through the dermis or flowing via the afferent lymphatic vessels (LV), it will add the contribution of DDC; which can also recognize, process, and express antigens in the context of MHC molecules classes I and II. These two populations of professional APC will initiate a large amplification of CD4+ and CD8+ T cells clones in the paracortex of CDLN. Some TCD4+ may in turn activate B cell cloning in the CDLN cortex. During antigen presentation, LC can direct Th1 or Th2 responses according with the types of cytokines and co-stimulatory factors released by LC and surrounding cells (Maldonado-López et al. 1999).

Once T cells are activated immunocompetent clone proliferation may occur towards a Th1 profile (secreting IL-2, IFN-α, TNF-α, promote inflammation, cytotoxicity, and delayed types II and IV hypersensitivity reactions); or towards a Th2 profile secreting IL-4, IL-5, IL-6, IL-10, IL-13, support humoral immunity and serve to down regulate the inflammatory actions of Th1 cells (Lebrec et al. 2001). Disruption of the Th1/Th2 balance may result in the loss of tolerance and promote destructive immune responses to self-tissues, exacerbated responses to drugs and autoimmune diseases ("horror autotoxicus") as proposed by Steinman (Steinman and Nussenzweig 2002).

The appearance of drug-induced delayed hypersensitivity (Types II or IV) will depend upon the fine tuning of the Th1/Th2 balance. Induction of tolerance is the basic mechanism by which over 95% of T cell clones derived to self antigens are deleted; and this could explain why the majority of patients do not exhibit ADR or CDR.

The idea that LC may play a role in down regulation of the cutaneous immune response is supported by four lines of evidence; first, immature human LC can accumulate in CDLN in patients with infections or malignancies in the absence of autoimmune diseases, such as vitiligo (Geissmann et al. 2002); second, recent papers indicate that mice lacking LC exhibit increased contact hypersensitivity (Kaplan et al. 2005); third, environmental stimulus at the skin can redirect the local and systemic immune system by means of up or down regulation of RANKL, (Loser et al. 2006), which is highly expressed on activated T cells and serves as a survival factor for DC, phagocytes and are also expressed in LC (Ali et al. 2007); and fourth, the early response to UV radiation is the depletion of LC and a reduction of epidermal antigen presenting function (Schwarz et al. 2005).

Recent therapeutic approaches for both autoimmunity or tolerance, involve the in vitro manipulation of bone marrow or peripheral blood precursors of DC with several cytokines cocktails, in order to obtain a DC population with a immature phenotype (frequently associated with tolerogenicity) or a DC population with a mature phenotype (normally referred as immunogenicity), in terms of MHC II, CD80, CD86, and CD40. The major cytokines used on DC precursor cultures include GM-CSF, TNF-α, IL-4, IL-10, TGF-β, and the use of ligands of different TLR as LPS (Uszynski and Hertl 2001). Hence, this can be a possibility to modulate LC activity into tolerogenic or immunogenic branches in situ; a situation that could be exploited for the benefit of those patients with repetitive CDR or under long drug treatments.

Other signals like the heat shock proteins and intercellular adhesion molecules (ICAM-1) can be expressed in the epidermal cells during severe drug eruption (Nishioka et al. 1999) or in response to common sensitizing agents, such as nickel, *p*-phenylenediamine, and urushiol, the antigen in poison ivy (Picardo et al. 1992); ensuing thus a very fine tunning of skin homeosthasis in response to drugs.

The efferent arm of the skin immune response begins with the exit of primed T cells from CDLN and their transit back to the skin via blood stream. In HEPV, T cells bind to E-selectin or P-selectin, expressed by endothelial cells, slowing transit through the vessel. Activation of these rolling T cells by various chemokines then stimulates T cells to stop and attach firmly to endothelial cells via integrins expressed on T cells. The homing mark of those lymphocytes that must arrive to skin is the cutaneous leukocyte antigen (CLA+) and some of the integrins like leukocyte factor antigen or very-late antigen 1. After firm binding, T cells can migrate through endothelial cells and become extravascular in the dermis. The extent of migration of these immunocompetent T cells on dermis or into epidermis varies as a function of the antigen originally encountered and the baseline physiopathological condition of the skin; for example, due to a preexisting disease.

Once activated T cells are in the skin they can recognize activating antigens and re-initiate the release of inflammatory CCL and CCR cascade from skin resident cells. In the same way, drug immunocompetent memory B cells or plasmatic cells are capable of arriving to cutaneous regions and release their Ig's, and trigger an inflammatory response via MA and EO newly recruited (Blanca et al. 2005).

In conclusion, epidermal DC may either drive tolerogenic as well as immunogenic responses by participating in both innate and acquired immune responses, and modulating both cellular and humoral immune responses. The actual speed with which afferent and efferent arms of SIS operate will determine both the occurrence as well as severity of ADR and/or CDR.

Tolerance to self or foreign antigens perpetuates homeosthasis and this may explain the fewer incidence of CDR. However, tolerance to foreign antigens may also contribute to the persistence of offending pathogens, such as viral or bacterial infections which are well documented enhancers of CDR; creating thus a condition of immune – dysregulation.

Based on this idea, the result of the combined presence of SMW and microbial infections very likely will contribute to enhanced CDR and ADR. The critical steps for activation of LC include the control of LC – KE epidermal interaction, i.e., by E-cadherin; the rate of LC migration towards CDLN, i.e., by IL-18; and the proper homeosthasis of the epicutaneous – epidermal environment. Whenever any of these are disrupted, the skin immune system is likely to launch an immune response whose final balance, immunogenic, or tolerogenic, will depend on patient's physiopathology. The sequence of events herein proposed to operate simultaneously might help to understand how chemical or physical agents, as well as epicutaneous microbial infections may prime epidermal modifications of skin permeability to drugs, enhancing thus the incidence and severity of ADR and CDR.

References

Ali A, Rautemaa R, Hietanen J, Beklen A, Konttinen Y (2007) A possible CD1a Langerhans cell-mast cell interaction in chronic hyperplastic candidosis. J Oral Pathol Med 36:329–336

Allan RS, Waithman J, Bedoui S, Jones CM, Villadangos JA, Zhan Y, Lew AM, Shortman K, Heath WR, Carbone FR (2006) Migratory dendritic cells transfer antigen to a lymph node-resident dendritic cell population for efficient CTL priming. Immunity 25:153–162

Ayala-García I, Hernández-Segura AM, Castell-Rodríguez AE, Alvarez-Pérez J, Hernández-Tellez B, Ramírez-González MD (2005) Participation of epidermal Langerhans cells in human pathology and their potential as targets for drug developmet: a review of literature. Proc West Pharmacol Soc 48:13–20

Beltraminelli HS, Lerch M, Arnold A, Bircher AJ, Haeusermann P (2005) Acute generalized exanthematous pustulosis induced by the antifungal terbinafine: case report and review of the literature. Br J Dermatol 152:780–783

Blanca M, Cornejo-Garcia JA, Torres MJ, Mayorga C (2005) Specificities of B cell reactions to drugs. The penicillin model. Toxicology 209:181–184

Bronnimann M, Yawalkar N (2005) Histopathology of drug-induced exanthems: is there a role in diagnosis of drug allergy? Curr Opin Allergy Clin Immunol 5:317–321

Brunton LL, Lazo JS, Parker KL (2006). Goodman and Gilman's the pharmacological basis of therapeutics, 11th edn. McGraw Hill, New York, USA, pp. 127–128, 1406–1424, 1741–1744

Burrell R, Flaherty DK, Sauers LJ (1992). Toxicology of the immune system: a human approach. VanNostrand Reinhold, New York, USA, pp. 235–292

Caux C, Dezutter-Damuyant C, Schmitt D, Banchereau J (1992) GM-CSF and TNF-alpha cooperate in the generation of dendritic Langerhans cells. Nature 360:258–261

Cheong C, Idoyaga J, Do Y, Pack M, Park SH, Lee H, Kang YS, Choi JH, Kim JY, Bonito A, Inaba K, Yamazaki S, Steinman RM, Park CG (2007) Production of monoclonal antibodies that recognize the extracellular domain of mouse Langerin/CD207. J Immunol Methods 324:48–62

Chu DH, Haake AR, Holbrook K, Loomis CA (2003) The structure and development of skin. In: Fitzpatrick's Dermatology in general medicine, 6th edn. McGraw Hill, New York, USA, pp. 58–88

Demirkan K, Bozkurt B, Karakaya G, Kalyoncu AF (2006) Anaphylactic reaction to drugs commonly used for gastrointestinal system diseases: 3 case reports and review of the literature. J Investig Allergol Clin Immunol 16:203–209

Demoly P, Hillaire-Buys D (2004) Classification and epidemiology of hypersensitivity drug reactions. Immunol Allergy Clin N Am 24:345–356

Descotes J, Choquet-Kastylevsky G (2001) Gell and Coombs's classification: is it still valid? Toxicology 158:43–49

FDA (2004) Serious adverse event definition. In: http://www.fad.gov/medwatch/report/DESK/ advent.htm. Updated on Jan 23th, 2004. Accessed on March 10th, 2008

Flacher V, Bouschbacher M, Verronese E, Massacrier C, Berthier-Vergnes O, DeSaint-Vis B, Caux C, Dezutter-Dambuyant C, Lebecque S, Valladau J (2006) Human Langerhans cells express a specific TLR profile and differentially respond to virus and Gram-positive bacteria. J Immunol 177:7959–7967

Geissmann F, Dieu-Nosjean MC, Dezutter C, Valladeau J, Kayal S, Leborgne M, Brousse N, Saeland S, Davoust J (2002) Accumulation of immature Langerhans cell in human lymph nodes draining chronically inflamed skin. J Exp Med 196:417–430

Ginhoux F, Tacke F, Angeli V, Bogunovic M, Loubeau M, Dai XM, Stanley ER, Randolph GJ, Merad M (2006) Langerhans cells arise from monocytes in vivo. Nat Immunol 7:265–273

Hacker C, Kirsch RD, Ju XS, Hieronymus T, Gust TC, Kuhl C, Jorgas T, Kurz SM, Rose-John S, Yokota Y, Zenke M (2003) Transcriptional profiling identifies Id2 function in dendritic cell development. Nat Immunol 4:380–386

Hammond-Thelin LA (2008) Cutaneous reactions related to systemic immunomodulators and targeted therapeutics. Dermatol Clin 26:121–159

Hengge UR, Ruzicka T, Schwartz RA, Cork MJ (2006) Adverse effects of topical glucocorticosteroids. J Am Acad Dermatol 54:1–15

Henri S, Siret C, Machy P, Kissenpfennig A, Malissen B, Leserman L (2007) Mature DC from skin and skin-draining LN retain ability to acquire and efficiently present targeted antigen. Eur J Immunol 37:1184–1193

Hertl-Yazdi MS, Hertl M (2005) Bullous drug reactions. Hautarzt 56:16–23

Ioulios P, Charalampos M, Efrossini T (2003) The spectrum of cutaneous reactions associated with calcium antagonists: a review of the literature and the possible etiopathogenic mechanisms. Dermatol Online J 9:6–11

Jones DH, Todd M, Craig TJ (2004) Early diagnosis is key in vancomycin-induced linear IgA bullous dermatosis and Stevens-Johnson syndrome. J Am Osteopath Assoc 104:157–163

Kanitakis J, Petruzzo P, Dubernard JM (2004) Turnover of epidermal Langerhans cells. N Eng J Med 351:2661–2662

Kaplan DH, Jenison MC, Sealand S, Shlomchik WD, Shlomchick MJ (2005) Epidemal Langerhans cell-deficient mice develop enhanced contact hypersensitivity. Immunity 23:611–620

Kissenpfennig A, Ait-Yahia S, Clair-Moninot V, Stossel H, Badell E, Bordat Y, Pooley JL, Lang T, Prina E, Coste I, Gresser O, Renno T, Winter N, Milon G, Shortman K, Romani N, Lebecque S, Malissen B, Sealand S, Douillard P (2005) Disruption of the langerin/CD207 gene abolishes Birbeck granules without a marked loss of Langerhans cells function. Mol Cell Biol 25:88–99

Knowles SR, Shear NH (2007) Recognition and management of severe cutaneous drug reactions. Dermatol Clin 25:245–253

Knowles SR, Shapiro LE, Shear NH (2003) Reactive metabolites and adverse drug reactions: clinical considerations. Clin Rev Allergy Immunol 24:229–238

Kobayashi KS, Flavell RA (2004) Shielding the double-edged sword: negative regulation of the innate immune system. J Leukoc Biol 75:428–433

Lebrec H, Kerdine S, Gaspard I, Pallardy M (2001) Th(1)/Th(2) responses to drugs. Toxicology 158:25–29

Litt JZ (2007) Litt's drug eruption reference manual, 13th edn. Informa Healthcare Pub, London, UK

Lopez S, Blanca-Lopez N, Cornejo-Garcia JA, Canto G, Torres MJ, Mayorga C, Blanca M (2007) Nonimmediate reactions to betalactams. Curr Opin Allergy Clin Immunol 7:310–316

Loser K, Mehling A, Loeser S, Apelt J, Kuhn A, Grabbe S, Schwarz T, Penninger JM, Beissert S (2006) Epidermal RANKL controls regulatory T-cell numbers via activation of dendritic cells. Nat Med 12:1372–1379

Lotze MT, Thomson AW (2001) Dendritic cells, 2th edn. Academic Press, San Diego, USA

Luther J, Glesby MJ (2007) Dermatologic adverse effects of antiretroviral therapy: recognition and management. Am J Clin Dermatol 8:221–233

Maestroni GJ (2004) Modulation of skin norepinephrine turnover by allergen sensitization: impact on contact hypersensitivity and T helper priming. J Invest Dermatol 122:119–124

Maldonado-López R, De Smedt T, Michel P, Godfroid J, Pajak B, Heirman C, Thielemans K, Leo O, Urbain J, Moser M (1999) CD8α+ and CD8α− subclasses of dendritic cells direct the development of distinct T helper cells in vivo. J Exp Med 189:587–592

Martin SF (2004) T lymphocyte-mediated immune responses to chemical haptens and metal ions: implications for allergic and autoimmune disease. Int Arch Allergy Immunol 134:186–198

Mertes PM, Laxenaire MC (2004) Adverse reactions to neuromuscular blocking agents. Curr Allergy Asthma Rep 4:7–16

Mockenhaupt M (2005) Severe cutaneous adverse drug reactions. Clinical features and epidemiology. Hautarzt 56:24–31

Mohamadzadeh M, Chen L, Schmaljohn AL (2007) How Ebola and Marburg viruses battle the immune system. Nat Rev Immunol 7:556–567

Naisbitt DJ, Pirmohamed M, Park BK (2007) Immunological principles of T-cell-mediated adverse drug reactions in skin. Expert Opin Drug Saf 6:109–124

Nikkels AF, Nikkels-Tassoudji N, Pierard GE (2006) Oral antifungal-exacerbated inflammatory flare-up reactions of dermatomycosis: case reports and review of the literature. Am J Clin Dermatol 7:327–331

Nishioka K, Groreishi M, Yokozeki H (1999) Heat shock proteins and skin diseases. Curr Opin Infect Dis 12:171–176

Orion E, Matz H, Wolf R (2005) The life-threatening complications of dermatologic therapies. Clin Dermatol 23:182–192

Peiser M, Koeck J, Kirschning CJ, Wittig B, Wanner R (2008) Human Langerhans cells selectively activated via Toll-like receptor 2 agonists acquire migratory and CD4+ T cell stimulatory capacity. J Leukoc Biol 83:1118–1127

Picardo M, Zompetta C, Marchese C, De Luca C, Faggioni A, Schmidt RJ, Santucci B (1992) Paraphenylenediamine, a contact allergen, induces oxidative stress and ICAM-1 expression in human keratinocytes. Br J Dermatol 126:450–455

Pichler WJ, Beeler A, Keller M, Lerch M, Posadas S, Schmid D, Spanou Z, Zawodniak A, Gerber B (2006) Pharmacological interaction of drugs with immune receptors: the p-I concept. Allergology Int 55:17–25

Pivarcsi A, Gombert M, Dieu-Nosjean MC, Lauerma A, Kubitza R, Meller S, Rieker J, Muller A, Da Cunha L, Haahtela A, Sonkoly E, Fridman WH, Alenius H, Kemeny L, Ruzicka T, Zlotnik A, Homey B (2004) CC chemokine ligand 18, an atopic dermatitis-associated and dendritic cell-derived chemokine, is regulated by staphylococcal products and allergen exposure. J Immunol 173:5810–5817

Randolph GJ, Ochando J, Partida-Sanchez S (2008) Migration of dendritic cell subsets and their precursors. Annu Rev Immunol 26:293–316

Riedl MA, Casillas AM (2003) Adverse drug reactions: types and treatment options. Am Fam Med 68:1781–1790

Rodriguez-Pena R, Antunez C, Martin E, Blanca-Lopez N, Mayorga C, Torres MJ (2006) Allergic reactions to beta-lactams. Expert Opin Drug Saf 5:31–48

Rodríguez Velasco JG, Torres Valdos JE, Montero Mora P, Juárez Morales DT, Rodríguez E, Almeida Arvizu VM (2006) Reactions to drugs. A review of literature. Rev Alerg Mex 53: 73–75

Romano A, Demoly P (2007) Recent advances in the diagnosis of drug allergy. Curr Opin Allergy Clin Immunol 7:299–303

Roosterman D, Goerge T, Schneider SW, Bunnett NW, Steinhoff M (2006) Neuronal Control of Skin Function: the Skin as a neuroimmunoendocrine organ. Physiol Rev 86:1309–1379

Roujeau JC (2006) Immune mechanisms in drug allergy. Allergology Int 55:27–33

Roychowdhury S, Svensson CK (2005) Mechanisms of drug-induced delayed-type hypersensitivity reactions in the skin. AAPS J 7:E834–E846

Saeki M, Saito Y, Nagano M, Teshima R, Ozawa S, Sawada J (2002) mRNA expression of multiple cytochrome p450 isozymes in four types of cultured skin cells. Int Arch Allergy Immunol 127:333–336

Sanborn RE, Sauer DA (2008) Cutaneous reactions to chemotherapy: commonly seen, less described, little understood. Dermatol Clin 26:103–119

Schmid-Wendtner MH, Korting HC (2006) The pH of the Skin Surface and Its Impact on the Barrier Function. Skin Pharmacol Physiol 19:296–302

Schoeters E, Verheyen GR, Nelissen I, Van Rompay AR, Hooyberghs J, Van Den Heuvel RL, Witters H, Schoeters GER, Van Tendeloo VFI, Berneman ZN (2007) Microarray analyses in dendritic cells reveal potential biomarkers for chemical-induced skin sensitization. Mol Immunol 44:3222–3233

Schwarz A, Maeda A, Kernebeck K, vanSteeg H, Beissert S, Schwarz T (2005) Prevention of UV radiation induced immunosuppression by IL-12 is dependent on DNA repair. J Exp Med 201:173–179

Segal AR, Doherty KM, Legott J, Zlotoff B (2007) Cutaneous reactions to drugs in children. Pediatrics 120(4):e1082–e1096

Senechal B, Elain G, Jeziorski E, Grondin V, Patey-Mariaud de Serre N, Jaubert F, Beldjord K, Lellouch A, Glorion C, Zerah M, Mary P, Barkaoui M, Emile JF, Boccon-Giboud L, Josset P, Debré M, Fischer A, Donadieu J, Geissman F (2007) Expansion of regulatory T cells in patients with Langerhans cell hystiocytosis. PLoS Med 4(8):1374–1384 (e253.doi:10.1371/journal.pmed.0040253)

Serbina NV, Pamer EG (2006) Monocyte emigration from bone marrow during bacterial infection requires signals mediated by chemokine receptor CCR2. Nat Immunol 7:311–317

Stein KR, Scheinfeld NS (2007) Drug-induced photoallergic and phototoxic reactions. Expert Opin Drug Saf 6:431–443

Steinman RM, Bancherau J (2007) Taking dendritic cells into medicine. Nature 449:419–426

Steinman RM, Nussenzweig MC (2002) Avoiding horror autotoxicus: The importance of dendritic cells in peripheral T cell tolerance. Proc Nat Acad Sci USA 99:351–358

Stoitzner P, Tripp CH, Eberhart A, Price KM, Jung JY, Bursch LS, Ronchesse F, Romani N (2006) Langerhans cells cross-present antigen derived from skin. Proc Natl Acad Sci USA 103:7783–7788

Sullivan JR, Shear NH (2002) Drug eruptions and other adverse drug effects in aged skin. Clin Geriatr Med 18:21–42

Tan EK, Grattan CE (2004) Drug – induced urticaria. Expert Opin Drug Saf 3:471–484

Thomas JA, Biggerstaff M, Sloane JP, Easton DF (1984) Immunological and histochemical analysis of regional variations of epidermal Langerhans cells in normal human skin. Histochem J 16:507–519

Uetrecht J (2005) Role of drug metabolism for breaking tolerance and the localization of drug hypersensitivity. Toxicology 209:113–118

Uetrecht J (2008) Idiosyncratic drug reactions: past, present and future. Chem Res Toxicol 21: 84–92

Uzan-Gafsou S, Bausinger H, Proamer F, Monier S, Lipsker D, Cazenave JP, Goud B, deLa SH, Hanau D, Salamero J (2007) Rab11A controls the biogenesis of Birbeck granules by regulating langerin recycling and stability. Mol Biol Cell 18:3169–3179

Uzinsky ST, Hertl M (2001) Novel therapeutic approaches in autoimmune skin disorders. In: Autoimune diseases of the skin. Pathogenesis, diagnosis and management. Springer Verlag, USA, pp. 337–364

Valeyrie-Allanore L, Sassolas B, Roujeau JC (2007). Drug-induced skin, nail and hair disorders. Drug Saf 30:1011–1030

Verdijk P, Dijkman R, Plasmeijer EI, Mulder AA, Zoutman WH, Mommaas AM, Tensen CP (2005) A lack of Birbeck granules in Langerhans cells is associated with a naturally occurring point mutation in the human Langerin gene. J Invst Dermatol 124:714–717

WHO (2007) International Statistical classification of diseases and related health problems. External causes of morbility and mortality (V01-Y98). Drugs, medicaments and biological substances causing adverse effects in therapeutic use (Y40-Y59). 10th edn. WHO, 2007. In: http://www.who.int/classifications/apps/icd10online Accessed on March 10th, 2008

Yawalkar N (2005) Drug-induced exanthems. Toxicology 209:131–134

Zaccara G, Franciotta D, Perucca E (2007) Idiosyncratic adverse reactions to antiepileptic drugs. Epilepsia 48:1223–44

Part III
Manipulation of Dendritic Cells for Immunotherapy

T Cell Regulatory Plasmacytoid Dendritic Cells Expressing Indoleamine 2,3 Dioxygenase

David J. Kahler and Andrew L. Mellor

Contents

Abstract Mature dendritic cells (DCs) are potent stimulators of T cells that recognize antigens presented by the DCs. In this chapter we describe mature DCs that suppress T cell responses to antigens they present due to expression of the intracellular enzyme indoleamine 2,3 dioxygenase (IDO). IDO-competent DCs are a subset of plasmacytoid DCs that can be induced to express IDO under certain inflammatory conditions in humans and mice. Though rare, IDO-expressing DCs acquire potent T cell suppressor activity that may predominate over the T cell stimulatory functions of all other antigen-presenting cells in physiologic environments due in part,

A.L. Mellor (✉)
Immunotherapy Center, Medical College of Georgia 1120, 15th Street, Augusta, GA 30912-2600, USA
amellor@mcg.edu

G. Lombardi, Y. Riffo-Vasquez (eds.), *Dendritic Cells,* Handbook of Experimental Pharmacology 188,

to cooperation with regulatory T cells. Thus, IDO-expressing DCs are critical regulators of adaptive immunity that contribute to a wide range of inflammatory disease processes. As such, manipulating IDO expression in DCs using IDO inhibitors or IDO inducers offers considerable opportunities to improve immunotherapies in a range of clinically-significant disease syndromes.

Abbreviations

1MT	1-methyl-tryptophan
HAA	3-Hydroxyanthranilic acid
APC	Antigen presenting cells
AF	Auto Fluorescent
BMDCs	Bone marrow-derived dendritic cells
CHOP	CCAAT/enhancer-binding protein homologous protein
COX2	Cyclooxygenase 2
CTLA4	Cytotoxic T-lymphocyte antigen 4
DT	Delayed type hypersensitivity
DCs	Dendritic cells
D-1MT	D-isomer of 1MT
EAE	Experimental autoimmune encephalitis
FACS	Fluorescence activated cell sorting
FSC	Forward scatter
GAS	Gamma interferon associated sites
GCN2	General control non-derepressible 2
GITR	Glucocorticoid-induced tumor necrosis factor receptor
IFNαβ	IFN type I
IFNγ	IFN type II
IHC	Immunohistochemistry
IDO	Indoleamine 2,3 dioxygenase
ISR	Integrated stress response
IFNAR	Interferon alpha receptor
IRF	Interferon regulatory factor
ISGF3	Interferon stimulated gene factor 3
ISRE	Interferon stimulated response elements
IFNs	Interferons
JAK	Janus activated kinase
L-1MT	L-isomer of 1MT
MACS	Magnetic activated cell sorting
mTOR	Mammalian target of rapamycin
MLRs	Mixed lymphocyte reactions
mAb	Monoclonal antibodies
MS	Multiple sclerosis
MDSCs	Myeloid-derived suppressor cells
mDC	Myeloid dendritic cell

NO	Nitric oxide
PBMC	Peripheral blood mononuclear cells
pDC	Plasmacytoid dendritic cell
PGE2	Prostaglandin E2
ROS	Reactive oxygen species
Tregs	Regulatory T cells
SSC	Side scatter
STAT	Signal transducer and activator of transcription
SOCS3	Suppressor of cytokine signaling 3
TCR	T cell receptor
TLR	Toll-like receptor
TDO	Tryptophan 2,3-dioxygenase
TDLNs	Tumor draining lymph nodes

1 Introduction

The notion that mature dendritic cells (DCs) induce clonal expansion and differentiation of T cells with effector functions is well established (Reis e Sousa 2006), as is the complementary notion that immature (or 'alternately activated') DCs induce weak or abortive T cell responses (Steinman et al. 2003; Morelli and Thomson 2007). In this chapter, we describe an under-appreciated aspect of DC immunobiology, the ability of some specialized DCs to promote active T cell suppression when fully mature. The mechanisms underlying active suppression by DCs are not well defined and are still under investigation, largely for technical reasons since assays to detect suppression mediated by DCs require careful optimization. Moreover, DCs specialized to mediate active T cell suppression represent a tiny minority of DCs that must be induced to acquire suppressive functions. Hence, these DCs are easy to overlook, unless cells from physiologic sources are treated and fractionated appropriately.

Despite their rarity, suppressive DCs may exert disproportionately potent effects in local tissue microenvironments by amplifying other regulatory mechanisms such as $CD4^{+}CD25^{+}$ regulatory T cells (Tregs) leading to dominant suppression that negates the T cell stimulatory functions of all other DCs and other antigen presenting cells (APCs) in the same local tissue milieu. One mechanism that has attracted considerable attention with regard to suppressive DCs involves expression of the intracellular enzyme indoleamine 2,3 dioxygenase (IDO) in specialized DCs, which acquire potent T cell suppressive functions as a consequence. For the purposes of this review, we focus exclusively on the IDO mechanism due to recent progress in understanding how IDO activity in specialized DCs promotes active T cell suppression. Though other mechanisms may also cause DCs to acquire suppressive functions we focus on the IDO mechanism to illustrate some key points about DCs with regulatory functions that may be applicable to other mechanisms.

Recent reviews summarize the extensive experimental evidence showing that IDO plays an important role in suppressing T cell immunity in murine models of infectious, autoimmune and allergic diseases, tumor growth, and survival of transplanted tissues and developing fetuses expressing alloantigens (Mellor and Munn 2004; Fallarino et al. 2007). Indeed, cells expressing IDO, including but not limited to DCs, may create and maintain immune privilege in selected tissues under homeostatic or inflammatory conditions (Jasperson et al. 2007; Mellor and Munn 2008). While the mechanistic basis of IDO-mediated effects on disease etiology is not fully understood, it is likely that IDO^+ DCs make critical contributions to a range of chronic inflammatory syndromes, especially those in which T cells contribute to disease etiology.

IDO-mediated T cell suppression by DCs may be clinically beneficial or detrimental according to which chronic inflammatory disease is under consideration. In cancer and chronic infectious diseases, lack of effective T cell immunity contributes to disease progression and persistence in otherwise immunocompetent individuals, suggesting that IDO^+ DCs may contribute to disease etiology. In contrast, aberrant T cell regulation allows excessive responses to healthy tissues and innocuous stimuli (such as commensal microorganisms or allergens) leading to autoimmune and allergic diseases, and host responses to donor alloantigens leads to rejection of healthy transplants, unless globally immunosuppressive drugs are used to prevent rejection. In these syndromes, IDO activity in DCs may be beneficial by slowing disease progression or transplant rejection, and artificially enhancing IDO expression (for example in DCs) may help shift the balance towards effective T cell suppression and long term tolerance.

After describing IDO biochemistry and molecular genetics, we summarize current knowledge about the identity of DCs competent to express IDO, and the signaling mechanisms that induce these specialized DCs to express IDO. Finally, we discuss the immunological significance of IDO-mediated T cell suppression by DCs, and how this knowledge might be exploited to improve immunotherapies to treat a range of chronic inflammatory diseases of clinical importance.

2 IDO Biochemistry

In this section we briefly describe the biochemistry of IDO including its substrates, downstream metabolites, and the cellular responses that occur following its activation. We identify compounds currently under investigation that reduce or inhibit IDO activity and end the section with a discussion of how an intracellular enzyme such as IDO might gain access to extracellular substrates and how decreased substrate is detected.

2.1 IDO Enzymology

Indoleamine 2,3-dioxygenase (IDO, EC1.13.11.17) is one of two conserved heme-containing enzymes in mammals that catalyze the initial and rate-limiting step in

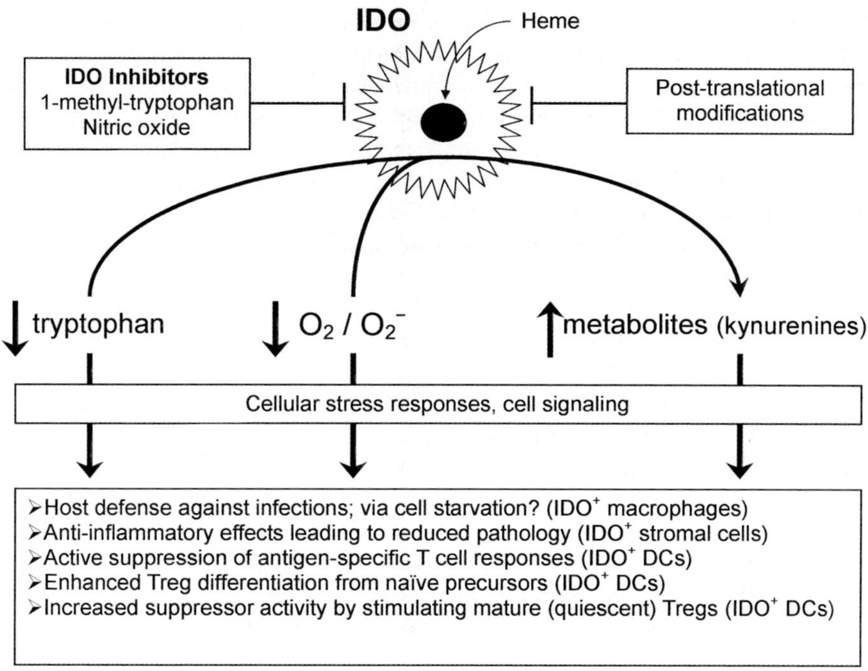

Fig. 1 IDO Biochemistry and Biology. Overview of the cellular responses to IDO activation resulting from decrease in tryptophan and reactive oxygen species and increased production of kynurenines. See text for details

oxidative degradation of the essential amino acid tryptophan along the kynurenine pathway (Taylor and Feng 1991; Mellor and Munn 1999). IDO degrades substrates containing indole rings such as (but not limited to) tryptophan (Fig. 1) and the neurotransmitter serotonin (Myint and Kim 2003). IDO gene expression is tightly regulated and is responsive to inflammatory signals such as interferons (IFNs). Hence, Toll-like receptor (TLR) ligands (such as LPS and CpGs) and other reagents that induce inflammation and IFN production also induce IDO expression.

Unlike IDO, tryptophan 2,3-dioxygenase (TDO, EC1.13.11.11) has substrate specificity for L-tryptophan only, is expressed exclusively in liver in response to glucocorticoids, and is thought to regulate dietary tryptophan intake to moderate tryptophan levels in serum (Salter et al. 1995; Liao et al. 2007). As no role for TDO in DCs has been described to date, we will not consider this enzyme further. As depicted in Fig. 1, in addition to catabolizing tryptophan cells expressing IDO consume reactive oxygen species (ROS) (Thomas and Stocker 1999), and generate downstream metabolites known collectively as kynurenines (Taylor and Feng 1991). Kynurenine itself is a stable metabolite produced by many IDO^+ cells, and the presence of kynurenine in serum or tissue culture supernatants is commonly used to evaluate IDO activity in cells, though some cells possess enzymes that catalyze further degradation and may not release kynurenine. Thus, biochemical changes brought about by IDO activity include tryptophan withdrawal (depletion), reduced oxidative stress and production of downstream tryptophan metabolites (kynurenines). These changes may influence cellular functions in various ways to bring about some well-documented effects of IDO activity such as inhibiting the spread of infectious microorganisms in macrophages, and activating counter-inflammatory mechanisms that ameliorate pathology, as well as suppressing T cell responses and stimulating Treg suppressor functions that have been described more recently (Fig. 1). In addition to affecting other cells in the same microenvironment, the biochemical changes brought about by IDO activity in DCs may also modify the phenotype, functions and differentiation/maturation status of DCs themselves via cell autonomous mechanisms.

2.2 IDO Inhibitors

Table 1 lists selected reagents that inhibit IDO enzyme activity directly, or have indirect inhibitory effects on IDO expression or enzyme activity by cells. Several synthetic tryptophan analogues inhibit IDO enzyme activity (Peterson et al. 1994), presumably by binding to the enzyme active site, which accepts the indole

Table 1 Reagents that inhibit or reduce enzyme IDO activity

Mode of Action	Reagent (inhibitor)	Reference
Competitive, inhibitor	1-Methyl-Tryptophan	Cady and Sono (1991), Agaugue et al. (2006), Hou et al. (2007), Metz et al. (2007)
	Brassinin	Gaspari et al. (2006), Banerjee et al. (2007)
	NSC 401366	Vottero et al. (2006)
Antioxidants	Epigallocatechingallate	Jeong et al. (2007)
	Rosmarinic acid	Lee et al. (2007)
	p-Coumaric acid	Kim et al. (2007)
	Pyrrolidine dithiocarbamate	Thomas and Stocker (1999), Thomas et al. (2001)
Metabolites	Nitric Oxide	Thomas et al. (1994, 2007), Samelson-Jones and Yeh (2006)
	Hydrogen peroxide	Poljak et al. (2006)
	Peroxynitrite	Fujigaki et al. (2006)
	N-chlorotaurine	Wirleitner et al. (2004)
Pharmacologic	Celecoxib	Basu et al. (2006)
	Zebularine	Liu et al. (2007)
Marine derived compounds	Exiguamine A	Brastianos et al. (2006)
	Garveia annulata	Pereira et al. (2006)

ring of substrates and substrate analogues (Sugimoto et al. 2006). For example, 1-methyl-tryptophan (1MT) is a competitive reversible IDO inhibitor commonly used in standard (cell-free) enzyme activity assays (Cady and Sono 1991; Sakurai et al. 2002; Travers et al. 2004; Hou et al. 2007; Ou et al. 2007). Surprisingly, the D-isomer of 1MT (D-1MT) was a less toxic, and more effective IDO inhibitor than the L-isomer of 1MT when tested in pre-clinical studies in mice as a method to block IDO activity in bioassays with indirect (but clinically relevant) readouts such as enhanced T cell stimulatory functions of DCs measured *ex vivo* and reduced tumor growth in vivo. D-1MT was also an effective IDO inhibitor in studies with human macrophages and DCs (Duluc et al. 2007; Hill et al. 2007b), though another report described results that were not consistent with this conclusion (Lob et al. 2007). Consequently, D-1MT is currently being evaluated as a potential tumor vaccine adjuvant treatment in cancer patients. It remains to be seen if the findings from pre-clinical studies are predictive of outcomes in human patients. This point notwithstanding, the novel paradigm that IDO activity may facilitate resistance of tumors and some chronic infections to T cell immunity in humans is driving interest in developing novel and more effective IDO inhibitors for clinical applications.

Brassinin (3-(S-methyldithiocarbamoyl)aminomethyl indole), a natural plant product, and its synthetic derivative, 5-bromobrassinin (5-Br-brassinin) are novel compounds that also inhibit IDO activity directly (Banerjee et al. 2007). An indole ring was not necessary for effective IDO inhibition, and substitution of the S-methyl group with large aromatic groups yielded reagents with more potent inhibitory effects than 1MT, at least in vitro (Gaspari et al. 2006). A non-indolic competitive IDO inhibitor, NSC 401366 (imidodicarbonimidic diamide N-methyl-N′-9-phenanthrenyl-monohydrochloride) was identified using a novel yeast based assay in which human IDO was expressed in a *Saccharomyces cerevisiae* tryptophan auxotroph. In this assay, yeast growth was restricted by limiting access to free tryptophan and inhibition of IDO by reagents under investigation restored yeast growth (Vottero et al. 2006). Although little is known about the biological function of NSC 401366, the assay itself may prove useful for screening and identifying new compounds with IDO inhibitory properties.

Another group of compounds exhibiting antioxidant properties inhibit IDO expression indirectly by interfering with cofactors required for enzymatic activity or signaling molecules upstream of IDO expression. Epigallocatechingallate, rosmarinic acid (a-ocaffeoyl-3,4-dihydroxyphenyl-lactic acid), and p-coumaric acid displayed IDO inhibitory properties in vitro using murine bone marrow-derived dendritic cells (BMDCs) or $CD11c^{+}CD8\alpha^{+}$ DCs harvested from tumor draining lymph nodes of mice injected with B16 melanoma cells (Youn et al. 2003; Jeong et al. 2007; Kim et al. 2007; Lee et al. 2007). These compounds inhibited IDO expression and function by blocking Cyclooxygenase 2 (COX2) or Prostaglandin E2 (PGE2) expression, reducing Signal Transducer and Activator of Transcription (STAT1) phosphorylation, and inhibiting the binding of activated STAT1 to the Interferon Regulatory Factor 1 (IRF1) promoter. Other antioxidants such as pyrrolidine dithiocarbamate, 2-mercaptoethanol, ebselen, and t-butyl hydroquinone have been reported to display IDO inhibitory properties (Thomas et al. 2001).

Some natural metabolites can also inhibit IDO activity. Nitric oxide (NO) inhibits IDO activity by binding irreversibly to the catalytic heme group (Thomas et al. 1994; Samelson-Jones and Yeh 2006). Exposure of recombinant human IDO to H_2O_2 in vitro caused oxidation of cysteine residues to sulfinic and sulfonic acids resulting in loss of enzymic activity but not tryptophan binding ability (Poljak et al. 2006). The peroxynitrite generator, 3-(4-morpholinyl) sydnonimine caused nitration of several tyrosine residues in recombinant human IDO leading to inactivation of IDO (Fujigaki et al. 2006). N-Chlorotaurine, the oxidation product of HOCl and intercellular taurine inhibits IDO in several murine models (Wirleitner et al. 2004).

Off target effects of two pharmacologic agents also inhibit IDO. The specific COX2 inhibitor Celecoxib reduced tumor associated IDO expression in a murine breast cancer model (Basu et al. 2006). Zebularine, a DNA methyl transferase inhibitor, was shown to induce IDO at high doses and inhibit IDO at low doses (Liu et al. 2007). Finally, some compounds isolated from marine organisms have IDO inhibitory activity. Exiguamine A isolated from the marine sponge *Neopetrosia exigua* (Brastianos et al. 2006), and fractions from crude extracts of the marine hydroid *Garveia annulata* were potent inhibitors of IDO (Pereira et al. 2006).

2.3 Tryptophan Transport and Tryptophanyl tRNA Synthetase

Because IDO is an intracellular enzyme, tryptophan must be present inside cells, or be transported into IDO^+ cells, to be degraded. This is an important consideration because T cells do not express IDO under physiologic conditions, and the ability of IDO^+ DCs to suppress T cell responses by removing tryptophan from the cytoplasm of T cells therefore requires explanation. Human monocyte-derived macrophages with IDO-mediated T cell suppressive functions express sodium-independent, tryptophan-specific transporters that may be critical for their T cell regulatory functions (Seymour et al. 2006). Likewise, transporters may allow IDO^+ DCs to acquire tryptophan from their immediate microenvironment. Speculatively, tryptophan transporters might be strategically distributed in immunologic synapses that form when T cells and DCs interact following recognition of cognate antigen, providing DCs with preferential access to free tryptophan from T cells. Such considerations, though technically difficult to verify (especially in physiologic settings) may explain why IDO^+ DCs may not need to fully deplete tryptophan from tissue microenvironments to influence T cell responses.

IFNγ treatment caused IDO-dependent tryptophan depletion in tissues of tumor-bearing mice, and induced expression of tryptophanyl-tRNA synthetase, the only tRNA synthetase gene that is responsive to inflammatory stimuli (Burke et al. 1995). These findings prompted speculation that tryptophan 'starvation' might negatively impact cell growth in the vicinity of IDO^+ cells; however, these effects did not fully explain how IFNγ slowed tumor growth in this experimental system. Another reason why tryptophan 'starvation' may not be the appropriate paradigm to explain IDO-mediated T cell suppression (Mellor and Munn 1999) emerged from evidence that T cells, in common with all cell types, detect reduced access to free amino acids via General Control Non-derepressible 2 (GCN2) kinase, which is triggered by increased binding of uncharged tRNAs to ribosomes (Dong et al. 2000). Thus, GCN2-kinase triggering may be highly sensitive to reduced tryptophan levels in the cell cytoplasm obviating the need to fully deplete tryptophan from cells or their immediate microenvironment to stimulate downstream responses, unless increased expression of tryptophanyl-tRNA synthetase protects cells from the anti-proliferative effects of tryptophan depletion (Burke et al. 1995).

3 IDO Molecular Genetics and Gene Expression

In this section we describe the molecular genetics of IDO and the recently identified IDO2 gene. We identify the tissues, cell types, and physiologic conditions under which IDO is expressed. Included in this section is a discussion of the growing list of agents and signaling pathways that have been identified to induce functional IDO.

3.1 IDO Genes

IDO genes are highly conserved in all mammalian species studied to date and they clearly evolved from ancestral genes related to the myoglobin gene. Recently, a second IDO gene (IDO2) was identified in mice and humans (Ball et al. 2007; Metz et al. 2007). In both species, IDO2 is closely linked to the previously identified IDO (IDO1) gene located in a syntenic region of chromosome 8. For the purposes of this review, we consider IDO as a single gene product, while acknowledging that IDO protein may be the product of IDO1, IDO2 or both genes. IDO1 and IDO2 genes exhibit similar but not identical patterns of regulated expression in response to inflammatory signals, and D-1MT inhibits enzyme activity of proteins encoded by IDO1 and IDO2 genes (Table 1). The biological significance of the two IDO genes is not yet clear, but some human ethnic groups possess relatively high frequencies (25–50%) of defective IDO2 alleles (Metz et al. 2007).

3.2 IDO Gene Expression

IDO is expressed constitutively in tissues with large mucosal surfaces (lungs, GI tract, maternal-fetal interface), and may be a consequence of inflammation at mucosal surfaces under homeostatic conditions (Yamamoto and Hayaishi 1967; Keith and Brownfield 1985; Munn et al. 1998). IDO expression also occurs at sites of infection and tumor growth, and in chronically inflamed tissues associated with allergic and autoimmune disease syndromes (Friberg et al. 2002; Hayashi et al. 2004;

Popov et al. 2006; Saxena et al. 2007). However, only a few cell types express IDO in these tissues. IDO is rarely, if ever, expressed by lymphoid cells under physiologic conditions, and IDO staining (assessed by immunohistochemical techniques) is largely confined to myeloid lineage cells (DCs, macrophages), and some stromal cells types such as epithelial cells lining blood vessels and some fibroblast-like cells. IDO+ cells always represent a small subset of any given cell type in tissues. Hence, lineage-specific factors that regulate the ability of cells to express IDO have not been defined and IDO appears to be regulated in large part by inflammatory cues (via IFNs) once cells have acquired competency to express IDO. It is important to emphasize that post-translational modifications, absence of co-factors such as hemin, and the presence of natural IDO inhibitors such as NO may compromise or inactivate IDO enzyme activity.

Hence, caution should be exercised in interpreting data based solely on methods that detect IDO mRNA or protein (Thomas et al. 2001; Braun et al. 2005). Typically, IDO enzyme activity is measured using HPLC techniques to detect kynurenine, a stable downstream metabolite produced by certain IDO$^+$ cell types. However, this method is not very sensitive, requiring relatively large numbers of cells, and relies on the assumption that IDO$^+$ cells secrete kynurenine as the end product of oxidative tryptophan catabolism. For the specific purpose of measuring IDO-mediated effects in DCs, more sensitive (albeit indirect) methods to detect IDO activity involve measuring T cell stimulatory functions of DCs (see Sect. 6).

3.3 IDO Inducers

Interferons are potent inducers of IDO gene transcription in specialized cell types competent to express IDO (Taylor and Feng 1991; Mellor and Munn 1999). We describe DC subsets specialized to express IDO ('IDO-competent DCs') in Sect. 4. IFNs are a large family of cytokines, divided into three classes (types I, II and III), which are produced during rapid innate immune responses to microbial infections, and at other sites of inflammation during normal tissue functions, or caused by extraneous factors such as tissue wounding and tumor growth (Pestka et al. 2004; Chelbi-Alix and Wietzerbin 2007). Human and murine IDO genes contain Interferon Stimulated Response Elements (ISRE) and Gamma Interferon Associated Sites (GAS) elements in the proximal promoter regions, which respond to type I and type II IFNs, respectively (Dai and Gupta 1990; Paguirigan et al. 1994; Sotero-Esteva et al. 2000; Decker et al. 2005).

The diversity of IFNα (type I) subtypes produced by cells at sites of infection or inflammation suggests that there is functional or cell-type specificity between subtypes, though little is known about such distinctions. Indeed, activation of different signaling pathways and responses were reported in DCs and T cells following in vitro treatment by different subtypes (Hilkens et al. 2003; van Boxel-Dezaire et al. 2006; Johnson and Scott 2007). For example, we observed IFNα 1–9 gene transcription in murine splenic CD19$^+$ pDCs treated with CpGs or a soluble form

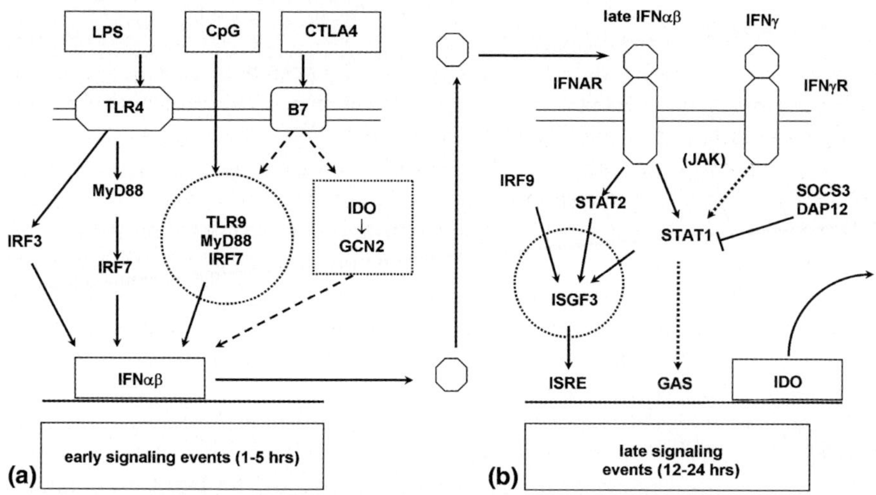

Fig. 2 Potential signaling events downstream of TLR and B7 ligation that induce IDO-competent pDCs to express IDO. (**a**) TLR4, TLR9 and B7 ligands stimulate IFNα transcription in pDCs via the distinct signaling pathways depicted (see text for details). (**b**) IFNα signaling through IFNAR induces formation of ISGF3 complexes containing activated STAT1–STAT2 heterodimers and IRF9 that act on ISRE motifs in IDO promoters. In contrast IFNγ induces IDO via STAT1-homodimers that bind to GAS elements. STAT-dependent signaling is suppressed by SOCS3 and DAP12 in most DCs

of Cytotoxic T-Lymphocyte Antigen 4 (CTLA4-Ig) (to ligate TLR9 or B7, respectively) prior to IDO expression (Baban et al. 2005; Manlapat et al. 2007). In contrast to IFNα, which is produced by many cell types (including pDCs) during innate immune responses, IFNγ (type II) is produced (for the most part) by lymphoid cells such as activated $CD4^+$ T cells during adaptive immune responses. Thus, DCs capable of expressing IDO may be responsive to a range of inflammatory cues at sites of tissue damage or infection, or in associated lymphoid tissues, that cause IFN release.

As depicted in Fig. 2, IFN type I (IFNαβ) and type II (IFNγ) induce IDO transcription via Janus Activated Kinase (JAK)/STAT signaling pathways that act on ISRE and GAS in IDO promoters, respectively (Platanias 2005). Under normal physiologic conditions few, if any, tissue DCs express IDO. However, when mice or splenocytes were treated with certain reagents that induce IDO (Table 2) a subset of DCs responded by expressing IDO and acquiring potent T cell suppressive functions. In many cases, the IDO inducers listed in Table 2 stimulated IDO expression indirectly by inducing IFNα production via MyD88/IRF7-dependent pathways that control IFNα expression in plasmacytoid DCs (pDCs). Thus, TLR ligands induced pDCs to express IFNα, which subsequently induced IDO-competent DCs to express IDO.

Similarly, soluble CTLA4 (CTLA4-Ig, a B7 ligand) induced IFNα production upstream of IDO, though in this case, IDO was also required upstream of IFNα production (Manlapat et al. 2007), revealing a cell (DC) autonomous feedback loop that presumably amplifies IDO expression via IFNα mediated signaling through its

Table 2 Reagents that induce IDO activity

Agent	Ligand	Receptor	Reference
Cytokines	IFNα/β	IFNAR1, IFNAR2	Baban et al. (2005)
	IFNγ	IFNG1, IFNGR2	Yasui et al. (1986)
	IL-10/TGFβ	IL-10R[a]	Finger and Bluestone (2002), Munn et al. (2002)
Fusion proteins	CTLA4-Ig	B71/2 (CD80/86)	Mellor et al. (2003, 2004), Fallarino et al. (2004), Baban et al. (2005), Fallarino et al. (2005), Manlapat et al. (2007)
	CD28-Ig[b]	B71/2 (CD80/86)	Fallarino et al. (2005)
	CD200-Ig	CD200R	Fallarino et al. (2004, 2005)
	GITR-Ig	GITRL	Grohmann et al. (2007)
	Anti B71/2 mAb	B71/2 (CD80/86)	Munn et al. (2004b)
TLR ligands	LPS	TLR4	Jung et al. (2007), Penberthy (2007)
	Resiquimod,R848	TLR7	Furset et al. (2007)
	CpG	TLR9	Mellor et al. (2005), Wingender et al. (2006), Manlapat et al. (2007)
PGE2			Braun et al. (2005), von Bergwelt-Baildon et al. (2006)
HDAC inhibitors SAHA/ITF2357			Reddy et al. (2007)

[a] IL10 (and TGFβ) sustains IDO expression in IFNγ activated mature DCs
[b] In conventional pDCs treated with siRNA to silence SOCS3

receptor (IFNAR). IFNγ also induced IDO expression in some DCs, such as CD8α^+ DCs, formerly known as lymphoid DCs (Fallarino et al. 2002b). These findings provide insights into the complex positive and negative signaling mechanisms that restrict IFN-mediated IDO expression to specialized cells in DC and other cell populations, though more studies will be needed to understand how IDO expression and IDO enzyme activity are regulated at the level of gene expression and post-translation, respectively.

4 IDO-Competent DCs

In this section, we describe DCs that can be induced to express functional IDO and acquire potent T cell suppressor functions as a consequence. DC phenotypes are heterogeneous, varying between tissues and dependent on DC maturation status. Moreover, it is difficult to draw parallels between DCs in mice and humans making it hard to draw firm conclusions from cross-species comparisons. Consequently, the primary focus of this section is on murine IDO-competent DCs, which have been defined in more detail than their counterparts in humans.

4.1 Murine IDO-Competent DCs

Two major DC subsets expressing the ubiquitous DC marker CD11c have been identified in mouse spleen (Table 3A). Myeloid DCs (mDCs) express relatively high levels of CD11c but do not express B220 (CD45R) or mPDCA1. Plasmacytoid DCs (pDCs) express both markers, but lower levels of CD11c than mDCs. Moreover, pDCs (but not mDCs) produce IFN type I in response to TLR ligation following microbial infection (Asselin-Paturel et al. 2001). IDO-competent DCs reside exclusively in the pDC subset, based on their morphologic appearance in tissues and on functional analyses of DC populations fractionated using the pDC specific-markers B220 and mPDCA1 (Fallarino et al. 2004, 2005, 2007; Baban et al. 2005). IDO-competent pDCs also exhibit phenotypes typical of mature DCs, expressing MHC and B7 molecules at relatively high levels compared to conventional pDCs and mDCs in spleen (Mellor et al. 2004).

Surprisingly, IDO^+ pDCs with T cell suppressor functions in tumor-draining lymph nodes (TDLNs) expressed the B cell marker CD19, a marker not previously associated with DCs (Munn et al. 2004a). Consistent with this finding, splenic IDO-competent pDCs also expressed CD19 (Baban et al. 2005; Mellor et al. 2005). $CD19^+$ pDCs are a rare DC subset representing only ~5–10% of total DCs (~10–20% of pDCs) in each tissue and only ~0.1–0.2% of total splenocytes (Fig. 3b), so that each mouse spleen typically yields only $\sim 10^5$ $CD19^+$ pDCs. Conventionally, pDCs have been defined as $CD19^{NEG}$, suggesting that $CD19^+$ pDCs represent a novel pDC subset that was over-looked, in part because CD19 is commonly used to segregate DCs from B cells. $CD19^+$ pDCs resemble conventional ($CD19^{NEG}$) pDCs in many ways, such as the ability to produce IFN type I following TLR ligation (Mellor et al. 2005; Manlapat et al. 2007).

Nevertheless, $CD19^+$ and $CD19^{NEG}$ pDCs are functionally, as well as phenotypically, distinct pDC subsets as IDO-competent pDCs reside exclusively in the $CD19^+$ pDC subset. For the purposes of the current discussion, the most important difference between rare $CD19^+$ pDCs and the more abundant conventional

Table 3A Phenotypic analyses of murine DC subsets

DC subset[a]	% Total DCs*	CD11c	B220 (CD45R)	CD8α	CD19	120G8	CCR6	B71/2 (CD80/86)	References
Myeloid (mDCs)	~50%	high	−	−	−	−	Int.	Inducible	Shortman and Naik (2007)
Plasmacytoid (pDCs)	~40%	low	+	+	−	+	Low	Inducible	Asselin-Paturel et al. (2003)
IDO-competent ($CD19^+$) pDCs	5–10%	high	+	+	+	−	High	high	Mellor et al. (2004, 2005), Baban et al. (2005), Manlapat et al. (2007)

[a] Based on analyses of murine splenic DCs

($CD19^{NEG}$) pDCs is the unique ability of $CD19^+$ pDCs from spleen and TDLNs to mediate IDO-mediated T cell suppression. Splenic $CD19^+$ pDCs also express CD8α, CD80, CD86, and the chemokine receptor CCR6 (Mellor et al. 2004; Manlapat et al. 2007), but $CD19^+$ pDCs do not express the conventional pDC markers 120G8 and mPDCA1 (Asselin-Paturel et al. 2003; Fallarino et al. 2005; Mellor et al. 2005).

4.1.1 Fractionation and Phenotypic Analyses of IDO-Competent PDCs

Two methods are widely used to fractionate DCs and DC subsets based on their affinity (or lack thereof) for specific monoclonal antibodies (mAb). Magnetic Activated Cell Sorting (MACS) is a rapid technique whereby cells labeled with mAb conjugated to magnetic beads are passed through a magnetic field to either enrich or deplete labeled cells from cell suspensions. In Fig. 3a, we show a typical dataset in which a standard MACS procedure yielded a cell population containing ~36% $CD11c^+$ cells (DCs) from a starting population of splenocytes containing only 7% DCs, representing a 5-fold enrichment for DCs. Note that carry over of $CD11c^{NEG}CD19^+$ and $CD11c^{NEG}CD19^{NEG}$ cells (mostly B and T cells, respectively) is significant, possibly due to interactions between DCs and T or B cells. Also, some cells in the $CD11c^+$ enriched population fall in the auto-fluorescent region (AF region, colored orange in Fig. 3a) and may not be DCs.

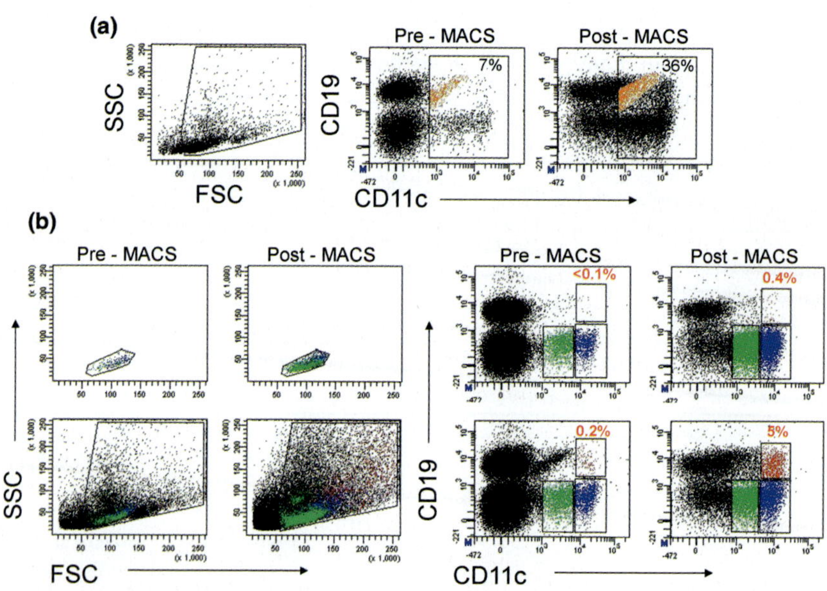

Fig. 3 Analysis of MACS Enriched $CD11c^+$ $CD19^+$ DC Populations. **(a)** Five-fold enrichment of $CD11c^+$ DCs resulting from typical MACS procedure. AF cells shown in *orange*. **(b)** Effects of strategic light scatter gating techniques to eliminate AF cells. Upper panels indicate elimination of $CD19^+$ IDO-competent DCs (shown in *red*). Application of wider light scatter gates reveals the location of $CD19^+$ pDCs. Conventional pDCs shown in *green* and myeloid mDCs shown in *blue*

Some investigators have reported significantly higher DC enrichment rates (up to 99% DCs) using more sophisticated procedures such as depleting T or B cells using CD5 or CD19 (Honda et al. 2005) or multiple rounds of MACS selection using mPDCA1 or CD8α following CD11c enrichment (Fallarino et al. 2004, 2005). In our experience, 'purified' populations of IDO-competent CD19$^+$ pDCs cannot be obtained via MACS techniques because they are extremely rare (even amongst DCs), and low recovery rates after each round of enrichment means that it is not feasible to use such methods to isolate IDO-competent CD19$^+$ pDCs. Moreover, sophisticated pre-enrichment techniques designed to deplete contaminating T or B cells using CD8α or CD19 also remove CD19$^+$ pDCs. These technical considerations aside, and for the reasons discussed in Sect. 4.1, MACS is still a useful technique for enriching CD19$^+$ pDCs from total splenocytes for further use in in vitro assays and IHC staining analyses (Mellor et al. 2004, 2005; Baban et al. 2005).

Fluorescence Activated Cell Sorting (FACS) is the second method by which DCs and DC subsets can be fractionated from total splenocytes. In this technique mAbs conjugated to fluorescent molecules allow specific DC subsets to be identified and sorted based on combinations of surface marker expression. However, careful optimization of enrichment protocols and sorting strategies is necessary as CD19$^+$ pDCs can be easily overlooked or inadvertently discarded during sorting procedures.

A common problem encountered during FACS is the presence of auto-fluorescent cells (AF) which complicate DC sorting because DCs display high forward and side (light) scatter (FSC, SSC) properties similar to naturally occurring AF cells. To address this problem, many investigators set precise initial sorting gates (based on FSC and SSC properties) to avoid collecting 'false positive' AF cells. While such gating techniques succeed in 'cleaning up' sorted cell populations, this approach can generate misleading outcomes because critical DC subsets may also be gated out with AF cells.

An example of this problem is shown in Fig. 3b using the pre- and post-MACS enrichment fractions shown in Fig. 3a to visualize the location of distinct DC subsets. Datasets in the upper panels of Fig. 3b show analyses of the light scatter (FSC, SSC) and phenotypic analyses (CD11c vs CD19) of total (pre-MACS) and DC-enriched (post-MACS) splenocytes, using precise a FSC and SSC analytic gating strategy designed to avoid AF cells. This strategy excludes almost all AF cells from DC populations, which contain large cohorts of CD19^{NEG} mDCs and conventional pDCs (CD11c^{HIGH} & CD11c^{LOW}, highlighted in blue & green, respectively), though contaminating lymphoid cells were also present.

However, the much rarer CD19$^+$CD11c^{HIGH} pDCs (highlighted in red) of major interest from the perspective of IDO-competent DCs were almost completely excluded by this restricted gating strategy. Thus, use of restricted sort gates will completely exclude IDO-competent pDCs from DC populations sorted by flow cytometry. In contrast, use of a much wider light scatter gate to analyze DC subsets revealed that CD19$^+$ pDCs were enriched ~25-fold following MACS. The key point is that CD19$^+$CD11c^{HIGH} pDCs were not excluded in this analysis because CD19$^+$ pDCs have relatively high light scatter properties compared to other DCs. Indeed, the pDC and mDC populations, as well as CD19$^+$ pDCs lie outside the region containing AF cells. Moreover, the common practice of using restrictive gating procedures to assess DC enrichment can lead to artificially inflated enrichment factors since restricted gating ignores the actual presence of contaminating cells in sorted populations.

In our studies on IDO-competent pDCs, we have consistently used FACS techniques to fractionate DC subsets prior to performing functional experiments to detect IDO-mediated T cell suppression by sorted DC subsets. In our hands, this approach circumvented some of the pitfalls associated with MACS separation techniques, and resulted in better enrichment of specific DC subsets.

4.1.2 Functional Analyses of IDO-Competent PDCs

A key attribute of CD19$^+$ pDCs is the potency of their T cell suppressor functions when induced to express IDO. We developed novel methods to measure the T cell suppressor functions of small numbers of sorted DCs. Briefly, sorted DCs were co-cultured in Mixed Lymphocyte Reactions (MLRs) with T cells of defined antigen-specificity from T cell receptor (TCR) transgenic mice and T cell proliferation was assessed using standard procedures. Parallel cultures containing IDO inhibitor (1MT) or excess tryptophan were included to determine if these manipulations rescued T cell responses suppressed by IDO$^+$ DCs due to IDO inhibition or preventing tryptophan depletion, respectively. Using this approach, we showed that FACS sorted splenic (CD11c^{HIGH}) DCs co-expressing B220, CD8α or CD19 contained IDO$^+$ pDCs after mice were pre-treated with B7 (CTLA4-Ig) and TLR9 (CpG) ligands to induce IDO (Mellor et al. 2004, 2005; Baban et al. 2005).

In contrast, CD11c^{HIGH} DCs that did not express these phenotypic markers (sorted from the same mice treated with IDO inducers) stimulated robust T cell proliferation that was not further enhanced by adding IDO inhibitor or excess tryptophan. For example, FACS sorted CD19^{NEG} splenocytes from mice treated with IDO inducers stimulated robust T cell proliferation, indicating that the T cell suppressive functions of CD19$^+$ pDCs predominated over the stimulatory functions of all other DCs (and other APCs) in unfractionated splenocyte populations, even though CD19$^+$ pDCs represent only a minor DC subset relative to CD19^{NEG} pDCs, which comprise 90–95% of all splenic DCs. Similar results were obtained with sorted DC subsets from TDLNs of melanoma bearing mice, showing that tumor growth induced IDO-competent pDCs to express functional IDO in TDLNs (Munn et al. 2004a).

The key point is that the presence of DCs with T cell stimulatory functions was not apparent unless rare CD19$^+$ pDCs were removed, even when IDO$^+$ pDCs were minor fractions amongst total DCs. This finding implies that the presence of residual or 'contaminating' CD19$^+$ pDCs may result in selected DC populations possessing IDO-dependent T cell suppressive functions, even though the majority of DCs in such populations do not express IDO. Hence, caution should be exercised when assigning IDO-dependent suppressive functions to all DCs present in unfractionated (or even fractionated) DC populations. Moreover, a few CD19$^+$ pDCs expressing IDO may establish and maintain suppressive tissue microenvironments, even though they are far outnumbered by other DCs. Hence, the presence of CD19$^+$ pDCs, and whether or not they are induced to express IDO, has profound implications for the outcome of T cell responses to antigenic stimuli following inflammation. In our experience, IDO-dependent T cell suppressive functions are more difficult to detect in DCs cultured from bone marrow or blood precursors, though some studies have reported such observations, especially amongst cultured human DCs (see Sect. 4.2).

Another method has been employed extensively by Grohmann and colleagues to assess IDO-dependent T cell suppressive functions of DCs, and involves adoptive transfer of DCs (pulsed with a peptide antigen) into mice and evaluating subsequent Delayed Type Hypersensitivity (DTH) responses by the classical immunological method of measuring foot-pad swelling (Grohmann et al. 2001a, b, 2003; Fallarino et al. 2007). This method has the advantage of measuring the actual immunizing and tolerizing properties of specific DC populations and fractionated DC subsets using a well-accepted in vivo model system. However, this experimental approach has the disadvantage of being an indirect measure of IDO-mediated T cell suppression, and this method may be prone to a number of extenuating circumstances that affect eventual outcomes. For example, it is unclear how to interpret observations based on treating small cohorts of donor DCs with IDO inhibitor before adoptive transfer, which then leads to enhanced DTH responses because the recipient mice contain a large excess of DCs and other cells, such as regulatory T cells, that are capable of influencing T cell responses. Though such outcomes may occur due to loss of direct T cell suppressive potential by treated DCs in recipient mice, it is also possible that IDO inhibitor modifies the viability or differentiation status of DCs, leading to completely different DTH outcomes not necessarily linked to loss of IDO activity.

Differences in the way that IDO-dependent T cell suppression is evaluated and in the way that DCs are prepared and fractionated make it difficult to compare results from one laboratory to another. This issue notwithstanding, there is now general agreement that murine IDO-competent DCs have plasmacytoid morphology, reside in the pDC subset, and produce IFNα when exposed to several ligands with IDO inducing properties (Table 2 and Fig. 2a). However, reported requirements for either IFN type I versus type II signaling to induce IDO expression in splenic DCs may (a) reflect key, biologically significant differences or (b) merely arise from differences in technical approaches (Fallarino et al. 2002b; Baban et al. 2005). Regarding the distinctive phenotype of IDO-competent pDCs, the discovery that CD19$^+$ pDCs from spleen and TDLNs were the only DC subset capable of mediating IDO-dependent T cell suppression represents corroborating evidence from two independent physiologic situations that IDO-competent DCs reside exclusively amongst the CD19$^+$ pDC subset in mice.

4.2 Human IDO-Competent DCs

Unlike their counterparts in mice, human IDO-competent DCs cannot be isolated directly from tissues. Instead, IDO$^+$ human DCs have been characterized by immunohistochemical analyses of tissue biopsy samples and by analyzing the functional

(T cell suppressive) status of DCs cultured from peripheral blood mononuclear cells (PBMCs). Variations between individual blood donors and DC preparation protocols complicate comparative data analyses between different laboratories. Consequently, there is little consensus, and lingering controversy about the identity and significance of human IDO-competent pDCs. These points notwithstanding, IDO^+ cells with plasmacytoid morphology (in some cases expressing DC markers) have been found in biopsies from a range of clinical tumors, in sentinel LNs draining sites of tumor growth and in granulomas caused by *Listeria* infection (Lee et al. 2003; Munn et al. 2004a; Munn and Mellor 2006; Popov et al. 2006), prompting speculation that IDO^+ cells may be DCs with T cell suppressor functions that inhibit anti-tumor immunity in cancer patients and help mediate an immunological 'standoff' between host and pathogen during chronic *Listeria* infections.

In early studies, functional analyses revealed that the majority of human DC cultures contained at least some DCs that suppressed T cell proliferation *ex vivo* via IDO, since adding IDO inhibitor significantly enhanced T cell responses (Hwu et al. 2000; Munn et al. 2002). Functional IDO activity was associated exclusively with DCs expressing the human pDC marker CD123 and the chemokine receptor CCR6 (Table 3B). Another group reported findings that were inconsistent with these initial reports (Terness et al. 2005). However, a recent report identified a human DC subset expressing IDO after culturing pBMCs with inactivated HIV-1, IFN type I or IFN type II (Boasso and Shearer 2007); DCs induced to express IDO by these agents expressed surface CD4, CD123, and BDCA2. In summary, the consensus is that human IDO-competent DCs can be detected amongst cultured PBMCs, provided that investigators adhere strictly to using specific protocols to prepare DCs and induce them to express IDO (Munn et al. 2005a). If correct, these findings suggest that there are particular requirements for differentiation and survival of human IDO-competent DCs in culture, which may have critical implications for clinical use

Table 3B Phenotypic analyses of human DC subsets

DC Subset[b]	CD11c	CD123	CCR6	CD4	BDCA2	References
Myeloid (mDCs)	+	–	?	+	–	Dzionek et al. (2000), Nair et al. (2004)
Plasmacytoid (pDCs)	–	+	?	+	+	Dzionek et al. (2000), Patterson et al. 2001), Hochrein et al. (2002), Janke et al. (2006), Cravens et al. (2007), Grage-Griebenow et al. (2007)
IDO-competent ($CD19^+$) pDCs	–	+	+	+	+	Munn et al. (2002), Boasso et al. (2005, 2007)

[b]Based on analyses of human DCs derived from pBMCs; leukocyte lineage (lin) negative (null for CD3, CD14, CD19, CD56) and HLA-DR, CD4 or CD33 positive

of cultured human DCs as vaccine adjuvants to stimulate anti-tumor immunity or, conversely, to suppress allo-responses to transplanted cells and tissues by recipient T cells.

4.3 IDO Induction in IDO-Competent PDCs

As key roles for IDO^+ DCs in disease progression have emerged from studies on murine models of human disease syndromes, it became important to identify physiologic mechanisms and artificial reagents that induce IDO-competent pDCs to express functional IDO. Reagents that induce DCs to express functional IDO were listed in Table 2 and, as discussed above, IFNs are positive regulators of IDO gene transcription via the JAK/STAT signaling mechanisms depicted in Fig. 2b (Platanias 2005). However post-translational factors also influence the ability of DCs to express functional IDO. For example, IFNγ induced splenic $CD8\alpha^+$ and $CD8\alpha^{NEG}$ DCs to express IDO protein, but only $CD8\alpha^+$ DCs acquired T cell suppressive functions (Grohmann et al. 2001a; Fallarino et al. 2002b). Most synthetic IDO inducing reagents listed in Table 2 bind to specific molecules expressed by DCs, including soluble CTLA4 (CTLA4-Ig), CD200-Ig and CpG-oligonucleotides, which ligate B7 (CD80/86) CD200-receptor and TLR9 respectively (Grohmann et al. 2002; Mellor et al. 2003, 2005; Fallarino et al. 2004). These reagents stimulated DCs to produce IFN, which then induced IDO expression, presumably via autocrine or paracrine signaling.

The biological significance of these molecular interactions which cause IDO-competent pDCs to express IDO are not clear and is the subject of ongoing research. However, B7 ligation leading to IDO induction may be linked to cooperative interactions between IDO-competent pDCs (which express B7 molecules) and Tregs, many of which express surface CTLA4. Indeed, Treg suppressor functions may depend on CTLA4 → B7 signaling from Tregs → pDCs (Fallarino et al. 2004; Mellor et al. 2004). The biological significance of IDO induction following ligation of TLRs is less obvious, though this response may be linked to counter-regulation of T cell responses during bacterial sepsis (Wingender et al. 2006).

Using mice with defective IFN signaling due to ablation of IFN type I (IFNAR) and type II (IFNγRα) receptors we found that IFN type I signaling was obligatory upstream of IDO following B7 ligation and TLR9 ligation (using CTLA4-Ig and CpGs, respectively), because IFNAR (but not IFNγRα) ablation abolished IDO induction in $CD19^+$ pDCs (Baban et al. 2005; Mellor et al. 2005). On further investigation, we confirmed that IFNα (but not IFNγ) induced selective STAT1 activation and functional IDO expression in splenic $CD19^+$ pDCs Requirements for IFN type I signaling to induce IDO were not consistent with previous reports that IFNγ induced IDO in DCs, (Grohmann et al. 2001a; Fallarino et al. 2002b) though different methods were used to prepare DCs, assess the requirements for IFN signaling and evaluate DC suppressor functions.

More recently, we discovered an obligatory requirement for cell autonomous IDO (and GCN2) upstream of IFNα expression by $CD19^+$ DCs following B7 ligation (Manlapat et al. 2007). The ability of CTLA4-Ig reagents to induce functional IDO expression depends on the structure of the Fc (Ig) domain and on the mouse strain used, suggesting that additional factors contribute to signaling processes that induce IDO following B7 ligation. In our experimental systems, a cytolytic isoform of CTLA4-IgG2a induced IDO expression in most mouse strains tested (except B6 mice), whereas a closely related non-cytolytic isoform (with mutated Fc binding and C1q binding domains) did not induce IDO (Mellor et al. 2004), suggesting that functionalities in the Fc domain were required to induce IDO. Moreover, a CTLA4-Ig3 isoform induced IDO in spleen of B6 mice, but failed to induce IDO in other mouse strains such as CBA mice (unpublished data).

The molecular basis for these disparities is currently unknown, but they may have important implications for the use of soluble CTLA4 in clinical settings, especially as human versions of CTLA4-Ig tested in mice and in the clinic did not induce IDO expression in mice, but may do so in (at least) some humans. We have also detected strain-specific disparities in IDO inducing properties of different sequence classes of CpGs, which ligate TLR9 (Table 4). Furthermore, CpGs exhibit sequence, strain, and dose specificity with respect to IFNα production (Blackwell and Krieg 2003; Vollmer et al. 2004a, b; Abel et al. 2005; Roberts et al. 2005; Booth et al. 2007; Martinson et al. 2007). While type B and C CpG sequences induced IFNα and IDO in most strains tested, type A CpGs only induced IFNα expression in DCs from BALB/c mice. Again, the molecular basis of these disparate responses to TLR ligands is unknown. The route of CpG administration was also critical since injecting CpGs into the tail vein induced IDO while intra-peritoneal injection of the same amount of CpGs did not induce IDO (Mellor et al. 2005; Wingender et al. 2006).

The mechanistic basis for the failure of IDO inducers to stimulate IDO expression in all DCs was investigated by Orabona and colleagues who reported that Suppressor of Cytokine Signaling 3 (SOCS3) and the molecular adapter DAP12 functioned as negative regulators of IDO transcription in most splenic DCs (Orabona et al. 2005a, b). CD28-Ig also induced IFNγ-dependent IDO expression through B7–1/B7–2 engagement but only in SOCS3-deficient pDCs (Fallarino et al. 2004, 2005). Treating pDCs with a soluble glucocorticoid-induced tumor necrosis factor receptor

Table 4 Strain-specific responses to three classes of TLR9 ligands (CpGs)

Mouse strain	Type A (2336)		Type B (1826)		Type C (2395)	
	IFNα[a]	IDO[b]	IFNα	IDO	IFNα	IDO
C57BL6/J	nt[c]	−	+	+	+	+
CBA	Nt	−	+	+	nt	+
BALB/c	+	−	+	+	−	+
129	Nt	−	+	−	+	+

[a] IFNα production assessed *ex vivo* (ELISA) following 5 h culture of CD11c$^+$ AMACS enriched DCs with indicated ligand

[b] IDO expression assessed (IHC) 24 h treatment in vivo (50–100 μg/mouse, i/v)

[c] Not tested

(GITR-Ig) induced IFNα-dependent IDO expression due to ligation of GITR ligand on pDCs via a non-canonical NF-κB mechanism, identifying a novel IDO induction pathway in DCs (Grohmann et al. 2007).

Human pDCs also expressed IDO following treatment with B7 ligands. Monocyte-derived DCs showed functional IDO expression following ligation of B7–1/B7–2 molecules on DCs by CTLA4/CD28 expressed by activated $CD4^+$ T cells (Munn et al. 2004b). In another study PBMCs expressing CD4 produced B7-dependent, functional IDO in response to CTLA4-Ig, but not CD28-Ig treatment (Boasso et al. 2005). Human ($CD4^+$, $CD123^+$, BDCA-2^+, BDCA-4^+) pDCs exposed to infectious or inactivated HIV expressed IDO, which was independent of IFN type I or type II signaling, but required the viral gp120 and cellular CD4 interaction (Boasso et al. 2007).

In summary, complex signaling mechanisms induce IDO-competent pDCs to express IDO, and prevent IDO up-regulation in other cells, including other DC subsets. The fact that IDO induction is tightly regulated and occurs only in minor DC subsets implies that there may be a critical need to regulate IDO induction and tailor this response to particular inflammatory conditions that prevail (or are induced) in some tissue microenvironments.

5 IDO-Mediated T Cell Suppression

In this section, we discuss how pDCs acquire potent and dominant T cell suppressor functions when induced to express IDO. IDO activity in DCs may influence how T cells respond to antigen stimuli in several ways. IDO may bring about cell autonomous changes in DCs themselves that (a) reduce their ability to stimulate clonal expansion of effector T cells and (b) enhance their ability to suppress T cell responses. Though emerging evidence supports this hypothesis (Hill et al. 2007a; Manlapat et al. 2007) it is not known how IDO activity modifies DC functions. Alternatively, T cells and Tregs may respond to activation signals from antigens expressed by IDO^+ DCs differently when T cells and Tregs experience the biochemical changes caused by IDO activity in DCs (Fig. 4). In the remainder of this section we discuss how IDO enzyme activity in DCs affects T cells and Tregs.

5.1 T Cell Suppression by IDO+ PDCs

Two basic hypotheses have been proposed to explain how IDO activity in DCs suppresses T cell responses when T cells are activated. First, T cells may sense and respond to reduced levels of free tryptophan and second, T cells may be sensitive to tryptophan metabolites produced by IDO^+ pDCs (Mellor and Munn 2004; Fallarino et al. 2007). There is evidence in support of each hypothesis, and these mechanisms are not mutually exclusive, though most studies were performed *ex vivo* and therefore it is not yet clear if findings are applicable to physiologic situations.

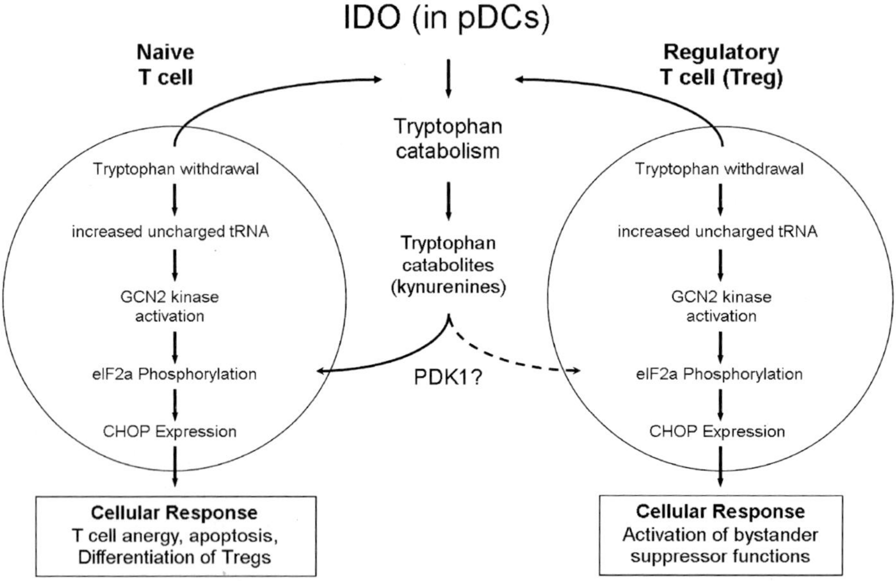

Fig. 4 IDO-mediated effects on T cells and Tregs. Tryptophan catabolism and the resulting metabolites produce different cellular responses in effector and regulatory T cells. See text for details

APCs (macrophages and DCs) expressing IDO cause activated T cells to undergo cell cycle arrest and apoptosis, and induced anergy if T cells survived (Munn et al. 1996, 1999, 2002, 2005b; Hwu et al. 2000; Grohmann et al. 2001a). Initial studies revealed that robust T cell proliferative responses to IDO^{+} APCs were restored by adding IDO inhibitor or excess tryptophan (Munn et al. 1999), suggesting that failure of T cells to undergo normal responses was due to active suppression by APCs, and was not a consequence of 'weak' T cell stimulation, which has been associated with immature APCs (Hackstein and Thomson 2004).

The finding that excess tryptophan rescued T cell proliferation provided a hint that tryptophan depletion was a key biochemical change that affected the way T cells responded to antigenic stimulation because adding excess tryptophan would increase consumption of ROS and production of downstream tryptophan metabolites. Consistent with this interpretation, human and murine T cells are highly sensitive to reduced access to free tryptophan during activation in the absence of APCs (Lee et al. 2002). T cells activated in chemically defined tryptophan-free medium underwent cell cycle arrest prior to S-phase (DNA synthesis). In contrast, T cells activated in medium without isoleucine and leucine began to incorporate thymidine, but stopped shortly after S-phase started, consistent with cessation of protein translation due to amino acid starvation. Thus, rather than tryptophan 'starvation', T cells appear to sense reduced access to tryptophan and trigger a response that shuts down cell cycle progression.

What mechanisms could account for such a response? The mammalian target of rapamycin (mTOR) and general control non-derepressible-2 (GCN2) kinase are two ribosome based mechanisms that sense and trigger cellular responses when cell access to amino acids is limited. Munn and colleagues performed comprehensive gene expression profile analyses that revealed a number of cell cycle control genes whose transcription rates were up-regulated significantly in activated T cells following abortive cell cycle arrest due to tryptophan deprivation (relative to control T cells) (Munn et al. 2005b). One such gene encodes CCAAT/enhancer-binding protein homologous protein (CHOP, aka GADD153), which is under strict transcriptional control by GCN2-kinase and has pro-apoptotic effects on cells (Harding et al. 2003; Wek et al. 2006; Puthalakath et al. 2007). To test the hypothesis that IDO-activity in DCs triggered GCN2-kinase activation in T cells, the effects of IDO$^+$ pDCs on T cells from GCN2-deficient (GCN2-KO) mice were evaluated. T cells from GCN2-KO mice responded normally to IDO$^+$ pDCs showing that intact GCN2 was essential for T cell susceptibility to the cell cycle inhibitory effects of IDO activity in DCs, and confirming that IDO-mediated effects on T cells were GCN2-dependent (Munn et al. 2005b). GCN2-kinase senses reduced access to amino acids when uncharged tRNA molecules bind to ribosomes (Fig. 4), which triggers GCN2-kinase activation and leads to a cascade of downstream responses known as the cellular integrated stress response (ISR) to amino acid withdrawal, which lead to cell cycle arrest and cessation of most (but not all) protein translation in cells (Dong et al. 2000; Harding et al. 2003). Interestingly, L-arginine depletion also induced GCN2-dependent T cell cycle arrest, suggesting that myeloid-derived suppressor cells (MDSCs), which express L-arginase, may also exploit the GCN2 mechanism to suppress T cell immunity in tumor microenvironments where MDSCs congregate (Rodriguez et al. 2007).

Though excess tryptophan completely abrogates the T cell suppressor functions of IDO$^+$ pDCs, certain downstream tryptophan metabolites enhance T cell apoptosis, and modify how T cells differentiate into effector T cells (Fallarino et al. 2002a; Frumento et al. 2002; Terness et al. 2002), suggesting that production of toxic metabolites may also contribute to IDO-mediated suppression. A recent study revealed that the downstream metabolite 3-Hydroxyanthranilic acid (HAA), which induces T cell apoptosis, inhibits NF-κB activation by binding to PDK1, an essential mediator of CD28-induced NF-κB activation in T cells activated by TCR engagement (Hayashi et al. 2007). Though it is not clear if IDO$^+$ pDCs produce sufficient HAA to affect T cell responses under physiologic conditions, administering HAA to mice alleviated experimentally induced asthma, providing support for the notion of using natural or synthetic tryptophan metabolites to treat chronic inflammatory disease syndromes with T cell involvement such as experimental autoimmune encephalitis (EAE), a murine model of multiple sclerosis (Platten et al. 2005). However, it is not known if natural tryptophan metabolites produced by IDO$^+$ cells also have palliative effects on chronic inflammatory diseases in physiologic settings.

5.2 IDO-Mediated Treg Differentiation and Activation

Though purified (sorted) IDO^+ pDCs suppress T cells that activate in response to antigens they present, the fact that IDO^+ pDCs constitute only a small fraction ($\sim$10% in mouse spleen and TDLNs) suggests that their suppressive functions ought to be subordinate to the stimulatory functions of other DCs in physiological microenvironments. Moreover, it is highly unlikely that T cells would preferentially recognize and respond to their cognate antigens displayed by the small subset of IDO-competent DCs, rather than the majority of other DCs present in inflamed tissue microenvironments. Hence, the ability of rare IDO^+ pDCs to mediate dominant suppression requires an explanation that does not rely exclusively on direct T cell suppression by IDO^+ pDCs themselves. Indeed, dominant suppression is not simply an artifact of in vitro culture systems because resident IDO^+ pDCs completely blocked T cell mediated destruction of splenic tissues following adoptive transfer of allo-specific T cells into mice treated with CTLA4-Ig to induce IDO (Mellor et al. 2003).

These considerations suggest that IDO^+ pDCs activate other T cell suppressive mechanisms. One candidate mechanism is $CD4^+$ $CD25^+$ Tregs, which are potent T cell suppressors in a range of clinically relevant syndromes, even though they also constitute only a minor subset ($\sim$5–10%) of $CD4^+$ T cells, a fact that contributed to Tregs being overlooked as sources of T cell suppression for some time (Sakaguchi 2005; Shevach et al. 2006). Key points about Tregs relevant to their potential interactions with IDO^+ pDCs are (a) the majority of Tregs are unique amongst T cells in expressing CTLA4 stably at the cell surface; (b) the proportions of effector T cells and Tregs that emerge from antigen-driven encounters with DCs depends on the functional (maturation) status of DCs (Mahnke et al. 2007); and (c) peripheral Tregs normally do not exhibit constitutive suppressor activity and 'resting' Tregs must be activated to acquire suppressor functions (Thornton et al. 2004).

As discussed previously, surface CTLA4 expression by Tregs provides a natural physiologic counterpart to the ability of synthetic soluble CTLA4 (CTLA4-Ig) to induce IDO expression in DCs by ligating B7 molecules (Grohmann et al. 2002; Mellor et al. 2003). Experimental evidence supporting this notion reveals that CTLA4 $\rightarrow$ B7 interactions between Tregs and IDO-competent (but IDO^{NEG}) DCs induce IDO expression in DCs (Fallarino et al. 2003; Mellor et al. 2004). Indeed, the T cell suppressive functions of cloned $CTLA4^+$ Tregs were completely dependent on DCs having an intact IDO1 gene and were blocked by adding anti-CTLA4 mAb (Mellor et al. 2004). If verified, the requirement for CTLA4 $\rightarrow$ B7 interactions to stimulate DCs to express IDO may have critical implications for understanding how anti-CTLA4 mAbs enhance T cell immunity to tumors in ongoing clinical trials in cancer patients (Peggs et al. 2006).

Immature DCs and certain DC subsets from some tissues (such as the GI tract) are more effective than the majority of DCs in promoting Treg differentiation. Little is currently known about mechanisms that influence how DCs promote Treg rather than effector T cell development. However, IDO activity in DCs may be one mechanism that favors Treg over effector T cell development, and experimental evidence supporting this hypothesis has emerged from several studies. For example, Fallarino et al. reported that IDO^+ DCs enhanced in vitro Treg differentiation from naïve CD4 precursors via the combined effects of GCN2-depdendent tryptophan depletion and tryptophan metabolites (Fallarino et al. 2006). Moreover, some promising new therapies to treat chronic inflammatory diseases in which enhanced Treg functions are likely to be beneficial may work, at least in part, by inducing DCs to express IDO. Thus, soluble CD40-Ig and CTLA4-Ig may facilitate allograft survival by inducing DCs to express IDO and promoting Treg differentiation, as well as blocking co-stimulation (Grohmann et al. 2002; Mellor et al. 2003; Guillonneau et al. 2007; Hill et al. 2007b). However, these synthetic reagents with immunosuppressive properties may also induce other cell types to express IDO that help suppress allograft rejection.

Even if the ability to promote increased Treg differentiation to control T cell responses is an important attribute of IDO^+ pDCs, this may not be sufficient to create suppressive microenvironments because mature Tregs are functionally quiescent and require additional activation signals (via the TCR) to stimulate suppressor functions (Thornton et al. 2004). Nevertheless, Tregs are constitutively activated and possessed potent suppressor functions when isolated from TDLNs of mice bearing melanomas, suggesting that tumor growth created physiologic conditions in which Tregs received activation signals. Consistent with this notion, IDO^+ pDCs from TDLNs activated quiescent splenic Tregs to acquire potent suppressor functions *ex vivo*, and this response was mediated via GCN2 since adding excess tryptophan and ablating GCN2 in Tregs blocked IDO-induced Treg activation (Sharma et al. 2007).

In this experimental system, the suppressor functions of IDO-activated Tregs were dependent on the PD-1 pathway because antibodies that blocked interactions between PD-1 and its ligands (PD-L1 and PD-L2) abrogated suppression completely. In contrast, splenic Tregs activated by standard mitogenic anti-CD3 treatment were less potent suppressors, and blockade of the PD-1 pathway had no effect on suppressor functions. Hence, dependence on PD-1 was a unique feature of IDO-activated Tregs. It remains to be seen if IDO^+ pDCs are also responsible (at least in part) for activating Tregs in other chronic inflammatory syndromes in which Tregs possess constitutive suppressor activity such as local sites of *Leishmania* infections (Peters and Sacks 2006), the GI-tract (Mrass and Weninger 2006) and the maternal-fetal interface during pregnancy (Hunt 2006), to name only a few syndromes in which pDCs expressing IDO may actively suppress T cell responses.

6 Summary and Conclusions

In this chapter, we describe subsets of pDCs specialized to express IDO, which acquire potent T cell suppressor functions when induced to express IDO. The discovery of IDO^+ pDCs is generating considerable interest in manipulating IDO expression to improve clinical outcomes in a wide range of chronic inflammatory syndromes, including cancer, chronic infections, autoimmune disease and transplantation. Clinical use of IDO inhibitors to enhance anti-tumor immunity is the subject of ongoing experimental trials, based on encouraging evidence that such treatments work in murine tumor models. If successful in humans, the use of IDO inhibitors to block IDO-mediated T cell suppression may be applicable to chronic infectious diseases in which T cell hypo-responsiveness is a major contributory factor to disease progression and persistence. Experimental evidence is also emerging in support of the hypothesis that increased IDO activity will suppress host T cell immunity allo-grafts following transplantation of healthy donor tissues. Hence, the ability of some DCs to express IDO offers considerable opportunities to improve immunotherapies in a wide range of disease syndromes that affect many people.

References

Abel K, Wang Y et al (2005) Deoxycytidyl-deoxyguanosine oligonucleotide classes A, B, and C induce distinct cytokine gene expression patterns in rhesus monkey peripheral blood mononuclear cells and distinct alpha interferon responses in TLR9-expressing rhesus monkey plasmacytoid dendritic cells. Clin Diagn Lab Immunol 12:606–621

Agaugue S, Perrin-Cocon L et al (2006) 1-Methyl-tryptophan can interfere with TLR signaling in dendritic cells independently of IDO activity. J Immunol 177:2061–2071

Asselin-Paturel C, Boonstra A et al (2001) Mouse type I IFN-producing cells are immature APCs with plasmacytoid morphology. Nat Immunol 2:1144–1150

Asselin-Paturel C, Brizard G et al (2003) Mouse strain differences in plasmacytoid dendritic cell frequency and function revealed by a novel monoclonal antibody. J Immunol 171:6466–6477

Baban B, Hansen AM et al (2005) A minor population of splenic dendritic cells expressing CD19 mediates IDO-dependent T cell suppression via type I IFN signaling following B7 ligation. Int Immunol 17:909–919

Ball HJ, Sanchez-Perez A et al (2007) Characterization of an indoleamine 2,3-dioxygenase-like protein found in humans and mice. Gene 396:203–213

Banerjee T, Duhadaway JB et al (2007) A key in vivo antitumor mechanism of action of natural product-based brassinins is inhibition of indoleamine 2,3-dioxygenase. Oncogene 27: 2851–2857

Basu GD, Tinder TL et al (2006) Cyclooxygenase-2 inhibitor enhances the efficacy of a breast cancer vaccine: role of IDO. J Immunol 177:2391–2402

Blackwell SE, Krieg AM (2003) CpG-A-induced monocyte IFN-gamma-inducible protein-10 production is regulated by plasmacytoid dendritic cell-derived IFN-alpha. J Immunol 170: 4061–4068

Boasso A, Herbeuval JP et al (2005) Regulation of indoleamine 2,3-dioxygenase and tryptophanyl-tRNA-synthetase by CTLA-4-Fc in human CD4+ T cells. Blood 105:1574–1581

Boasso A, Herbeuval JP et al (2007) HIV inhibits CD4+ T-cell proliferation by inducing indoleamine 2,3-dioxygenase in plasmacytoid dendritic cells. Blood 109:3351–3359

Boasso A, Shearer GM (2007) How does indoleamine 2,3-dioxygenase contribute to HIV-mediated immune dysregulation. Curr Drug Metab 8:217–223

Booth JS, Nichani AK et al (2007) Innate immune responses induced by classes of CpG oligodeoxynucleotides in ovine lymph node and blood mononuclear cells. Vet Immunol Immunopathol 115:24–34

Brastianos HC, Vottero E et al (2006) Exiguamine A, an indoleamine-2,3-dioxygenase (IDO) inhibitor isolated from the marine sponge Neopetrosia exigua. J Am Chem Soc 128:16046–16047

Braun D, Longman RS et al (2005) A two-step induction of indoleamine 2,3 dioxygenase (IDO) activity during dendritic-cell maturation. Blood 106:2375–2381

Burke F, Knowles RG et al (1995) The role of indoleamine 2,3-dioxygenase in the anti-tumour activity of human interferon-gamma in vivo. Int J Cancer 60:115–122
Cady SG, Sono M (1991) 1-Methyl-DL-tryptophan, beta-(3-benzofuranyl)-DL-alanine (the oxygen analog of tryptophan), and beta-[3-benzo(b)thienyl]-DL-alanine (the sulfur analog of tryptophan) are competitive inhibitors for indoleamine 2,3-dioxygenase. Arch Biochem Biophys 291:326–333
Chelbi-Alix MK, Wietzerbin J (2007) Interferon, a growing cytokine family: 50 years of interferon research. Biochimie 89:713–718
Cravens PD, Hayashida K et al (2007) Human peripheral blood dendritic cells and monocyte subsets display similar chemokine receptor expression profiles with differential migratory responses. Scand J Immunol 65:514–524
Dai W, Gupta SL (1990) Regulation of indoleamine 2,3-dioxygenase gene expression in human fibroblasts by interferon-gamma. Upstream control region discriminates between interferon-gamma and interferon-alpha. J Biol Chem 265:19871–19877
Decker T, Muller M et al (2005) The Yin and Yang of type I interferon activity in bacterial infection. Nat Rev Immunol 5:675–687
Dong J, Qiu H et al (2000) Uncharged tRNA activates GCN2 by displacing the protein kinase moiety from a bipartite tRNA-binding domain. Mol Cell 6:269–279
Duluc D, Delneste Y et al (2007) Tumor-associated leukemia inhibitory factor and IL-6 skew monocyte differentiation into tumor-associated macrophage-like cells. Blood 110:4319–4330
Dzionek A, Fuchs A et al (2000) BDCA-2, BDCA-3, and BDCA-4: Three Markers for Distinct Subsets of Dendritic Cells in Human Peripheral Blood. J Immunol 165:6037–6046
Fallarino F, Asselin-Paturel C et al (2004) Murine plasmacytoid dendritic cells initiate the immunosuppressive pathway of tryptophan catabolism in response to CD200 receptor engagement. J Immunol 173:3748–3754
Fallarino F, Gizzi S et al (2007) Tryptophan catabolism in IDO+ plasmacytoid dendritic cells. Curr Drug Metab 8:209–216
Fallarino F, Grohmann U et al (2003) Modulation of tryptophan catabolism by regulatory T cells. Nat Immunol 4:1206–1212
Fallarino F, Grohmann U et al (2002a) T cell apoptosis by tryptophan catabolism. Cell Death Differ 9:1069–1077
Fallarino F, Vacca C et al (2002b) Functional expression of indoleamine 2,3-dioxygenase by murine CD8 alpha(+) dendritic cells. Int Immunol 14:65–68
Fallarino F, Grohmann U et al (2006) the combined effects of tryptophan starvation and tryptophan catabolites down-regulate T cell receptor {zeta}-chain and induce a regulatory phenotype in naive T cells. J Immunol 176:6752–6761
Fallarino F, Orabona C et al (2005) Ligand and cytokine dependence of the immunosuppressive pathway of tryptophan catabolism in plasmacytoid dendritic cells. Int Immunol 17:1429–1438
Finger EB, Bluestone JA (2002) When ligand becomes receptor[—]tolerance via B7 signaling on DCs. Nat Immunol 3:1056–1057
Friberg M, Jennings R et al (2002) Indoleamine 2,3-dioxygenase contributes to tumor cell evasion of T cell-mediated rejection. Int J Cancer 101:151–155
Frumento G, Rotondo R et al (2002) Tryptophan-derived catabolites are responsible for inhibition of T and natural killer cell proliferation induced by indoleamine 2,3-dioxygenase. J Exp Med 196:459–468
Fujigaki H, Saito K et al (2006) Nitration and inactivation of IDO by peroxynitrite. J Immunol 176:372–379
Furset G, Floisand Y et al (2007) Impaired expression of indoleamine 2, 3-dioxygenase in monocyte-derived dendritic cells in response to Toll-like receptor-7/8 ligands. Immunology 123:263–271
Gaspari P, Banerjee T et al (2006) Structure-activity study of brassinin derivatives as indoleamine 2,3-dioxygenase inhibitors. J Med Chem 49:684–692

Grage-Griebenow E, Loseke S et al (2007) Anti-BDCA-4 (neuropilin-1) antibody can suppress virus-induced IFN-alpha production of plasmacytoid dendritic cells. Immunol Cell Biol 85:383–390
Grohmann U, Bianchi R et al (2003) Functional plasticity of dendritic cell subsets as mediated by CD40 versus B7 activation. J Immunol 171:2581–2587
Grohmann U, Fallarino F et al (2001a) IL-6 inhibits the tolerogenic function of CD8 alpha + dendritic cells expressing indoleamine 2,3-dioxygenase. J Immunol 167:708–714
Grohmann U, Fallarino F et al (2001b) CD40 ligation ablates the tolerogenic potential of lymphoid dendritic cells. J Immunol 166:277–283
Grohmann U, Orabona C et al (2002) CTLA-4-Ig regulates tryptophan catabolism in vivo. Nat Immunol 3:1097–1101
Grohmann U, Volpi C et al (2007) Reverse signaling through GITR ligand enables dexamethasone to activate IDO in allergy. Nat Med 13:579–586
Guillonneau C, Hill M et al (2007) CD40Ig treatment results in allograft acceptance mediated by CD8CD45RC T cells, IFN-gamma, and indoleamine 2,3-dioxygenase. J Clin Invest 117:1096–1106
Hackstein H, Thomson AW (2004) Dendritic cells: emerging pharmacological targets of immunosuppressive drugs. Nat Rev Immunol 4:24–34
Harding HP, Zhang Y et al (2003) An integrated stress response regulates amino acid metabolism and resistance to oxidative stress. Mol Cell 11:619–633
Hayashi T, Beck L et al (2004) Inhibition of experimental asthma by indoleamine 2,3-dioxygenase. J Clin Invest 114:270–279
Hayashi T, Mo JH et al (2007) 3-Hydroxyanthranilic acid inhibits PDK1 activation and suppresses experimental asthma by inducing T cell apoptosis. Proc Natl Acad Sci USA 104:18619–18624
Hilkens CM, Schlaak JF et al (2003) Differential responses to IFN-alpha subtypes in human T cells and dendritic cells. J Immunol 171:5255–5263
Hill JA, Feuerer M et al (2007a) Foxp3 transcription-factor-dependent and -independent regulation of the regulatory T cell transcriptional signature. Immunity 27:786–800
Hill M, Tanguy-Royer S et al (2007b) IDO expands human CD4 + CD25high regulatory T cells by promoting maturation of LPS-treated dendritic cells. Eur J Immunol 37:3054–3062
Hochrein H, O'Keeffe M et al (2002) Human and mouse plasmacytoid dendritic cells. Hum Immunol 63:1103–1110
Honda K, Yanai H et al (2005) IRF-7 is the master regulator of type-I interferon-dependent immune responses. Nature 434:772–777
Hou DY, Muller AJ et al (2007) Inhibition of indoleamine 2,3-dioxygenase in dendritic cells by stereoisomers of 1-methyl-tryptophan correlates with antitumor responses. Cancer Res 67: 792–801
Hunt JS (2006) Stranger in a strange land. Immunol Rev 213:36–47
Hwu P, Du MX et al (2000) Indoleamine 2,3-dioxygenase production by human dendritic cells results in the inhibition of T cell proliferation. J Immunol 164:3596–3599
Janke M, Witsch EJ et al (2006) Eminent role of ICOS costimulation for T cells interacting with plasmacytoid dendritic cells. Immunology 118:353–360
Jasperson LK, Bucher C et al (2007) Indoleamine 2,3-dioxygenase is a critical regulator of acute GVHD lethality. Blood 111:3257–3265
Jeong YI, Jung ID et al (2007) (-)-Epigallocatechin gallate suppresses indoleamine 2,3-dioxygenase expression in murine dendritic cells: evidences for the COX-2 and STAT1 as potential targets. Biochem Biophys Res Commun 354:1004–1009
Johnson LM, Scott P (2007) STAT1 expression in dendritic cells, but not T cells, is required for immunity to Leishmania major. J Immunol 178:7259–7266
Jung ID, Lee CM et al (2007) Differential regulation of indoleamine 2,3-dioxygenase by lipopolysaccharide and interferon gamma in murine bone marrow derived dendritic cells. FEBS Lett 581:1449–1456
Keith IM, Brownfield MS (1985) Evidence for presence of kynurenine in lung and brain of neonate hamsters. Histochemistry 83:465–471

Kim SI, Jeong YI et al (2007) p-Coumaric acid inhibits indoleamine 2, 3-dioxygenase expression in murine dendritic cells. Int Immunopharmacol 7:805–815

Lee GK, Park HJ et al (2002) Tryptophan deprivation sensitizes activated T cells to apoptosis prior to cell division. Immunology 107:452–460

Lee HJ, Jeong YI et al (2007) Rosmarinic acid inhibits indoleamine 2,3-dioxygenase expression in murine dendritic cells. Biochem Pharmacol 73:1412–1421

Lee JR, Dalton RR et al (2003) Pattern of recruitment of immunoregulatory antigen-presenting cells in malignant melanoma. Lab Invest 83:1457–1466

Liao M, Pabarcus MK et al (2007) Impaired dexamethasone-mediated induction of tryptophan 2,3-dioxygenase in heme-deficient rat hepatocytes: Translational control by a hepatic eIF2{alpha} kinase, the heme-regulated inhibitor (HRI). J Pharmacol Exp Ther 33:979–989

Liu H, Xue ZT et al (2007) Low dose Zebularine treatment enhances immunogenicity of tumor cells. Cancer Lett 257:107–115

Lob S, Konigsrainer A et al (2007) Levo- but not dextro-1-methyl tryptophan abrogates the IDO activity of human dendritic cells. Blood 111:2152–2154

Mahnke K, Johnson TS et al (2007) Tolerogenic dendritic cells and regulatory T cells: a two-way relationship. J Dermatol Sci 46:159–167

Manlapat AK, Kahler DJ et al (2007) Cell-autonomous control of interferon type I expression by indoleamine 2,3-dioxygenase in regulatory CD19+ dendritic cells. Eur J Immunol 37: 1064–1071

Martinson JA, Tenorio AR et al (2007) Impact of class A, B and C CpG-oligodeoxynucleotides on in vitro activation of innate immune cells in human immunodeficiency virus-1 infected individuals. Immunology 120:526–535

Mellor AL, Munn DH (1999) Tryptophan catabolism and T-cell tolerance: immunosuppression by starvation? Immunol Today 20:469–473

Mellor AL, Munn DH (2004) IDO expression by dendritic cells: tolerance and tryptophan catabolism. Nat Rev Immunol 4:762–774

Mellor AL, Munn DH (2008) Creating immune privilege: active local suppression that benefits friends, but protects foes. Nat Rev Immunol 8:74–80

Mellor AL, Baban B et al (2003) Cutting edge: induced indoleamine 2,3 dioxygenase expression in dendritic cell subsets suppresses T cell clonal expansion. J Immunol 171:1652–1655

Mellor AL, Chandler P et al (2004) Specific subsets of murine dendritic cells acquire potent T cell regulatory functions following CTLA4-mediated induction of indoleamine 2,3 dioxygenase. Int Immunol 16:1391–1401

Mellor AL, Baban B et al (2005) Cutting edge: CpG oligonucleotides induce splenic CD19+ dendritic cells to acquire potent indoleamine 2,3-dioxygenase-dependent T cell regulatory functions via IFN Type 1 signaling. J Immunol 175:5601–5605

Metz R, Duhadaway JB et al (2007) Novel Tryptophan Catabolic Enzyme IDO2 Is the Preferred Biochemical Target of the Antitumor Indoleamine 2,3-Dioxygenase Inhibitory Compound D-1-Methyl-Tryptophan. Cancer Res 67:7082–7087

Morelli AE, Thomson AW (2007) Tolerogenic dendritic cells and the quest for transplant tolerance. Nat Rev Immunol advanced online publication 7:610–621

Mrass P, Weninger W (2006) Immune cell migration as a means to control immune privilege: lessons from the CNS and tumors. Immunol Rev 213:195–212

Munn DH, Mellor AL (2006) The tumor-draining lymph node as an immune-privileged site. Immunol Rev 213:146–158

Munn DH, Pressey J et al (1996) Selective activation-induced apoptosis of peripheral T cells imposed by macrophages. A potential mechanism of antigen-specific peripheral lymphocyte deletion. J Immunol 156:523–532

Munn DH, Zhou M et al (1998) Prevention of allogeneic fetal rejection by tryptophan catabolism. Science 281:1191–1193

Munn DH, Shafizadeh E et al (1999) Inhibition of T cell proliferation by macrophage tryptophan catabolism. J Exp Med 189:1363–1372

Munn DH, Sharma MD et al (2002) Potential regulatory function of human dendritic cells expressing indoleamine 2,3-dioxygenase. Science 297:1867–1870

Munn DH, Sharma MD et al (2004a) Expression of indoleamine 2,3-dioxygenase by plasmacytoid dendritic cells in tumor-draining lymph nodes. J Clin Invest 114:280–90

Munn DH, Sharma MD et al (2004b) Ligation of B7-1/B7-2 by human CD4+ T cells triggers indoleamine 2,3-dioxygenase activity in dendritic cells. J Immunol 172:4100–4110

Munn DH, Mellor AL et al (2005a) Dendritic cells have the option to express IDO-mediated suppression or not. Blood 105:2618

Munn DH, Sharma MD et al (2005b) GCN2 kinase in T cells mediates proliferative arrest and anergy induction in response to indoleamine 2,3-dioxygenase. Immunity 22:633–642

Myint AM, Kim YK (2003) Cytokine-serotonin interaction through IDO: a neurodegeneration hypothesis of depression. Med Hypotheses 61:519–525

Nair MP, Schwartz SA et al (2004) Drug abuse and neuropathogenesis of HIV infection: role of DC-SIGN and IDO. J Neuroimmunol 157:56–60

Orabona C, Belladonna ML et al (2005a) Cutting edge: silencing suppressor of cytokine signaling 3 expression in dendritic cells turns CD28-Ig from immune adjuvant to suppressant. J Immunol 174:6582–6586

Orabona C, Tomasello E et al (2005b) Enhanced tryptophan catabolism in the absence of the molecular adapter DAP12. Eur J Immunol 35:3111–3118

Ou X, Cai S et al (2007) Enhancement of dendritic cell-tumor fusion vaccine potency by indoleamine-pyrrole 2,3-dioxygenase inhibitor, 1-MT. J Cancer Res Clin Oncol 134:525–533

Paguirigan AM, Byrne GI et al (1994) Cytokine-mediated indoleamine 2,3-dioxygenase induction in response to Chlamydia infection in human macrophage cultures. Infect Immun 62: 1131–1136

Patterson S, Rae A et al (2001) Plasmacytoid dendritic cells are highly susceptible to human immunodeficiency virus type 1 infection and release infectious virus. J Virol 75:6710–6713

Peggs KS, Quezada SA et al (2006) Principles and use of anti-CTLA4 antibody in human cancer immunotherapy. Curr Opin Immunol 18:206–213

Penberthy WT (2007) Pharmacological targeting of IDO-mediated tolerance for treating autoimmune disease. Curr Drug Metab 8:245–266

Pereira A, Vottero E et al (2006) Indoleamine 2,3-dioxygenase inhibitors from the Northeastern Pacific Marine Hydroid Garveia annulata. J Nat Prod 69:1496–1499

Pestka S, Krause CD et al (2004) Interferons, interferon-like cytokines, and their receptors. Immunol Rev 202:8–32

Peters N, Sacks D (2006) Immune privilege in sites of chronic infection: leishmania and regulatory T cells. Immunol Rev 213:159–179

Peterson AC, Migawa MT, Martin MJ, Hamaker LK, Czerwinski KM, Zhang W, Arend RA, Fisette PL, Ozaki Y, Will JA, Brown RR, Cook JM (1994) Evaluation of functionalized tryptophan derivatives and related compounds as competitive inhibitors of indoleamine 2,3-dioxygenase. Med Chem Res:531–544

Platanias LC (2005) Mechanisms of type-I- and type-II-interferon-mediated signalling. Nat Rev Immunol 5:375–386

Platten M, Ho PP et al (2005) Treatment of autoimmune neuroinflammation with a synthetic tryptophan metabolite. Science 310:850–855

Poljak A, Grant R et al (2006) Inhibition of indoleamine 2,3 dioxygenase activity by H2O2. Arch Biochem Biophys 450:9–19

Popov A, Abdullah Z et al (2006) Indoleamine 2,3-dioxygenase-expressing dendritic cells form suppurative granulomas following Listeria monocytogenes infection. J Clin Invest 116: 3160–3170

Puthalakath H, O'Reilly LA et al (2007) ER stress triggers apoptosis by activating BH3-only protein Bim. Cell 129:1337–1349

Reddy P, Sun Y et al (2007) 35: Histone deacetylase inhibitors induce indoleamine 2, 3-dioxygenase and modulate dendritic cell functions. Biol Blood Marrow Transplant 13: 15–16

Reis e Sousa C (2006) Dendritic cells in a mature age. Nat Rev Immunol 6:476–483

Roberts TL, Sweet MJ et al (2005) Cutting Edge: Species-Specific TLR9-Mediated Recognition of CpG and Non-CpG Phosphorothioate-Modified Oligonucleotides. J Immunol 174:605–608
Rodriguez PC, Quiceno DG et al (2007) L-arginine availability regulates T-lymphocyte cell-cycle progression. Blood 109:1568–1573
Sakaguchi S (2005) Naturally arising Foxp3-expressing CD25 + CD4+ regulatory T cells in immunological tolerance to self and non-self. Nat Immunol 6:345–352
Sakurai K, Zou JP et al (2002) Effect of indoleamine 2,3-dioxygenase on induction of experimental autoimmune encephalomyelitis. J Neuroimmunol 129:186–196
Salter M, Hazelwood R et al (1995) The effects of a novel and selective inhibitor of tryptophan 2,3-dioxygenase on tryptophan and serotonin metabolism in the rat. Biochem Pharmacol 49: 1435–1442
Samelson-Jones BJ, Yeh SR (2006) Interactions between nitric oxide and indoleamine 2,3-dioxygenase. Biochemistry 45:8527–8538
Saxena V, Ondr JK et al (2007) The countervailing actions of myeloid and plasmacytoid dendritic cells control autoimmune diabetes in the nonobese diabetic mouse. J Immunol 179:5041–5053
Seymour RL, Ganapathy V et al (2006) A high-affinity, tryptophan-selective amino acid transport system in human macrophages. J Leukoc Biol 80:1320–1327
Sharma MD, Baban B et al (2007) Plasmacytoid dendritic cells from mouse tumor-draining lymph nodes directly activate mature Tregs via indoleamine 2,3-dioxygenase. J Clin Invest 117:2570–2582
Shevach EM, DiPaolo RA et al (2006) The lifestyle of naturally occurring CD4 + CD25 + Foxp3+ regulatory T cells. Immunol Rev 212:60–73
Shortman K, Naik SH (2007) Steady-state and inflammatory dendritic-cell development. Nat Rev Immunol 7:19–30
Sotero-Esteva WD, Wolfe D et al (2000) An indoleamine 2,3-dioxygenase-negative mutant is defective in stat1 DNA binding: differential response to IFN-gamma and IFN-alpha. J Interferon Cytokine Res 20:623–632
Steinman RM, Hawiger D et al (2003) Dendritic cell function in vivo during the steady state: a role in peripheral tolerance. Ann N Y Acad Sci 987:15–25
Sugimoto H, Oda S et al (2006) Crystal structure of human indoleamine 2,3-dioxygenase: catalytic mechanism of O2 incorporation by a heme-containing dioxygenase. Proc Natl Acad Sci USA 103:2611–2616
Taylor MW, Feng GS (1991) Relationship between interferon-gamma, indoleamine 2,3-dioxygenase, and tryptophan catabolism. Faseb J 5:2516–2522
Terness P, Bauer TM et al (2002) Inhibition of allogeneic T cell proliferation by indoleamine 2,3-dioxygenase-expressing dendritic cells: mediation of suppression by tryptophan metabolites. J Exp Med 196:447–457
Terness P, Chuang JJ et al (2005) Regulation of human auto- and alloreactive T cells by indoleamine 2,3-dioxygenase (IDO)-producing dendritic cells: too much ado about IDO? Blood 105:2480–2486
Thomas SR, Stocker R (1999) Antioxidant activities and redox regulation of interferon-gamma-induced tryptophan metabolism in human monocytes and macrophages. Adv Exp Med Biol 467:541–552
Thomas SR, Mohr D et al (1994) Nitric oxide inhibits indoleamine 2,3-dioxygenase activity in interferon-gamma primed mononuclear phagocytes. J Biol Chem 269:14457–14464
Thomas SR, Salahifar H et al (2001) Antioxidants inhibit indoleamine 2,3-dioxygenase in IFN-gamma-activated human macrophages: posttranslational regulation by pyrrolidine dithiocarbamate. J Immunol 166:6332–6340
Thomas SR, Terentis AC et al (2007) Post-translational regulation of human indoleamine 2,3-dioxygenase activity by nitric oxide. J Biol Chem 282:23778–23787
Thornton AM, Piccirillo CA et al (2004) Activation requirements for the induction of CD4 + CD25+ T cell suppressor function. Eur J Immunol 34:366–376
Travers MT, Gow IF et al (2004) Indoleamine 2,3-dioxygenase activity and L-tryptophan transport in human breast cancer cells. Biochim Biophys Acta 1661:106–112

van Boxel-Dezaire AH, Rani MR et al (2006) Complex modulation of cell type-specific signaling in response to type I interferons. Immunity 25:361–372
Vollmer J, Jurk M et al (2004a) CpG oligodeoxynucleotides stimulate IFN-gamma-inducible protein-10 production in human B cells. J Endotoxin Res 10:431–438
Vollmer J, Weeratna R et al (2004b) Characterization of three CpG oligodeoxynucleotide classes with distinct immunostimulatory activities. Eur J Immunol 34:251–262
von Bergwelt-Baildon MS, Popov A et al (2006) CD25 and indoleamine 2,3-dioxygenase are up-regulated by prostaglandin E2 and expressed by tumor-associated dendritic cells in vivo: additional mechanisms of T-cell inhibition. Blood 108:228–237
Vottero E, Balgi A et al (2006) Inhibitors of human indoleamine 2,3-dioxygenase identified with a target-based screen in yeast. Biotechnol J 1:282–288
Wek RC, Jiang HY et al (2006) Coping with stress: eIF2 kinases and translational control. Biochem Soc Trans 34:7–11
Wingender G, Garbi N et al (2006) Systemic application of CpG-rich DNA suppresses adaptive T cell immunity via induction of IDO. Eur J Immunol 36:12–20
Wirleitner B, Neurauter G et al (2004) Down-regulatory effect of N-chlorotaurine on tryptophan degradation and neopterin production in human PBMC. Immunol Lett 93:143–149
Yamamoto S, Hayaishi O (1967) Tryptophan Pyrrolase of Rabbit Intestine. d- and l-tryptophan-cleaving enzyme or enzymes. J. Biol. Chem. 242:5260–5266
Yasui H, Takai K et al (1986) Interferon enhances tryptophan metabolism by inducing pulmonary indoleamine 2,3-dioxygenase: its possible occurrence in cancer patients. Proc Natl Acad Sci USA 83:6622–6626
Youn J, Lee KH et al (2003) Beneficial effects of rosmarinic acid on suppression of collagen induced arthritis. J Rheumatol 30:1203–1207

Aspirin and the Induction of Tolerance by Dendritic Cells

Matthew Buckland and Giovanna Lombardi

Contents

Abstract Tolerance is maintained by central and peripheral regulatory mechanisms and is essential to prevent autoimmunity. In the setting of solid organ or haematopoietic transplantation, the indirect pathway of allorecognition is a significant driver of chronic rejection. Chronic rejection proceeds despite effective immunosuppressive therapy, therefore achieving immunological tolerance to control the indirect pathway is a desirable goal. Tolerance induction may be achieved by vaccination with modified antigen presenting cells (APCs). Mature dendritic cells (DCs) are potent APCs, but immature DCs have been shown to have a reduced allo-stimulatory capacity and can be tolerogenic. Drug treatment has been shown to decrease the allostimulatory capacity of DC compared to immature DC. Dexamethasone and vitamin D3 have been established as having potent effects on dendritic cell immunogenicity.

M. Buckland (✉)
Immunoregulation Laboratory, Department of Nephrology and Transplantation, 5th Floor Thomas Guy House, Guys Hospital Campus, Kings College London School of Medicine, Guys, Kings College and St Thomas Hospitals, London SE1 9RT, UK
matthew.buckland@kcl.ac.uk

G. Lombardi, Y. Riffo-Vasquez (eds.), *Dendritic Cells,* Handbook of Experimental Pharmacology 188,

The effects of Aspirin, a non-steroidal anti-inflammatory, on DCs have not previously been so extensively studied and here we will review the work which has been carried out using Aspirin to induce tolerogenic DCs.

We have examined the mechanisms of tolerance induction using human DCs and T cells. It has been possible to demonstrate that in aspirin treated, human DCs there is inhibition of the nuclear factor K-B (NFKB) signalling pathway, modified cytokine production, reduced expression of co-stimulatory molecules (CD40, CD80, and CD86) and increased expression of immunoglobulin-like transcript-3 (ILT3). The decreased expression of co-stimulatory molecules is maintained following cytokine or lipopolysaccharide (LPS) challenge. Drug treatment of DCs increases the expression of immunoglobulin-like transcript 3 (ILT3) when compared with immature DCs (iDCs), and these high levels of expression are maintained when the cells are challenged with a maturational stimulus. Aspirin also reduces the allo-stimulatory capacity of human DCs, and induces hypo-responsiveness and regulatory activity in responder T cells. These regulatory T-cells were $CD4^+$ $CD25^+$ $FOXP3^+$ and by studying $CD25^-$ or CD45RA populations, it was possible to determine that these regulatory T cells were generated de novo rather than requiring the expansion of naturally occurring Tregs.

Aspirin continues therefore to be of interest with regard its wider effects on immune regulation, other than that mediated by direct inhibition of cyclo-oxygenase, in particular its ability to induce tolerogenic DCs at therapeutic concentrations in humans.

1 Introduction

1.1 Tolerogenic Dendritic Cells

There are several lines of evidence that suggest that dendritic cells (DCs) may be a useful tool in achieving transplantation tolerance. One key feature of DCs is their excellent capacity for migration to T cell areas of recipient lymphoid tissue (Austyn and Larsen 1990; Larsen et al. 1990). This capacity of DCs to migrate to the sites of initiation of rejection offers the opportunity to directly inhibit allospecific T cell activation. DC expression of death-inducing ligands [e.g. Fas ligand (FasL; CD95L) or tumour necrosis factor (TNF)-like receptor apoptosis-inducing ligand (TRAIL)] might also allow direct deletion of alloreactive T cells. In mice, both classic myeloid ($CD8a^-$) and 'lymphoid-related' ($CD8a^+$) DCs promote apoptosis of alloreactive T cells via expression of FasL (Suss and Shortman 1996; Lu et al. 1997). In addition, there is now experimental evidence to suggest that DCs in the steady state (in the absence of deliberate exposure to maturation signals) can tolerize peripheral $CD4^+$ and $CD8^+$ T cells by inducing deletion, anergy or regulation, depending on the model system studied (Steinman and Nussenzweig 2002; Steinman et al. 2003). It is thought that, this is an important physiological process designed to limit the pool of autoreactive T cells which might otherwise cause disease. It should be noted that steady state DCs in lymph nodes may present a tissue-specific self-antigen under noninflammatory conditions without fully deleting autoreactive T cells or inducing active autoimmunity (Scheinecker et al. 2002).

The definition of what constitutes a tolerogenic dendritic cell remains elusive. Since we traditionally refer to DCs by their state of maturity, it is tempting to try and place tolerogenic DCs at one or other end of the maturity spectrum.

Pathogen matured DCs prime T cells with effective antigen presentation and co-stimulation, facilitate their escape from $CD4^{+}$ $CD25^{+}$ T cell mediated suppression (Pasare and Medzhitov 2003). It should therefore follow that maturation is not desirable in the generation of tolerogenic DCs, however, CD40 triggering of glucocorticoid treated DCs has been shown to promote IL-10 and regulatory T cell production (Rea et al. 2000).

In-vitro, immature DCs (iDCs) tend to demonstrate limited antigen presentation capacity, however, in-vivo within secondary lymphoid organs, iDCs have a unique capacity to process and present antigens without exposure to maturational stimuli (Inaba et al. 1998; Steinman et al. 2003; Wilson and Villadangos 2004). In this case, immature type DCs would be ideal to induce anergy to self-antigens, thus an immature phenotype may be tolerogenic. Following maturation, however, iDCs are more effective at presenting antigen on major histocompatibility (MHC) class II. When a matured DC interacts with a T-cell that recognizes a pathogen derived antigenic sequence, this is likely to be a higher affinity interaction than one with an autoreactive T-cell (since low affinity clones are the ones that are likely to escape negative selection) (Nossal 1994). High affinity T cells are therefore more likely to be activated by iDCs than their low affinity counterparts. Taken together, it would appear that both mature and iDCs could induce tolerance and that, this is dependent on the context of the interaction with a T cell, both the type of responder cell and the location of the interaction (e.g. lymph node or tissue).

Tolerance may be induced by DCs which invoke anergy in responder T-cells, but may also arise due to the expansion or de novo generation of regulatory T-cell subsets. Because anergy is often the consequence of sub-optimal co-stimulation, there has been a tendency to apply the terms immature and tolerogenic DCs synonymously. However, since the expansion or induction of regulatory T-cell subsets requires activation and adequate co-stimulation, it may be anomalous to apply the terms mature or immature to DCs which have a distinct functional capacity (Reis e Sousa 2006).

To overcome the difficulties apparent from the maturity dichotomy as applied to tolerogenic dendritic cells, the concept of them as separate subset of DCs has emerged (Fazekas de St Groth 1998).

To be able to identify tolerogenic DCs separately from immature and mature DCs functionally may be useful since phenotypically they may fall into neither category. Tolerogenic DCs can express substantial levels of co-stimulatory molecules and other maturation markers (Albert et al. 2001; Menges et al. 2002). The converse is also true; the expression of a particular co-stimulatory molecule or cytokine does not necessarily lead to immunity. In an antigen specific model, DCs from $CD40^{-/-}$ and $CD40L^{-/-}$ mice did not elicit $CD4^{+}$ or $CD8^{+}$ T cell immunity, even though the DCs presented antigen on MHC Class I and II, and expressed high levels of CD80/86. In addition the indirect activation of DCs by inflammatory mediators results in the usual phenotypic markers of a mature DC, and whilst able to support the clonal expansion of $CD4^+$ T cells, they are not capable of polarising the T cell response, i.e. they do not form interferon-γ (IFNγ) producing effector cells in an otherwise Th1 (helper T-cell type 1) model (Sporri and Reis e Sousa 2005).

Tolerogenic dendritic cells therefore create a unique problem of definition. They cannot be simply classified by their cell surface phenotype or cytokine profile, although these may be suggestive. The capacity to induce tolerance, i.e. a functional test, is required to determine the capacity of these cells. This may require an in-vitro or in-vivo approach. The traditional paradigm of signal 1 and signal 2 may require additional thought in the context of tolerogenic DCs. Whilst the B-7 family of molecule members CD80 and CD86 are traditionally thought of as archetypal providers of signal 2, they also provide a negative signal via cytotoxic T-lymphocyte antigen-4 (CTLA-4). Similarly, other cell surface molecules such as OX40 ligand, 4–1BB ligand and CD70 all contribute to immunity but can also have an inhibitory effect on T cell activation (Watts 2005). The outcome of an immune response in terms of memory and deletional tolerance is possibly dependent on the size and site of the antigen exposure and the number of cells that survive the secondary contraction phase of immunity (Zinkernagel 2000).

In the quest for a tolerogenic DC, it appears likely that we are seeking a cell that has the appropriate quantitative differences in expression of cell surface and secreted molecules. Tolerogenic capacity may even be related to DC longevity, since the time available to provide the appropriate signals to expand a limited pool of regulatory T cells may also be crucial (Hou and Van Parijs 2004).

Whether tolerogenic DCs are themselves innate or induced has in part been answered by the use of DC-specific inducible expression of T cell epitopes by recombination or DIETER mice (Probst et al. 2005). In their experiments Probst et al. demonstrated that steady state DCs can induce $CD8^+$ T cell tolerance to cytomegalovirus (CMV) dominant epitopes in-vivo but that in the presence of CD40 stimulation immunity reliably occurs. These results suggest that for some DCs at least, tolerance is the default setting and that it should be possible by pharmacological means to either to enhance or retain this state (still often referred to as immaturity).

1.2 Aspirin

Aspirin is a member of the non-steroidal anti-inflammatory agent (NSAID) class of drugs. It is used clinically for its analgesic, antipyretic, anti-platelet and anti-inflammatory actions. Hippocrates wrote about a bitter powder extracted from willow bark that could ease aches and pains and reduce fevers. This remedy is also mentioned in texts from ancient Sumeria, Egypt and Assyria. Native Americans claim to have used it for headaches, fever, sore muscles, rheumatism, and chills.

The Reverend Edward Stone, a vicar from Chipping Norton, Oxfordshire England, noted in 1763 that the bark of the willow was effective in reducing a fever. The active extract of the bark, called salicin, after the Latin name for the White willow (Salix alba), was isolated to its crystalline form in 1828 by Henri Leroux, a French pharmacist, and Raffaele Piria, an Italian chemist, who then succeeded in separating out the acid in its pure state. Salicin is highly acidic when in a saturated solution with water (pH = 2.4), hence salicylic acid. This chemical was also isolated from meadowsweet flowers (genus Filipendula, formerly classified in the genus Spiraea) by German researchers in 1839. While their extract was somewhat effective, it also caused digestive problems such as irritated stomach and diarrhoea, and even death when consumed in high doses. In 1853, a French chemist named Charles Frederic Gerhardt neutralized salicylic acid by buffering it with sodium (sodium salicylate) and acetyl chloride, creating acetosalicylic anhydride. In 1897, Arthur Eichengrun and Felix Hoffmann, a research assistant at Friedrich Bayer and Co. in Germany, derivatized one of the hydroxyl functional groups in salicylic acid with an acetyl group (forming the acetyl ester), which greatly reduced the negative effects. This was the first synthetic drug, and the start of the pharmaceuticals industry.

NSAIDs mediate their effects by inhibition of prostaglandin and thromboxane synthesis by the enzyme cyclo-oxygenase (COX), the demonstration of which led to the Nobel prize in medicine or physiology for John Robert Vane (Smith et al. 1994; Vane et al. 1994; Vella et al. 1997). COX has two distinct enzymatic sites, involved sequentially in the conversion of arachidonic acid to prostaglandins and thromboxanes, which mediate various events, including vasodilatation and inflammatory-associated events (Marnett and Kalgutkar 1999). NSAIDs inhibit entry of arachidonic acid into the upper part of the channel which forms part of the COX site (Picot et al. 1994). However, aspirin is the only NSAID to do so in an irreversible manner (Smith et al. 1994), by acetylation of the enzyme (Roth and Siok 1978). It has also been suggested of aspirin that, in addition to inhibition of prostaglandin synthesis, it may favour production of the mediator 15- hydroxyeicosatetraenoic (15-HETE) by one form of the COX enzyme, COX2, with unknown consequences (Smith et al. 1994).

Two forms of the COX enzyme are recognised. COX1 is constitutively expressed and contributes to the protective effects of prostaglandins on the gut mucosa (Kargman et al. 1996; Cohn et al. 1997). COX2 is induced and associated with inflammatory events (Herschman 1999). Additional roles have been defined for these receptors including a role for COX-2 mediators in oral tolerance (Newberry et al. 1999).

In macrophage or aortic endothelial cell lines, the IC50 for inhibition of prostaglandin synthesis by aspirin was $0.3 +/- 0.2\,\mu g\ ml^{-1}$ for COX1 and $50 +/- 10\,\mu g\ ml^{-1}$ for COX2, demonstrating a predominant COX1 effect (Smith and Willis 1971; Mitchell et al. 1993). By comparison, indomethacin which is a reversible competitive inhibitor of COX1 and COX2 has IC50 values of $0.01 +/- 0.001\,\mu g/ml$ for COX1 and $0.6 +/- 0.08\,\mu g\ ml^{-1}$ for COX2 (Akarasereenont et al. 1994).

2 Immunoregulatory Effects of Aspirin

2.1 In Vitro Effects of Aspirin

Expression of COX1 and COX2 has been determined directly on human DCs by immunoblot or flow cytometry (Whittaker et al. 2000), whilst in mice selective inhibition and immunoblots have provided equivalent evidence (Harizi et al. 2001). The effect of prostanoids on DCs depends in part on their state of activation and site of exposure. In peripheral tissues, prostaglandin-E2 (PGE_2) appears to have stimulatory effects on iDCs. In addition to its potential to modulate the maturation, IL-12-producing capacity, and Th-cell-polarizing ability of DCs, there is evidence that PGE_2 affects other chemokine receptor expression and apoptosis of these professional antigen presenting cells (APC). For instance, PGE_2 inhibits the production of inflammatory chemokines CCL3 and CCL4 in mouse bone-marrow derived DCs (Jing et al. 2003). By decreasing chemokine release, PGE_2 may act as an anti-inflammatory agent preventing excessive accumulation of activated immune cells. Previous data have reported that PGE_2 may act on cells in a paracrine manner, and plays a crucial role in cell to cell interaction. For example, monocyte-derived PGE_2 has suppressive effects on APC function of DCs in vivo. In fact, using indomethacin, Bjercke et al. provided evidence that the superior APC function of DCs may, at least in part, be attributed to the higher PGE_2 production by monocytes (Bjercke and Gaudernack 1985).

Since prostanoids such as PGE_2 have been shown to enhance DC maturation (Jonuleit et al. 1997; Rieser et al. 1997; Vieira et al. 2000; Whittaker et al. 2000), it is no surprise that aspirin has been shown to inhibit human DC immunostimulatory function. Three recent papers have looked at the effect of aspirin on DC (Matasic et al. 2000; Hackstein et al. 2001; Ho et al. 2001) and stimulated this investigation into the ability of aspirin to create tolerogenic DC. Matasic and colleagues (Matasic et al. 2000) demonstrated that aspirin inhibits human DC maturation and immunostimulatory function. Aspirin in combination with the maturing factors TNFα, IL-1α and PGE_2 was shown to decrease DC immunostimulatory capacity compared to mDC, although it was increased above that of iDC. The cell surface expression of MHC class I, class II, CD80, CD83 and CD86 were similarly decreased. In addition NF-κB activation and IL-12 secretion were also inhibited by aspirin treatment. Additional findings with other COX inhibitors, notably indomethacin (COX1/2), ketoprofen (COX1) and NS-398 (COX2) that had no discernible effect on DCs function suggest that aspirin may mediate its effects via a COX independent mechanism.

Hackstein and colleagues (Hackstein et al. 2001) suggested that whilst aspirin promotes initial DC development and functional activity, it freezes them at an immature state. This conclusion is drawn from data concerning morphology, phenotype, migration, endocytosis, allo-stimulatory capacity and resistance to maturational stimuli. The aspirin treated, murine bone marrow derived DCs, demonstrated reduced levels of CD40, CD80, CD86 and MHC class II which was only marginally increased with LPS. These DCs expressed lower levels of NF-κB, did not produce IL-10 and only low level IL-12 which was again unaffected by LPS stimulation. Hackstein et al. also demonstrated that aspirin modified DCs could migrate to lymph nodes and that they had endocytic capacity as determined by fluorescein isothiocyanate (FITC)-dextran uptake. In a further paper by Ho et al., the time-course of aspirin effects was shown to be rapid, with decreased LPS induced IL-12 and IL-10 in human DCs after just 3 h of aspirin exposure (Ho et al. 2001). TNFα production was also inhibited in aspirin DCs by either LPS or IL-12 stimulation.

Collectively these papers suggest that aspirin may generate a favourable tolerogenic phenotype in DCs in a COX independent fashion.

2.2 In-Vivo Effects of Aspirin

Little has been published on the in-vivo effects of aspirin modified DCs. Angus Thomson has studied the effects of aspirin on DC migration and the ability to stimulate a direct type hypersensitivity (Hackstein et al. 2001). Whilst Trinitrobenzenesulfonic acid (TNBS)-pulsed, purified bone marrow derived myeloid DC, induced strong contact hypersensitivity responses in C57BL/10J mice after rechallenge with the model hapten 7 days later, aspirin-treated DC failed to elicit a significant immune response. In fact, the responses of animals sensitized with TNBS-pulsed, aspirin-treated DC were similar to those of non-sensitized mice. Our own experiments support this data. When carboxyfluorescein succinimidyl ester (CFSE) labelled D011.10 mice are injected with Balb/C bone marrow derived DCs labelled with lipophilic fluorochrome PKH96, they co-locate to the spleen, but failed to proliferate when compared with mature DCs, as determined by dilution of CFSE by flow cytometry (unpublished data). In transplantation studies in mice, we were however only able to demonstrate a survival advantage for skin allografts when an indirect only model of CBK ($H2^k + K^b$) allografts were transplanted onto CBA/Ca recipients that were thymectomised and CD8 depleted. Since the indirect pathway is the main driver of chronic rejection, this approach remains of interest.

3 Mechanisms of Tolerance by Aspirin DCs

What comprises a tolerogenic dendritic cell remains open to debate. It would appear that perhaps the best approach is to define these cells by function, since they are likely to possess a varied phenotype and whilst it is useful to compare them to iDCs (which possess tolerogenic capacity), they are best considered as a discrete entity (Reis e Sousa 2006). Aspirin DCs appear to fulfil this functionally and possess a number of phenotypic features, some of which are predictable and some unexpected for cells with this type of function. The next sections will focus on how the available data from work on human cells, may be interpreted to explain the regulatory function that aspirin DCs induce in responder T cells.

3.1 Co-Inhibitory Molecules and Phenotypic Features

Aspirin DCs possess low levels of co-stimulatory molecules (Matasic et al. 2000; Buckland et al. 2006b), but it is likely that in a model of anergy or regulation induced by impaired co-stimulation, there will be a threshold of activation for T cells without which they will undergo apoptosis. Aspirin DCs fulfil the role of a "co-stimulation deficient" APC, but they are capable of limited up-regulation of these molecules when challenged with maturational stimuli, suggesting that they retain responsiveness to their environment (Buckland et al. 2006b). The finding of this and similar studies are summarised in Table 1.

The role of class II invariant peptide (CLIP) expression in the process of T cell activation is intriguing. Little is known about how CLIP may interact at the immunological synapse in order to down-regulate immune responses, but this may

Table 1 Phenotypic and functional effects of aspirin on human monocyte derived dendritic cells

Phenotypic marker or function	EFFECT
Maturation marker	
CD80	Unaffected
CD83	Decreased
CD86	Decreased
CD40	Decreased
Inhibitory molecule expression	
ILT-3	Increased
PDL-1	Increased
Antigen uptake	
Mannose receptor	Reduced
Macropinocytosis	Unchanged
Cytokine production	
IL-1	Unchanged
IL-10	Decreased
IL-12	Increased
TNFα	Increased
Transcription factors	
NF-κB nuclear translocation	Reduced
ERK activity	Reduced
T-cell activation	
Direct allorseponses	Reduced
Indirect alloresponses	Reduced

Compiled from the author's unpublished data and references (Matasic et al. 2000; Weissmann et al. 2002; Jing et al. 2003; Buckland et al. 2006b)

be a function of competing with T-cell receptor (TCR) ligands to reduce cognate interactions (Rohn et al. 2004). We have demonstrated on aspirin DCs that CLIP is significantly increased as a proportion of all MHC class II, the elevated expression may well be important in regulating the level of antigen specific signals T cells acquire, affecting their level of activation, by out-competing for allo-antigen.

The precise role of cell surface molecules such as ILT-3 and programmed death ligand-1 (PDL-1) in the induction of tolerance has not yet been fully elucidated. The ligand for ILT-3 is not yet known, but the presence of the intracellular inhibitory tyrosine motifs (ITIMs) is associated with a blunting of the usual Ca^{2+} flux and tyrosine phosphorylation activity in responder T cells, consistent with inhibitory function (Cella et al. 1997). In a recent publication studying the effect of Vitamin D3 on DCs, wherein naïve T cells were tolerized by repeated rounds of stimulation in the presence of anti-ILT3, it was demonstrated that naïve T cells exposed to iDCs are ILT-3 dependent for regulation, whereas those exposed to Vitamin D3 DCs were not (Penna et al. 2005; see also Chapter by Adorini and Penna). We have demonstrated that both whole $CD4^+$ and $CD4^+$ $CD25^-$ T cells expressed similar levels of FOXP3 after a single round of stimulation and are ILT-3 independent, which may well correlate with the activation requirements and cytokine profiles of these two different cell populations (Buckland et al. 2006a,b). As well as significant ILT-3 expression on aspirin DCs, we saw modest levels of PDL-1 (intermediate between that observed on immature and TNF-α, IL-1α and PGE_2 [TIP] activated DCs). PDL-1 also possesses an ITIM domain and mice deficient in its ligand PD-1 are unable to control immune responses (Nishimura et al. 1998, 1999, 2001). Expression of PDL-1 is therefore expected to be greatest on mature DCs; however, its expression even at low levels on DCs which have a tolerogenic phenotype is likely to contribute to the signalling required to divert responder T cells to a regulatory phenotype. Additional work studying the mechanisms of $CD8^+$ T cell deletion during induction of tolerance to the direct pathway show that PDL-1 and CTLA4 dependent mechanisms are involved (Iwakoshi et al. 2000; Ito et al. 2003), thus the induction of PDL-1 on tolerogenic DCs may be a key step in the deletion of allo-reactive $CD8^+$ T cells which are central to the direct alloresponse.

3.2 Antigen Processing and Functional Capacity of Aspirin DCs

Whilst other approaches to the generation of tolerogenic DCs have previously been described (Steinbrink et al. 1997; Lu et al. 1999; Penna and Adorini 2000; Yoshimura et al. 2001; Akiyama et al. 2002; Tan et al. 2005b), the differentiation of DCs as determined by loss or gain of surface markers such as CD14 and CD11c is also frequently inhibited (Griffin 2000) and this may result in cells that are less effective in inducing tolerance in vivo. We have also demonstrated that aspirin treated DCs, which are $CD14^-CD11c^{hi}$, retain the capacity to efficiently process antigen by two endocytic pathways (Buckland et al. 2006a), this is important if such DCs are to be used to induce indirect pathway tolerance, when recipient DCs are modified and they need to retain their capacity to process and present antigens.

3.3 Signaling Pathways and Novel Mechanisms

In human mDCs treated with aspirin, we have demonstrated NFκB inhibition, which is in keeping with previous observations as to the effect of aspirin on endothelial cells (Pierce et al. 1996; Buckland et al. 2006b) and DCs (Matasic et al. 2000). The mechanism described is the prevention of NFκB translocation to the nucleus and this would be consistent with the reduction in phosporylated – IKB (pIKB) which was found (Tan et al. 2005b). See also the Chapter by Adorini and Penna for comparative discussion on signalling effects on DCs by Vit D receptor analogues.

The observation that immature and aspirin DCs appeared to support IFNγ production by naïve T cells stimulated the decision to investigate Indoleamine 2,3-dioxygenase (IDO) production by these cells (unpublished data). Previously IFNγ was demonstrated to be the most reliable method of upregulating IDO expression on DCs (Mellor and Munn 2004). We found that iDCs do not express IDO, that it is potently induced by TIP as a maturational stimulus and that aspirin treatment inhibits this up-regulation, although not completely. These findings suggest that in aspirin DCs, IDO is not the key determinant of inducing a tolerant state; the significant upregulation on TIP DCs would be consistent with high levels of IDO providing a very potent negative stimulus to counterbalance or terminate immune responses. More recently is has been demonstrated that kynurenine pathways independent of IDO may also play a part in tolerogenesis and this should be studied further with aspirin DCs (Belladonna et al. 2006).

3.4 T Cell Responses to Aspirin DCs

Consistent with the observed phenotype and signalling changes, aspirin treated DCs were observed to be less potent allogeneic stimuli than iDCs (Matasic et al. 2000; Buckland et al. 2006a,b). We have shown this effect with whole, naïve and $CD4^+$ $CD25^-$ responder T cells (Table 2). Cytokine production from the mixed lymphocyte reaction (MLR) from the whole $CD4^+$ population was suppressed compared with mature DCs and was the same as that observed when iDCs were used as the allogeneic stimulus. In addition to experiments with naïve T cells, when studying $CD25^+$ depleted $CD4^+$ T cells it was still possible to induce regulation, suggesting that these regulatory T cells do not arise from the naturally occurring $CD4^+$ $CD25^+$ T cell pool. When naïve T cells respond to aspirin DCs, the production of IFNγ was maintained, but we also observed IL-5 production. The T cells from the aspirin DC co-cultures were anergic and regulated the alloresponse of other T cells in an allo-specific manner. The addition of IL-2 reversed the anergy, thus these cells have not all been forced toward activation induced cell death. Regardless of the starting population (Whole $CD4^+$ or $CD4^+$ $CD25^-$) following co-culture with aspirin or iDCs, these allo-regulatory T cells are $CD25^{hi}$ and express the forkhead transcription factor FOXP3 (Table 2). FOXP3 is not abrogated by the presence of anti-ILT3 during the generation of regulatory T cells, consistent with their maintained capacity

Table 2 Aspirin favours the induction of regulatory T-cells

Features of aspirin treated DCs favouring tregs
Inhibit IDO
Upregulate ILT-3
Downregulate CD83,CD86, CD40
Maintain PDL-1 expression
Features of T-cells that encounter aspirin DCs
Reduced Th1 development
Hyporesponsive to direct and indirect pathway stimulation
Refractory to rechallenge
Increased CTLA-4 expression
Increased PD-1 expression
Enhanced $CD4^{+}$ $CD25^{+}$ $FoxP3^{+}$ supressor T-cells

Compiled from the author's own unpublished work and that in references (Matasic et al. 2000; Buckland et al. 2006a,b)

to regulate. The high levels of intracellular CTLA4 and the expression of PD-1 on the resultant regulatory T cells, alongside elevated intracellular IL-10 are consistent with the transwell findings that regulation is both contact and soluble factor mediated.

There has been much focus on the capacity of DCs to induce IL-10 producing regulatory cells (Jonuleit et al. 2000; Menges et al. 2002; Levings et al. 2005; Tan et al. 2005a), by the paracrine or autocrine secretion of IL-10. Other authors also cite evidence for the induction of contact dependent Tregs (Sato et al. 2003). Much of the evidence for the requirement of IL-10 is indirect and from the production of cytokine in DC-T cell co-culture, and in the case of naïve T cells derived from cord blood, much of this IL-10 derives from the T cells themselves (Rainsford and Reen 2002). In aspirin treated DCs challenged by maturational stimuli, we saw inhibition of IL-10 and a concomitant rise in IL-12, TNFα and IL-1β, whereas Matasic et al. reported decreased IL-12 production to stimulation with TIP (Matasic et al. 2000). IDCs produce IL-10 in an autocrine fashion, and become less sensitive to its effects as they mature (De Smedt et al. 1997), this IL-10 is in turn inhibitory on the production of IL-12 (Xia and Kao 2003). The regulation of IL-10 production is mediated in part through ERK and p38 MAP kinase pathways (Xia and Kao 2003). Aspirin has been shown to inhibit ERK activity via inhibition of mEK (proximal regulator of ERK) in neutrophils (Weissmann et al. 2002). The concomitant blockade of NF-κB and ERK by aspirin in DCs would facilitate the inhibition of IL-10 with a concomitant increase in IL-12, whilst preventing the related phenotypic maturation of the DCs. This particular phenotype may explain the observed efficiency in inducing regulation in naïve T cells, by IL-12 supporting IFNγ production and facilitating cell cycle progression in regulatory cells, thus avoiding activation induced cell death. This picture is analogous to the observations that IFNγ is essential in the development of operational tolerance to alloantigen in vivo in a murine model (Sawitzki et al. 2005).

Taken together the data suggest that the regulatory T cells induced by aspirin DCs belong to the $CD4^+$ $CD25^+$ $FOXP3^+$ subset and that whilst IL-10 may not be necessary for their induction, in keeping with previous observations they do produce Il-10 which is one of several requirements for suppression. Perhaps novel to this subset of regulatory T cells is the parallel induction of high CTLA4 and PD-1, which allows redundancy in the regulatory mechanism, ensuring that a regulatory phenotype is maintained.

3.5 15-Hydroxyeicosatetraenoic Acid and Lipoxins

Aspirin is of particular interest in the pharmacological manipulation of DCs because it has preferential activity via COX-2, and has been shown to favour the production of the mediator 15-HETE (Meade et al. 1993). 15-HETE has been shown to inhibit mitogen induced proliferation of murine splenocytes and T cells (Bailey et al. 1982; Low et al. 1984). A direct effect has also been demonstrated for 15-HETE on the induction of suppressor T cells. Pre-treatment of mice with 15-HETE before immunization with allogeneic splenocytes, resulted in suppression of the allo-response as determined by subsequent in-vitro re-challenge (Aldigier et al. 1984). Subsequently Mexmain et al. demonstrated that 15-HETE treated thymocytes inhibited the proliferation of allo-stimulated splenocytes and that this suppression was associated with a rise in cGMP in the thymocytes (Mexmain et al. 1985).

In addition aspirin has been shown to stimulate the production of lipoxins which exert anti-inflammatory effects via DC cytokine production (Parkinson 2006). Lipoxin A4 (LXA4) modulates innate and acquired immune responses through induction of suppressor of cytokine signalling-2 (SOCS-2) expression (Machado et al. 2006). The SOCS proteins are thought to regulate cytokine receptor–triggered signal transduction by docking to the intracellular domains of their receptors or by facilitating proteosome-dependent degradation of transcription factors, thereby preventing activation of downstream signalling elements. The mechanisms for induction of SOCS-2 and its 'molecular targets,' as well as the mode of inhibition by which it mediates suppression, are not known (Machado et al. 2006). Aspirin triggered lipoxins (ATL) share the same receptors and mediate the same biological effects as those observed with LXA4, thus a further mechanism for the action of aspirin may be via lipoxin synthesis from DCs, but this is yet to be determined (Hachicha et al. 1999).

4 Conclusions

Tolerogenic DCs have a wide range of potential therapeutic applications including allogeneic transplantation and autoimmunity. Whilst the direct pathway of alloreactivity is dominant early in transplantation, the frequency of responder T cells diminishes with time and this process is well controlled with short-term high dose immunosuppressive therapy. The indirect pathway of allo-reactivity is by contrast poorly controlled with drug therapies alone, the frequency of responders tends to increase with time and the need for immunosuppressive therapy is currently for the life of the graft, with all the attendant risks. It has been demonstrated that DCs modified by pharmacological agents such as aspirin, can be maintained in a tolerogenic state and that in-vitro they can be used to generate regulatory T cells, in-vivo there is some evidence that they can delay indirect pathway mediated graft loss.

Given the wide use of aspirin in prevention of acute ischemic events in patients with coronary artery disease and as an anti-pyretic or analgesic, it would be desirable to further dissect the potential for aspirin in affecting chronic inflammatory processes, including atherosclerosis, autoinflammatory and alloresponses via its effects on DCs.

References

Akarasereenont P, Mitchell JA, Thiemermann C, Vane JR (1994) Relative potency of nonsteroid anti-inflammatory drugs as inhibitors of cyclooxygenase-1 or cyclooxygenase-2. Br J Pharmacol 112(suppl):183

Akiyama Y, Shirasugi N, Aramaki O, Matsumoto K, Shimazu M, Kitajima M, Ikeda Y, Niimi M (2002) Intratracheal delivery of a single major histocompatibility complex class I peptide induced prolonged survival of fully allogeneic cardiac grafts and generated regulatory cells. Hum Immunol 63:888–892

Albert ML, Jegathesan M, Darnell RB (2001) Dendritic cell maturation is required for the cross-tolerization of $CD8^+$ T cells. Nat Immunol 2:1010–1017

Aldigier JC, Gualde N, Mexmain S, Chable-Rabinovitch H, Ratinaud MH, Rigaud M (1984) Immunosuppression induced in vivo by 15 hydroxyeicosatetraenoic acid (15 HETE). Prostaglandins Leukot Med 13:99–107

Austyn JM, Larsen CP (1990) Migration patterns of dendritic leukocytes. Implications for transplantation. Transplantation 49:1–7

Bailey JM, Bryant RW, Low CE, Pupillo MB, Vanderhoek JY (1982) Regulation of T-lymphocyte mitogenesis by the leukocyte product 15-hydroxy-eicosatetraenoic acid (15-HETE). Cell Immunol 67:112–120

Belladonna ML, Grohmann U, Guidetti P, Volpi C, Bianchi R, Fioretti MC, Schwarcz R, Fallarino F, Puccetti P (2006) Kynurenine pathway enzymes in dendritic cells initiate tolerogenesis in the absence of functional IDO. J Immunol 177:130–137

Bjercke S, Gaudernack G (1985) Dendritic cells and monocytes as accessory cells in T-Cell responses in man .2. Function as antigen-presenting cells. Scand J Immunol 21:501–508

Buckland M, Jago C, Fazekesova H, George A, Lechler R, Lombardi G (2006a) Aspirin modified dendritic cells are potent inducers of allo-specific regulatory T-cells. Int Immunopharmacol 6:1895–1901

Buckland M, Jago CB, Fazekasova H, Scott K, Tan PH, George AJ, Lechler R, Lombardi G (2006b) Aspirin-treated human DCs up-regulate ILT-3 and induce hyporesponsiveness and regulatory activity in responder T cells. Am J Transplant 6:2046–2059

Cella M, Dohring C, Samaridis J, Dessing M, Brockhaus M, Lanzavecchia A, Colonna M (1997) A novel inhibitory receptor (ILT3) expressed on monocytes, macrophages, and dendritic cells involved in antigen processing. J Exp Med 185:1743–1751

Cohn SM, Schloemann S, Tessner T, Seibert K, Stenson WF (1997) Crypt stem cell survival in the mouse intestinal epithelium is regulated by prostaglandins synthesized through cyclooxygenase-1. J Clin Invest 99:1367–1379

De Smedt T, Van Mechelen M, De Becker G, Urbain J, Leo O, Moser M (1997) Effect of interleukin-10 on dendritic cell maturation and function. Eur J Immunol 27:1229–1235

Fazekas de St Groth B (1998) The evolution of self-tolerance: a new cell arises to meet the challenge of self-reactivity. Immunol Today 19:448–454

Griffin MD (2000) Potent inhibition of dendritic cell differentiation and maturation by vitamin D analogs. Biochem Biophys Res Commun 270:701–708

Hachicha M, Pouliot M, Petasis NA, Serhan CN (1999) Lipoxin (LX)A(4) and aspirin-triggered 15-epi-LXA(4) inhibit tumor necrosis factor 1 alpha-initiated neutrophil responses and trafficking: Regulators of a cytokine-chemokine axis. J Exp Med 189:1923–1929

Hackstein H, Morelli AE, Larregina AT, Ganster RW, Papworth GD, Logar AJ, Watkins SC, Falo LD, Thomson AW (2001) Aspirin inhibits in vitro maturation and in vivo immunostimulatory function of murine myeloid dendritic cells. J Immunol 166:7053–7062

Harizi H, Juzan M, Grosset C, Rashedi M, Gualde N (2001) Dendritic cells issued in vitro from bone marrow produce PGE(2) that contributes to the immunomodulation induced by antigen-presenting cells. Cell Immunol 209:19–28

Herschman HR (1999) Function and regulation of prostaglandin synthase 2. Adv Exp Med Biol 469:3–8

Ho LJ, Chang DM, Shiau HY, Chen CH, Hsieh TY, Hsu YL, Wong CS, Lai JH (2001) Aspirin differentially regulates endotoxin-induced IL-12 and TNF-alpha production in human dendritic cells. Scand J Rheumatol 30:346–352

Hou WS, Van Parijs LA (2004) Bcl-2-dependent molecular timer regulates the lifespan and immunogenicity of dendritic cells. Nat Immunol 5:583–589

Inaba K, Turley S, Yamaide F, Iyoda T, Mahnke K (1998) Efficient presentation of phagocytosed cellular fragments on the MHC class II products of dendritic cells. J Exp Med 188:2163

Ito T, Nayer A, Yagita H, Auchincloss JH, Sayegh MH, Najafian N (2003) The role of inhibitory costimulatory pathway PD-1 in regulating alloimmune responses in vivo. Am J Transplant 3:169

Iwakoshi NN, Mordes JP, Markees TG, Phillips NE, Rossini AA, Greiner DL (2000) Treatment of allograft recipients with donor-specific transfusion and anti-CD154 antibody leads to deletion of alloreactive $CD8^+$ T cells and prolonged graft survival in a CTLA4-dependent manner. J Immunol 164:512–521

Jing H, Vassiliou E, Ganea D (2003) Prostaglandin E2 inhibits production of the inflammatory chemokines CCL3 and CCL4 in dendritic cells. J Leukoc Biol 74:868–879

Jonuleit H, Kuhn U, Muller G, Steinbrink K, Paragnik L, Schmitt E, Knop J, Enk AH (1997) Pro-inflammatory cytokines and prostaglandins induce maturation of potent immunostimulatory dendritic cells under fetal calf serum-free conditions. Eur J Immunol 27:3135–3142

Jonuleit H, Schmitt E, Schuler G, Knop J, Enk AH (2000) Induction of interleukin 10-producing, nonproliferating CD4(+) T cells with regulatory properties by repetitive stimulation with allogeneic immature human dendritic cells. J Exp Med 192:1213–1222

Kargman S, Charleson S, Cartwright M, Frank J, Riendeau D, Mancini J, Evans J, O'Neill G (1996) Characterization of prostaglandin G/H synthase 1 and 2 in rat, dog, monkey, and human gastrointestinal tracts. Gastroenterology 111:445–454

Larsen CP, Steinman RM, Witmer-Pack M, Hankins DF, Morris PJ, Austyn JM (1990) Migration and maturation of langerhans cells in skin transplants and explants. J Exp Med 172:1483–1493

Levings MK, Gregori S, Tresoldi E, Cazzaniga S, Bonini C, Roncarolo MG (2005) Differentiation of Tr1 cells by immature dendritic cells requires IL-10 but not $CD25^+CD4^+$ Tr cells. Blood 105:1162–1169

Low CE, Pupillo MB, Bryant RW, Bailey JM (1984) Inhibition of phytohemagglutinin-induced lymphocyte mitogenesis by lipoxygenase metabolites of arachidonic acid: structure-activity relationships. J Lipid Res 25:1090–1095

Lu L, Qian S, Hershberger PA, Rudert WA, Lynch DH, Thomson AW (1997) Fas ligand (CD95L) and B7 expression on dendritic cells provide counter-regulatory signals for T cell survival and proliferation. J Immunol 158:5676–5684

Lu L, Lee WC, Takayama T, Qian S, Gambotto A, Robbins PD, Thomson AW (1999) Genetic engineering of dendritic cells to express immunosuppressive molecules (viral IL-10, TGF-beta, and CTLA4Ig). J Leukoc Biol 66:293–296

Machado FS, Johndrow JE, Esper L, Dias A, Bafica A, Serhan CN, Aliberti J (2006) Anti-inflammatory actions of lipoxin A4 and aspirin-triggered lipoxin are SOCS-2 dependent. Nat Med 12:330–334

Marnett LJ, Kalgutkar AS (1999) Cyclooxygenase 2 inhibitors: discovery, selectivity and the future. Trends Pharmacol Sci 20:465–469

Matasic R, Dietz AB, Vuk-Pavlovic S (2000) Cyclooxygenase-independent inhibition of dendritic cell maturation by aspirin. Immunology 101:53–60

Meade EA, Smith WL, DeWitt DL (1993) Differential inhibition of prostaglandin endoperoxide synthase (cyclooxygenase) isozymes by aspirin and other non-steroidal anti-inflammatory drugs. J Biol Chem 268:6610–6614

Mellor AL, Munn DH (2004) IDO expression by dendritic cells: tolerance and tryptophan catabolism. Nat Rev Immunol 4:762–774

Menges M, Rossner S, Voigtlander C, Schindler H, Kukutsch NA (2002) Repetitive injections of dendritic cells matured with tumor necrosis factor induce antigen-specific protection of mice from autoimmunity. J Exp Med 195:15–21

Mexmain S, Cook J, Aldigier JC, Gualde N, Rigaud M (1985) Thymocyte cyclic AMP and cyclic GMP response to treatment with metabolites issued from the lipoxygenase pathway. J Immunol 135:1361–1365

Mitchell JA, Akarasereenont P, Bishop-Bailey D, Wood EG, Thiemermann C, Vane JR (1993) Aspirin is a more potent inhibitor of prostacyclin biosynthesis by endothelial cells than by LPS-treated J774 macrophages. Br J Pharmacol 109(suppl):2

Newberry RD, Stenson WF, Lorenz RG (1999) Cyclooxygenase-2-dependent arachidonic acid metabolites are essential modulators of the intestinal immune response to dietary antigen. Nat Med 5:900–906

Nishimura H, Minato N, Nakano T, Honjo T (1998) Immunological studies on PD-1 deficient mice: implication of PD-1 as a negative regulator for B cell responses. Int Immunol 10:1563–1572

Nishimura H, Nose M, Hiai H, Minato N, Honjo T (1999) Development of lupus-like autoimmune diseases by disruption of the PD-1 gene encoding an ITIM motif-carrying immunoreceptor. Immunity 11:141–151

Nishimura H, Okazaki T, Tanaka Y, Nakatani K, Hara M, Matsumori A, Sasayama S, Mizoguchi A, Hiai H, Minato N, Honjo T (2001) Autoimmune dilated cardiomyopathy in PD-1 receptor-deficient mice. Science 291:319–322

Nossal GJV (1994) Negative selection of lymphocytes. Cell 76:229–239

Parkinson JF (2006) Lipoxin and synthetic lipoxin analogs: an overview of anti-inflammatory functions and new concepts in immunomodulation. Inflamm Allergy Drug Targets 5:91–106

Pasare C, Medzhitov R (2003) Toll pathway-dependent blockade of $CD4^+CD25^+$T cell-mediated suppression by dendritic cells. Science 299:1033–1036

Penna G, Adorini L (2000) 1 Alpha,25-dihydroxyvitamin D3 inhibits differentiation, maturation, activation, and survival of dendritic cells leading to impaired alloreactive T cell activation. J Immunol 164:2405–2411

Penna G, Roncari A, Amuchastegui S, Daniel KC, Berti E, Colonna M, Adorini L (2005) Expression of the inhibitory receptor ILT3 on dendritic cells is dispensable for induction of $CD4^+Foxp3^+$ regulatory T cells by 1,25-dihydroxyvitamin D3. Blood 106:3490–3497

Picot D, Loll PJ, Garavito RM (1994) The X-ray crystal structure of the membrane protein prostaglandin H2 synthase-1. Nature 367:243–249

Pierce JW, Read MA, Ding H, Luscinskas FW, Collins T (1996) Salicylates inhibit I kappa B-alpha phosphorylation, endothelial-leukocyte adhesion molecule expression, and neutrophil transmigration. J Immunol 156:3961–3969

Probst HC, McCoy K, Okazaki T, Honjo T, van den Broek M (2005) Resting dendritic cells induce peripheral $CD8^+$ T cell tolerance through PD-1 and CTLA-4. Nat Immunol 6:280–286

Rainsford E, Reen DJ (2002) Interleukin 10, produced in abundance by human newborn T cells, may be the regulator of increased tolerance associated with cord blood stem cell transplantation. Br J Haematol 116:702–709

Rea D, van Kooten C, van Meijgaarden KE, Ottenhoff TH, Melief CJ, Offringa R (2000) Glucocorticoids transform CD40-triggering of dendritic cells into an alternative activation pathway resulting in antigen-presenting cells that secrete IL-10. Blood 95:3162–3167

Reis e Sousa C (2006) Dendritic cells in a mature age. Nat Rev Immunol 6:476–483

Rieser C, Bock G, Klocker H, Bartsch G, Thurnher M (1997) Prostaglandin E2 and tumor necrosis factor alpha cooperate to activate human dendritic cells:synergistic activation of interleukin 12 production. J Exp Med 186:1603–1608

Rohn TA, Boes M, Wolters D, Spindeldreher S, Muller B, Langen H, Ploegh H, Vogt AB, Kropshofer H (2004) Upregulation of the CLIP self peptide on mature dendritic cells antagonizes T helper type 1 polarization. Nat Immunol 5:909–918

Roth GJ, Siok CJ (1978) Acetylation of the NH2-terminal serine of prostaglandin synthetase by aspirin. J Biol Chem 253:3782–3784

Sato K, Yamashita N, Yamashita N, Baba M, Matsuyama T (2003) Regulatory dendritic cells protect mice from murine acute graft-versus-host disease and leukemia relapse. Immunity 18: 367–379

Sawitzki B, Kingsley CI, Oliveira V, Karim M, Herber M, Wood KJ (2005) IFN-[Gamma] production by alloantigen-reactive regulatory T cells is important for their regulatory function in vivo. J Exp Med 201:1925–1935

Scheinecker C, McHugh R, Shevach EM, Germain RN (2002) Constitutive presentation of a natural tissue autoantigen exclusively by dendritic cells in the draining lymph node. J Exp Med 196:1079–1090

Smith JB, Willis AL (1971) Aspirin selectively inhibits prostaglandin production in human platelets. Nat New Biol 231:235–237

Smith WL, Meade EA, DeWitt DL (1994) Pharmacology of prostaglandin endoperoxide synthase isozymes-1 and -2. Ann N Y Acad Sci 714:136–142

Sporri R, Reis e Sousa C (2005) Inflammatory mediators are insufficient for full dendritic cell activation and promote expansion of $CD4^+$ T cell populations lacking helper function. Nat Immunol 6:163–170

Steinbrink K, Wolfl M, Jonuleit H, Knop J, Enk AH (1997) Induction of tolerance. by IL-10-treated dendritic cells. J Immunol 159:4772–4780

Steinman RM, Nussenzweig MC (2002) Avoiding horror autotoxicus: the importance of dendritic cells in peripheral T cell tolerance. Proc Natl Acad Sci USA 99:351

Steinman RM, Hawiger D, Nussenzweig MC (2003) Tolerogenic dendritic cells. Annu Rev Immunol 21:685–711

Suss G, Shortman K (1996) A subclass of dendritic cells kills CD4 T cells via Fas/Fas-ligand-induced apoptosis. J Exp Med 183:1789–1796

Tan PH, Beutelspacher SC, Wang YH, McClure MO, Ritter MA, Lombardi G, George AJ (2005a) Immunolipoplexes: an efficient, nonviral alternative for transfection of human dendritic cells with potential for clinical vaccination. Mol Ther 11:790–800

Tan PH, Sagoo P, Chan C, Yates JB, Campbell J, Beutelspacher SC, Foxwell BM, Lombardi G, George AJ (2005b) Inhibition of NF-kappa B and oxidative pathways in human dendritic cells by antioxidative vitamins generates regulatory T cells. J Immunol 174:7633–7644

Vane JR, Mitchell JA, Appleton I, Tomlinson A, Bishop-Bailey D, Croxtall J, Willoughby DA (1994) Inducible isoforms of cyclooxygenase and nitric-oxide synthase in inflammation. Proc Natl Acad Sci USA 91:2046–2050

Vella JP, Spadafora-Ferreira M, Murphy B, Alexander SI, Harmon W, Carpenter CB, Sayegh MH (1997) Indirect allorecognition of major histocompatibility complex allopeptides in human renal transplant recipients with chronic graft dysfunction. Transplantation 64:795–800

Vieira PL, de Jong EC, Wierenga EA, Kapsenberg ML, Kalinski P (2000) Development of Th1-inducing capacity in myeloid dendritic cells requires environmental instruction. J Immunol 164:4507–4512

Watts TH (2005) TNF/TNFR family members in costimulation of T cell responses. Annu Rev Immunol 23:23–68

Weissmann G, Montesinos MC, Pillinger M, Cronstein BN (2002) Non-prostaglandin effects of aspirin III and salicylate: inhibition of integrin-dependent human neutrophil aggregation and inflammation in COX 2- and NF kappa B (P105)-knockout mice. Adv Exp Med Biol 507: 571–577

Whittaker DS, Bahjat KS, Moldawer LL, Clare-Salzler MJ (2000) Autoregulation of human monocyte-derived dendritic cell maturation and IL-12 production by cyclooxygenase-2-mediated prostanoid production. J Immunol 165:4298–4304

Wilson NS, Villadangos JA (2004) Lymphoid organ dendritic cells: beyond the Langerhans cells paradigm. Immunol. Cell Biol 82:91–98

Xia CQ, Kao KJ (2003) Suppression of interleukin-12 production through endogenously secreted interleukin-10 in activated dendritic cells: involvement of activation of extracellular signal-regulated protein kinase. Scand J Immunol 58:23–32

Yoshimura S, Bondeson J, Foxwell BM, Brennan FM, Feldmann M (2001) Effective antigen presentation by dendritic cells is NF-kappaB dependent: coordinate regulation of MHC, co-stimulatory molecules and cytokines. Int Immunol 13:675–683

Zinkernagel RM (2000) Localization dose and time of antigens determine immune reactivity. Semin Immunol 12:163–171

Use of Rapamycin in the Induction of Tolerogenic Dendritic Cells

Ryan Fischer, Heth R. Turnquist, Timuçin Taner, and Angus W. Thomson

Contents

Abstract Rapamycin (RAPA), a macrocyclic triene antibiotic pro-drug, is a clinically-utilized 'tolerance-sparing' immunosuppressant that inhibits the activity of T, B, and NK cells. Furthermore, maturation-resistance and tolerogenic properties of dendritic cells (DC) can be supported and preserved by conditioning with RAPA. Propagation of murine bone marrow (BM)-derived myeloid DC (mDC) in clinically relevant concentrations of RAPA (RAPA-DC) generates phenotypically immature

---

A.W. Thomson (✉)
University of Pittsburgh, W1544 Biomedical Science Tower, 200 Lothrop Street, Pittsburgh, PA 15213, USA
thomsonaw@upmc.edu

G. Lombardi, Y. Riffo-Vasquez (eds.), *Dendritic Cells,* Handbook of Experimental Pharmacology 188,

DC with low levels of MHC and significantly reduced co-stimulatory molecules (especially CD86), even when exposed to inflammatory stimuli. RAPA-DC are weak stimulators of T cells and induce hyporesponsiveness and apoptosis in allo-reactive T cells. An interesting observation has been that RAPA-DC retain the ability to stimulate and enrich the regulatory T cells (Treg). Presumably as a result of these properties, alloantigen (alloAg)-pulsed recipient-derived DC are effective in subverting anti-allograft immune responses in rodent transplant models, making them an attractive subject for further investigation of their tolerance-promoting potential.

Abbreviations

Ag	Antigen
AlloAg	AlloAg
BM	Bone marrow
CCR	C-C motif receptor
CNI	Calcineurin inhibitor
CSA	Cyclosporine
CTL	Cytotoxic T lymphocyte
CTR-DC	Control, BM-derived DC
DC	Dendritic cell
FKBP12	FK506-binding protein 12
GM-CSF	Granulocyte/macrophage colony-stimulating factor
GVHD	Graft-versus-host disease
iDC	Immature DC
LPS	Lipopolysacchride
mDC	Myeloid DC
MHC	Major histocompatibility complex
MLR	Mixed leukocyte reaction
MMF	Mycophenolate mofetil
mTOR	Mammalian target of rapamycin
MTX	Methotrexate
NK	Natural killer
RAPA	Rapamycin
RAPA-DC	RAPA-conditioned, BM-derived DC
TCR	T-cell receptor
Th	T helper
Tr1	Treg type-1
Treg	Regulatory T cell
VEGF	Vascular endothelial growth factor

1 Introduction

Diverse subsets of dendritic cells (DC) exist in the circulation, lymphoid and non-lymphoid tissues; however, most experimental studies and therapeutic protocols in rodents, primates and humans have focused on either myeloid (m)DC or plasmacytoid (p)DC (Morelli and Thomson 2007; Ueno et al. 2007). It is understood that endogenous DC play critical roles in the induction and regulation of immune responses (Banchereau and Steinman 1998; Banchereau et al. 2000; Morelli and Thomson 2003; Steinman et al. 2003; Morelli and Thomson 2007; Lotze and Thomson 2001). These rare, ubiquitously-distributed, migratory leukocytes are derived from $CD34^+$ hematopoietic stem cells, and were originally named for their branching (i.e. dendritic), shape. DC convey antigen (Ag) from peripheral sites, such as skin, or other non-lymphoid tissues, to T cells in secondary lymphoid organs, the sites for the generation of immunity and tolerance. They are extremely well-equipped for Ag capture, processing and presentation to rare T cells expressing specific receptors that recognize Ag peptides bound to major histocompatability complex (MHC) molecules. Under steady-state, non-inflammatory conditions in lymphoid and non-lymphoid tissues, including the commonly-transplanted organs (kidney, heart, liver and skin), DC reside as "immature" antigen presenting cells (Austyn et al. 1994; Larsen et al. 1994; Woo et al. 1994; Coates et al. 2004). Immature DC (iDC) are at best, poor stimulators of T cells, readily inducing anergy or apoptosis in naïve T cells (Morelli and Thomson 2007; Zheng et al. 2008) and inactivating or deleting memory and effector $CD8^+$ T cells (Kenna et al. 2008). iDC express few surface MHC and accessory molecules (e.g. CD40, CD54 [ICAM-1], CD80 [B7–1], or CD86 [B7–2]), but constitutively express programmed cell death ligand 1 (PD-L1 = B7–H1), an inhibitor of T cells.

iDC act as immunological sensors alerting for potentially dangerous microbes, by directly recognizing microbial components or by receiving signals formulated by the innate immune system. iDC expression of Toll-like (TLR), nucleotide oligomerization domain (NOD) receptors, and receptor for advanced glycation end products (RAGE), enables sensing of pathogen-associated molecular patterns (PAMPs) and endogenously-arising damage-associated molecular patterns (DAMPs) (Lotze et al. 2007; Ueno et al. 2007). Triggering of these receptors directs DC "maturation," that is, increased surface expression of MHC, accessory, and co-stimulatory molecules. Upon maturation, DC up-regulate the expression of the chemokine (C-C motif) receptor 7 (CCR7; Sallusto et al. 1998). CCR7 enhances trafficking of DC to T cell areas of secondary lymphoid tissues (i.e. spleen and lymph nodes) in response to the CCR7 ligands, CCL19 or CCL21. Once in the secondary lymphoid tissue, mature DC present Ag peptides bound to MHC class II molecules to $CD4^+$ T helper (Th) cells. To generate cytotoxic T lymphocytes (CTL), DC must present Ag peptides complexed with MHC class I molecules to $CD8^+$ T cells, a process known as "cross-presentation." Such cross-presentation allows DC to induce CTL responses to immune complexes, non-replicating forms of microbes and vaccines, and dying cells (Jensen 2007).

1.1 DC and Promotion of Transplant Tolerance

Evidence implicating DC as the main immunological stimulus for graft rejection was provided by the "parking" experiments of Lechler and Batchelor (Lechler and Batchelor 1982). However, DC may also regulate immune reactivity towards tolerant states and graft acceptance by a variety of mechanisms. These mechanism are most likely not mutually inclusive and include immune deviation (i.e. skewing of T cells to the T helper 2 (Th2) phenotype), inducing or stimulating immune regulation (i.e. induction of regulatory T cells (Treg), such as Foxp3$^+$ CD4$^+$ CD25$^+$ (Fehervari and Sakaguchi 2004) or Treg type-1 (Tr1) cells that make IL-10 (Levings et al. 2005)), and in *bona fide* tolerance, (i.e. deletion or anergy). A wealth of details regarding the regulation of T cells by DC is available in existing reviews (Banchereau and Steinman 1998; Thomson and Lu 1999; Lechler et al. 2001; Lu and Thomson 2001; Morelli et al. 2001; Coates and Thomson 2002; Morelli and Thomson 2003; Steinman et al. 2003; Morelli and Thomson 2007).

Over the past several years, many studies have unveiled the mechanisms by which different subsets of DC induce or maintain tolerance in vivo. Some of these mechanisms have been exploited for the generation of tolerogenic DCs in vitro which, when transferred, induce donor-specific tolerance for therapeutic purposes. Tolerogenic DC are characteristically immature, expressing low surface MHC molecules, a low ratio of co-stimulatory to inhibitory signals, and an impaired ability to synthesize Th1 cell-driving or inflammatory cytokines (Morelli and Thomson 2007). Various anti-inflammatory and immunosuppressant agents have been used to manipulate in vitro-propagated DC. Included are IL-10 and transforming growth factor-β1 (TGF-β1), prostaglandin E2, histamine, and vitamin D3, among others. Additionally, numerous clinically approved or experimental immunosuppressive drugs such as corticosteroids, cyclosporine (CSA), tacrolimus (or FK506), mycophenolate mofetil (MMF), and sanglifehrin A have been used to target DC differentiation and function (Morelli and Thomson 2007).

Of special interest to our lab has been the immune modulator RAPA. This immunosuppressant inhibits the mammalian target of rapamycin (mTOR), a serine or threonine kinase, and impairs the maturation and T cell allostimulatory function of DC. RAPA-conditioned mDC (RAPA-DC) do not display the typical CD86 upregulation induced by TLR ligands (Turnquist et al. 2008) or CD40 (Turnquist et al. 2007). RAPA-DC can enrich the naturally occurring T Treg, whereas their ability to expand CD4$^+$ effector T cells is markedly impaired (Turnquist et al. 2007). Finally, when host-derived RAPA-DC are pulsed with donor antigens and administered to the host prior to transplantation, donor heart graft survival can be prolonged indefinitely (Taner et al. 2005), especially when combined with a short course of RAPA (Turnquist et al. 2007). We will discuss RAPA, its effects on DC and other immune cells, and the therapeutic potential of RAPA-DC in this chapter.

2 Rapamycin

2.1 Discovery and Development

RAPA is a macrocyclic triene antibiotic pro-drug with immunosuppressant properties (Sehgal 1998). RAPA was discovered as a product of the bacterium *Streptomyces hygroscopicus* in a soil sample from Rapa Nui, an island better known as Easter Island. Originally developed as an anti-fungal agent, potent immunosuppressant and anti-proliferative actions prompted investigations into its use as an agent to prevent solid organ rejection. In 1999, it received FDA approval for the prophylaxis of kidney transplant rejection in patients aged 13 years or older (Saunders et al. 2001). Both the immunosuppressive and antiproliferative activities of RAPA are well established, and it is widely used in kidney transplantation and emerging as a treatment for certain oncologic disorders (Kahan and Camardo 2001; Montaner 2007; Altman and Platanias 2008).

2.2 Biochemistry and Mechanism of Actions

RAPA is similar in structure to FK506, and like FK506, forms a complex with the intracellular immunophilin FK506-binding protein 12 (FKBP12) (Sehgal 2003). Unlike FK506, however, the RAPA-FKBP12 gain-in-function complex does not inhibit calcineurin phosphatase activity. Instead, the RAPA-FKBP12 inhibits the function of the mTOR (Sehgal 2003). mTOR is highly conserved, and through the integration of signals arising from growth factors, nutrients, cytokines and cellular stress, regulates critical physiological events, including mRNA translation, cell size, autophagy, and growth (Hay and Sonenberg 2004; Wullschleger et al. 2006; Gao et al. 2007). Downstream targets of mTOR include cyclin D1, MYC avian myelocytomatosis viral oncogene homolog, and hypoxia-inducible factor-1α (Hartford and Ratain 2007). The continued dissection of mTOR regulation of cell activity, including that of innate and adaptive immune cells, is an active and rapidly evolving field.

2.3 Clinical Utilization of RAPA

The well-characterized effects of RAPA on the immune system have obvious implications for numerous immune-mediated conditions, including, but not limited to, graft rejection, autoimmune disease, and graft-versus-host disease (GVHD). Initially, RAPA was considered for its potent activity against *Candida* and *Aspergillus* species though its immunosuppressant effects limited any treatment potential (Hartford and Ratain 2007). The field of transplantation exploited those effects, by using RAPA for the prevention of kidney allograft rejection. RAPA has unique anti-atherogenic and anti-neoplastic properties, can promote immunological tolerance (Li et al. 1999; Wells et al. 1999), and reduces the incidence or severity of chronic allograft nephropathy (Groth et al. 1999; Augustine et al. 2007). RAPA has been shown to prolong allograft survival in many animal models, including solid organ transplantation, bone marrow transplantation and pancreatic islet cell grafting (Sehgal 2003). In humans, the drug was studied initially as an adjunct to CSA and steroids to prevent acute rejection in kidney transplant recipients (Kahan et al. 1999; MacDonald 2001). Subsequent studies have shown its efficacy when combined with a variety of other immunosuppressive agents. RAPA has been long-regarded as a "renal-sparing agent," capable of ameliorating calcineurin inhibitor (CNI)-induced renal toxicity when patients where converted from CNI to RAPA (Sehgal 2003). RAPA's side effect profile, which includes impaired wound healing and hepatic artery thrombosis, has limited its efficacy in *de novo* transplantations.

The anti-proliferative effects of RAPA have been exploited in other areas of medicine. Recent reports have identified RAPA as a potential treatment option in tuberous sclerosis, Huntington disease, and lupus (Lui et al. 2008; Meikle et al. 2008; Zeng et al. 2008). RAPA is also effective for patients with coronary artery stenosis. RAPA-eluting stents, FDA-approved in 2002, show an ability to prevent re-stenosis in coronary angioplasty, without significant changes in mortality or stent-related complications (Gurm et al. 2008). The inhibition of mTOR with RAPA, and its subsequent effect on proliferation, is also a target for anti-cancer drugs in post-transplant malignancies. Guba et al. (Guba et al. 2005) demonstrated the inhibition of primary and metastatic tumor growth by anti-angiogenesis. Conversion to RAPA from MMF, CNI, or azathioprine treatment (and maintained prednisone therapy) in a series of renal allograft recipients resulted in regression of Kaposi's sarcoma and large B cell lymphoma, without compromising graft function (Boratynska et al. 2007). RAPA has also been evaluated for its ability to inhibit GVHD following unrelated or matched related allogeneic stem cell transplant. Following chemotherapy and total body irradiation, patients receiving RAPA and FK506 in place of methotrexate (MTX) as prophylaxis for GVHD had rapid engraftment, a low incidence of GVHD, minimal toxicity, and excellent survival (Cutler et al. 2007).

3 Effects of RAPA on Non-Immune Cells

Due to the central and extensive role of mTOR in cell biology, the effects of RAPA are not limited to cells of the immune system. RAPA inhibits smooth muscle and endothelial cell proliferation, with implications for its use in controlling chronic allograft rejection (Sehgal 2003). Indeed, RAPA arrests the progression of graft vascular disease in a non-human primate model (Ikonen et al. 2000) and slows cardiac transplant vasculopathy in humans (Mancini et al. 2003). Its inhibition of vascular endothelial growth factor (VEGF) has been purported as a potential explanation of its anti-angiogenic properties (Guba et al. 2005).

4 Effects of RAPA on Immune Effector Cells

Inhibition of mTOR results in suppression of cytokine-driven cell proliferation, ribosomal protein synthesis, translation initiation, and cell cycle arrest in the G_1 phase (Raught et al. 2001; Sehgal 2003). Hence, RAPA blocks alloAg- and IL-2-induced T cell proliferation, and lippolysaccharide (LPS) or mitogen-induced B cell proliferation and immunoglobulin production.

4.1 B Cells

RAPA suppresses B cell activity, inhibiting their proliferation and differentiation into plasma cells (Aagaard-Tillery and Jelinek 1994; Kim et al. 1994). RAPA suppresses LPS-induced proliferation of B cells through a calcium-independent pathway. It also inhibits IL-2-dependent and independent proliferation of purified normal human B lymphocytes stimulated with *Staphylococcus aureus* (SA) and soluble CD40L in mid-G1 phase of the cell cycle. Relatedly, RAPA prevents SA and IL-2- or IL-6-dependent differentiation into antibody-producing cells, thereby decreasing the production of immunoglobulins M, G, and A (Luo et al. 1992; Sehgal 2003). There is also recent evidence that RAPA decreases the incidence of donor-specific antibodies in a porcine model of arterial transplantation. This effect is accompanied by a reduction of graft infiltration by macrophages (Rigol et al. 2008).

4.2 T Cells

Unlike other commonly-used immunosuppressive agents, such as the calcineurin inhibitors, which prevent activation-induced cell death by blocking TCR signaling, RAPA allows TCR signaling, but instead impedes CD28 and cytokine/growth factor receptor signaling (Lai and Tan 1994; Mondino and Mueller 2007). Thus, TCR-stimulated T cells undergo apoptosis or become anergic, even in the presence of co-stimulation or proinflammatory cytokines (Wells et al. 1999; Mondino and Mueller 2007). This supports tolerance induction in animal models (Li et al. 1999; Wells et al. 1999; Blaha et al. 2003).

In an early rodent cardiac allograft model, it was observed that RAPA treatment reduced, but did not abolish the induction of Th1 cytokines and preserved the expression of Th2-type cytokines (Wasowska et al. 1996). However, Bundick et al. (Bundick et al. 1995) observed that RAPA inhibited the induction of Th2-polarized chronic GVHD in a murine BM transplant model. RAPA preserves T cell ability to produce IL-2, and seems not to affect negative thymic selection of autoreactive T cells, leaving some immune function intact, and preventing a predilection to autoimmunity produced in mice given a syngeneic bone marrow transplant and treated with CSA (Vogelsang and Hess 1993). Also, the influence of RAPA on memory T cells (Tmem) is equally unclear and has been an area of limited study. Pearl et al. (Pearl et al. 2005) showed that T cell depletion following transplantation facilitates reduced immunosuppressive needs. Naïve T cells and T cells with potential regulatory function were not prevalent following depletion. Instead, post-deletional T cells are of a specific memory phenotype and demonstrate resistance to the effects of RAPA (Pearl et al. 2005).

4.3 Regulatory T Cells

It has been demonstrated repeatedly that both human and mouse Treg (both naturally occurring $CD4^+$ $CD25^+$ $Foxp3^+$ and Tr1 cells) are comparatively insensitive to RAPA compared to naïve effector populations. There is strong evidence for their induction, expansion, and function in the presence of RAPA (Battaglia et al. 2005, 2006a,b,c; Game et al. 2005; Coenen et al. 2006). Of significance, is the recent finding that RAPA can allow the selective expansion of murine naturally-occurring $CD4^+$ $CD25^+$ $Foxp3^+$ Treg, that prevent pancreatic islet allograft rejection (Battaglia et al. 2005). Moreoever, RAPA and IL-10 allow the induction of Tr1 cells that mediate islet transplant tolerance (Battaglia et al. 2006b).

In human studies, RAPA has proven capable of expanding $CD4^+$ $CD25^{hi}$ allosuppressive Treg in culture conditions (Game et al. 2005; Coenen et al. 2006). Relatedly, the Treg facilitating capacity of RAPA was supported when kidney transplant recipients given alemtuzumab induction and maintained on MMF, and receiving either low-dose CSA or RAPA as an adjunct therapy were compared. Those who received RAPA were found to have four-fold higher Treg ($CD4^+$, $CD25^{hi}$) counts than their counterparts which received CSA (Ruggenenti et al. 2007). RAPA also may select for the development of $CD8^+$ $CD103^+$ Treg cells (Uss et al. 2007). When peripheral mononuclear cells isolated from healthy human donors were incubated with allogeneic cells in a five-day MLR in the presence of RAPA, the cells showed an increased level of CD103 expression on $CD8^+$ T cells. CD103 directs T cells to their ligand, E-cadherin, found on renal tubular epithelial cells, among other epithelial cells. $CD8^+$ $CD103^+$ Treg are found in late renal allograft rejection, and are capable of suppressing T cell proliferation in MLR (Uss et al. 2007). Mechanisms behind the preferential expansion of Treg with RAPA remain elusive, though a recent report implicates the serine/threonine kinase, Pim 2 (Basu et al. 2008). Pim 2 was found to be constitutively expressed in freshly isolated resting Tregs, but not in $CD4^+$ $CD25^-$ T effector cells. Its expression was noted to confer resistance to the apoptotic affects of RAPA on Treg.

4.4 Natural Killer Cells

A paucity of data exists as to how innate cells, including natural killer (NK) cells, are affected by the administration of RAPA. It has been demonstrated that in the first 24 h post-transplant, >70% of the lymphocytes in rat liver allografts are NK cells (Obar et al. 2005). Of current relevance is the recent observation that RAPA, unlike CSA or FK506, inhibits NK cell function and NK numbers in vivo (Wai et al. 2008).

5 Immunodulatory Effects of RAPA on Endogenous and BM-Derived DC

There is now considerable evidence that RAPA profoundly impacts rodent and human DC generation, maturation, and typical T cell stimulatory function (Hackstein et al. 2003; Monti et al. 2003; Woltman et al. 2003; Taner et al. 2005; Turnquist et al. 2007; Horibe et al. 2008; Ikeguchi et al. 2008). The *ex vivo* propagation of murine BM-derived mDC in clinically-relevant concentrations of RAPA (RAPA-DC) generates phenotypically iDC with low levels of MHC class II and significantly reduced co-stimulatory molecules (CD40, CD80 and CD86; Fig. 1) compared to the control (CTR-DC) counterparts. This inhibition is IL-4 dependent in murine systems, and can be antagonized by FKBP12 competition (Hackstein et al. 2003). A reduced expression of CD86 persists and decreased allostimulatory capacity persits, even when RAPA-DC are exposed to inflammatory stimuli, such as bacterial LPS, CpG, and CD40 ligation (Turnquist et al. 2008; Hackstein et al. 2003; Taner et al. 2005; Turnquist et al. 2007). This maturation resistance is due, in part, to enhanced expression of ST2L (Turnquist et al. 2008; Brint et al. 2004), a negative regulator of TLR and CD40 signaling (Turnquist et al. 2008; Brint et al. 2004).

5.1 *Cytokine Production by RAPA-DC*

Horibe et al. (Horibe et al. 2008) recently demonstrated decreased production of IL-6 and IL-10 by murine RAPA-DC in response to LPS stimulation, when compared to control (CTR)-DC, generated in the absence of RAPA. While IL-10 production is reduced consistently in RAPA-DC, production of IL-12 by RAPA-DC is more variable, ranging from decreased production to no difference in production when compared to CTR-DC (Monti et al. 2003; Horibe et al. 2008). Our work has shown that DC exposed to RAPA in vivo have a diminished ability to produce IL-12 and TNF-α in response to IL-4 stimulation (Hackstein et al. 2003). Likewise, when generated in culture with RAPA for an extended period, RAPA-exposed DC display decreased expression of IL-12p40 following stimulation with agonistic anti-CD40 mAb (Turnquist et al. 2007). However, it appears that an inhibited production of the IL-12-regulating cytokine, IL-10, by DC exposed to RAPA briefly before LPS stimulation, results in increased IL-12 production by human and murine BM-derived mDC (Ohtani et al. 2008). Thus, regulation of IL-12 production by RAPA-exposed DC and the functional impact of secreted IL-12 is an area that needs further examination.

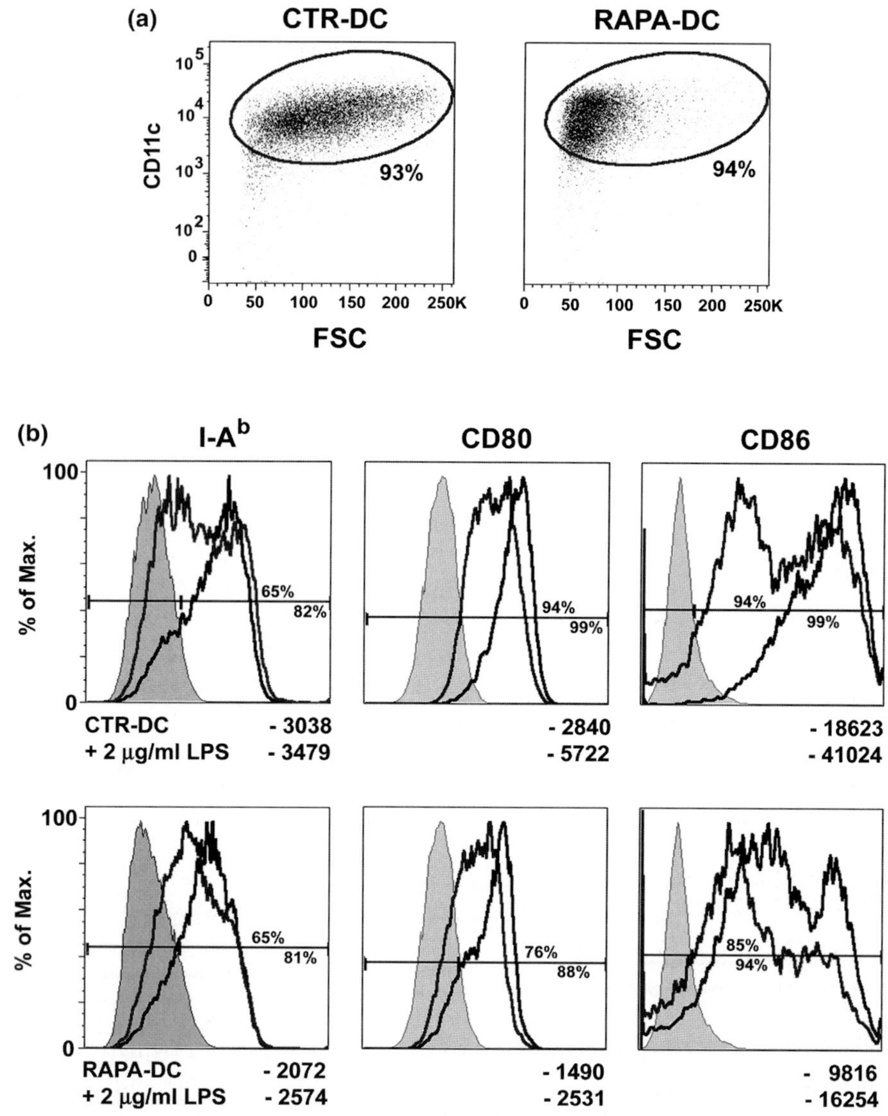

Fig. 1 Phenotypic analysis of RAPA-DC. **(a)** BM-derived DC were generated from C57BL/10 mice with GM-CSF and IL-4 ($1{,}000\,\mathrm{U\,ml^{-1}}$), in the presence (RAPA-DC) of $10\,\mathrm{ng\,ml^{-1}}$ RAPA or in medium alone (control [CTR]-DC). Both CTR-DC and RAPA-DC were purified based on CD11c expression to $>90\%$ from 7 day cultures, and stimulated as indicated for 18 h as indicated with LPS ($2\,\mu\mathrm{g\,ml^{-1}}$). RAPA-DC, compared to CTR-DC are a much more homogenous population with significantly reduced size DC. **(b)** RAPA-DC tend to express lower MHC class II (I-A^b) and greatly reduced CD80 and CD86 compared to CTR-DC. Likewise, compared to CTR-DC, RAPA-DC display inhibited expression of MHC II, CD80, and CD86 following exposure to pro-inflammatory stimuli, such as LPS. Data presented are gated on CD11c$^+$ cells and numbers indicate mean fluorescent intensity (MFI) for each group. *Shaded histograms* = isotype control, *grey histogram* = unstimulated DC, *black histogram* = LPS stimulated

5.2 RAPA-DC and Antigen Presentation

Clinically relevant concentrations of RAPA inhibit macropinocytosis and endocytosis by mouse BM-derived DC, both in vitro and in vivo (Hackstein et al. 2002). Similar changes in phenotype and function have been reported for RAPA-treated human monocyte-derived DC (Monti et al. 2003). RAPA-DC were also shown to express decreased levels of uptake of Ag receptors (mannose receptor, CD32, CD46, and CD91), contributing to decreased endocytosis of labeled dextran (Monti et al. 2003). The precise mechanism behind the inhibition of endocytosis in unclear, but may be related to RAPAs relationship with the p70 S6 kinase, which complexes with the endocytosis-inhibiting Rho Family G proteins Cdc42 and Rac1 (Chou and Blenis 1996). In spite of the impaired endocytosis, alloAg presentation by DC is not blocked through conditioning with RAPA (Taner et al. 2005). Relatedly, DC grown in the presence of RAPA, do not exhibit modifications of MHC class I or II antigen processing pathways (Lee et al. 2005). These pathways, however, are inhibited by the administration of CSA and FK506 (Lee et al. 2005).

5.3 Migration by RAPA-DC

Another important observation has been that both human and murine mDC generated in RAPA, upregulate CCR7 comparable to control counterparts and exhibit unhindered migration to CCL19 and CCL21 and secondary lymphoid tissue (Taner et al. 2005; Sordi et al. 2006; Turnquist et al. 2007). The ability of RAPA-conditioned DC to retain CCR7 expression or regulation and migrate in vivo to the secondary lymphoid tissue, while maintaining a low expression of CD86 and diminished allostimulatory capacity, has important implications for their function as cellular therapy (i.e. 'negative' vaccines; Chaussabel and Banchereau 2005) for prevention of transplant rejection.

5.4 RAPA-DC Stimulation of T Cells

RAPA-DC are weak stimulators of T cells (Fig. 2) and induce hyporesponsiveness (Hackstein et al. 2003; Taner et al. 2005) and apoptosis (Turnquist et al. 2007) in alloreactive T cells. It has been demonstrated that T cells from the spleens of C3H ($H2^k$) mice, primed in vivo by syngeneic RAPA-DC pulsed with alloAg from B10 ($H2^b$) mice, showed markedly reduced proliferative responses to secondary stimulation by both the direct (B10 DC) and indirect (B10 Ag-pulsed C3H DC) pathways (Taner et al. 2005). This response was alloAg-specific, as third party (BALB/c, $H2^d$) DC were able to induce strong responses in the T cell population (Taner et al. 2005). In a rat model of vascularized skin transplantation, T cells derived from skin transplant recipients pre-treated with donor-derived RAPA-DC and induction immunotherapy (lymphocyte depletion and transient CSA

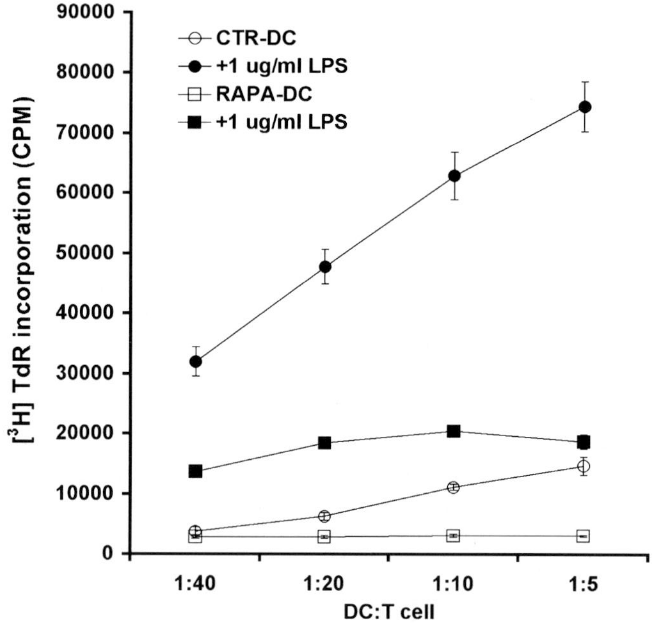

Fig. 2 RAPA-DC display a resistance to functional maturation. As described in Fig. 1, BM-derived DC were generated from BALB/c mice, purified and stimulated for 18 h with 1 μg ml^{-1} LPS. When used as stimulators in 72 h MLR, RAPA-DC displayed markedly reduced allostimulatory activity utilizing bulk B10 T cells as responders

therapy) showed long-term hyporesponsiveness to donor APC. Up to 150 days after transplant, T cells from these animals showed significantly decreased production of IFN-γ and IL-10 after a 4-day MLR when compared to T cells from transplanted animals that had received CTR-DC or donor BM cells (Horibe et al. 2008).

Various reports provide strong evidence that certain DC subsets and pharmacologically-modified DC can expand/induce Treg, with potential for therapy in transplantation (Walsh et al. 2004; Morelli and Thomson 2007). An interesting recent observation has been that RAPA-DC retain the ability to stimulate and enrich for Treg (Turnquist et al. 2007). By contrast, CTR-DC, although able to expand Treg, favor the expansion of non-Treg (Turnquist et al. 2007), especially when the CTR-DC are matured. Importantly, these Treg from RAPA, but not CTR-DC cultures were potent allogAg-specific suppressors of effector proliferation in vitro (Turnquist et al. 2007).

6 RAPA-DC as 'Negative Cellular Vaccines'

Consistent with the above characteristics, alloAg-pulsed, recipient-derived DC have been shown to subvert anti-allograft immune responses in rodent transplant models. We have found that a single systemic infusion of recipient-derived, donor alloAg-pulsed RAPA-DC delivered to mice before transplantation of a fully MHC mismatched heart, prolongs allograft survival significantly (Taner et al. 2005). When the RAPA-DC are given repeatedly without immunosuppression (Taner et al. 2005), or a single infusion is combined with short-term, low dose RAPA (Turnquist et al. 2007) indefinite graft survival is observed. More recently, alloAg-pulsed, recipient derived RAPA-DC, combined with transient immunosuppression (anti-lymphocyte serum and CSA) promoted long-term graft survival in Lewis rats across a full MHC barrier when delivered systemically pre- (Ikeguchi et al. 2008) or post-transplant (Horibe et al. 2008). In these studies, as well as in the previous heart transplant model, $CD4^+$ $Foxp3^+$ T cells were easily identifiable in the long-surviving grafts. Significantly, resistance to transplant rejection could be transferred to naïve animals by infusing $CD4^+$ cells isolated from mice vaccinated with RAPA-DC and with long-surviving heart grafts (Turnquist et al. 2007). These studies provide support for the therapeutic capacity of RAPA-conditioned, BM-derived DC and underscores the potential of RAPA-DC as negative cellular vaccines. It appears that these DC may have the capacity to abrogate/regulate immune responses in an Ag-specific manner, thus inhibiting immune responses to foreign- or self-Ag, while preserving immune responses to unrelated Ag or microbes.

7 Concluding Remarks

DC are uniquely specialized antigen presenting cells that play critical roles in the induction and regulation of immune responses. Their inherent tolerogenic potential is now well-documented. Pharmacologic conditioning of DC with numerous agents has proven successful in creating maturation-resistant, tolerogenic DC. RAPA-conditioned, maturation-resistant DC represent clinically-applicable vectors ('negative cellular vaccines') that can be loaded with donor Ag, with potential for assessment of their therapeutic potential. Future examinations will need to further delineate mechanisms behind experimental observations, and to begin the translation of these technologies to the bedside. We are standardizing culture conditions to generate human RAPA-DC, and have demonstrated that pharmacologically modified non-human primate DC can be generated in numbers that appear clinically relevant to human therapy (Zahorchak et al. 2007). A model in which Ag-pulsed recipient-derived RAPA-DC might be exploited for the induction of tolerance would have a wide range of applications, not only in the field of transplantation (especially for live-donor transplants), but also in the regulation of autoimmunity, GVHD, and other immune-driven disorders.

Acknowledgements Many of studies described were supported by National Institutes of Health (NIH) grants to A.W.T. (R01AI41011 and R01AI60994). In addition, H.R.T. was aided through support from non-concurrent fellowships from the American Society of Transplantation and the NIH (T32CA082084 and F32AI072940).

References

Aagaard-Tillery KM, Jelinek DF (1994) Inhibition of human B lymphocyte cell cycle progression and differentiation by rapamycin. Cell Immunol 156:493–507

Altman JK, Platanias LC (2008) Exploiting the mammalian target of rapamycin pathway in hematologic malignancies. Curr Opin Hematol 15:88–94

Augustine JJ, Bodziak KA, Hricik DE (2007) Use of sirolimus in solid organ transplantation. Drugs 67:369–391

Austyn JM, Hankins DF, Larsen CP, Morris PJ, Rao AS, Roake JA (1994) Isolation and characterization of dendritic cells from mouse heart and kidney. J Immunol 152:2401–2410

Banchereau J, Steinman RM (1998) Dendritic cells and the control of immunity. Nature 392: 245–252

Banchereau J, Briere F, Caux C, Davoust J, Lebecque S, Liu YJ, Pulendran B, Palucka K (2000) Immunobiology of dendritic cells. Annu Rev Immunol 18:767–811

Basu S, Golovina T, Mikheeva T, June CH, Riley JL (2008) Cutting edge: Foxp3-mediated induction of pim 2 allows human T regulatory cells to preferentially expand in rapamycin. J Immunol 180:5794–5798

Battaglia M, Stabilini A, Roncarolo MG (2005) Rapamycin selectively expands $CD4^+$ $CD25^+$ $FoxP3^+$ regulatory T cells. Blood 105:4743–4748

Battaglia M, Stabilini A, Draghici E, Gregori S, Mocchetti C, Bonifacio E, Roncarolo MG (2006a) Rapamycin and interleukin-10 treatment induces T regulatory type 1 cells that mediate antigen-specific transplantation tolerance. Diabetes 55:40–49

Battaglia M, Stabilini A, Draghici E, Migliavacca B, Gregori S, Bonifacio E, Roncarolo MG (2006b) Induction of tolerance in type 1 diabetes via both CD4 + CD25 + T regulatory cells and T regulatory type 1 cells. Diabetes 55:1571–1580

Battaglia M, Stabilini A, Migliavacca B, Horejs-Hoeck J, Kaupper T, Roncarolo MG (2006c) Rapamycin promotes expansion of functional CD4 + CD25 + FOXP3+ regulatory T cells of both healthy subjects and type 1 diabetic patients. J Immunol 177:8338–8347

Blaha P, Bigenzahn S, Koporc Z, Schmid M, Langer F, Selzer E, Bergmeister H, Wrba F, Kurtz J, Kiss C, Roth E, Muehlbacher F, Sykes M, Wekerle T (2003) The influence of immunosuppressive drugs on tolerance induction through bone marrow transplantation with costimulation blockade. Blood 101:2886–2893

Boratynska M, Watorek E, Smolska D, Patrzalek D, Klinger M (2007) Anticancer effect of sirolimus in renal allograft recipients with de novo malignancies. Transplant Proc 39:2736–2739

Brint EK, Xu D, Liu H, Dunne A, McKenzie AN, O'Neill LA, Liew FY (2004) ST2 is an inhibitor of interleukin 1 receptor and Toll-like receptor 4 signaling and maintains endotoxin tolerance. Nat Immunol 5:373–379

Bundick RV, Craggs RI, Holness E (1995) The effect of cyclosporin A, FK506, and rapamycin on the murine chronic graft-versus-host response–an in vivo model of Th2-like activity. Clin Exp Immunol 99:467–472

Chaussabel D, Banchereau J (2005) Dendritic cells, therapeutic vectors of immunity and tolerance. Am J Transplant 5:205–206

Chou MM, Blenis J (1996) The 70 kDa S6 kinase complexes with and is activated by the Rho family G proteins Cdc42 and Rac1. Cell 85:573–583

Coates PT, Thomson AW (2002) Dendritic cells, tolerance induction and transplant outcome. Am J Transplant 2:299–307

Coates PT, Duncan FJ, Colvin BL, Wang Z, Zahorchak AF, Shufesky WJ, Morelli AE, Thomson AW (2004) In vivo-mobilized kidney dendritic cells are functionally immature, subvert alloreactive T-cell responses, and prolong organ allograft survival. Transplantation 77:1080–1089

Coenen JJ, Koenen HJ, van Rijssen E, Hilbrands LB, Joosten I (2006) Rapamycin, and not cyclosporin A, preserves the highly suppressive $CD27^+$ subset of human $CD4^+$ $CD25^+$ regulatory T cells. Blood 107:1018–1023

Cutler C, Li S, Ho VT, Koreth J, Alyea E, Soiffer RJ, Antin JH (2007) Extended follow-up of methotrexate-free immunosuppression using sirolimus and tacrolimus in related and unrelated donor peripheral blood stem cell transplantation. Blood 109:3108–3114

Fehervari Z, Sakaguchi S (2004) Control of Foxp3 + CD25 + CD4+ regulatory cell activation and function by dendritic cells. Int Immunol 16:1769–1780

Game DS, Hernandez-Fuentes MP, Lechler RI (2005) Everolimus and basiliximab permit suppression by human CD4 + CD25+ cells in vitro. Am J Transplant 5:454–464

Gao W, Lu Y, El Essawy B, Oukka M, Kuchroo VK, Strom TB (2007) Contrasting effects of cyclosporine and rapamycin in de novo generation of alloantigen-specific regulatory T cells. Am J Transplant 7:1722–1732

Groth CG, Backman L, Morales JM, Calne R, Kreis H, Lang P, Touraine JL, Claesson K, Campistol JM, Durand D, Wramner L, Brattstrom C, Charpentier B (1999) Sirolimus (rapamycin)-based therapy in human renal transplantation: similar efficacy and different toxicity compared with cyclosporine. Sirolimus European Renal Transplant Study Group. Transplantation 67:1036–1042

Guba M, Yezhelyev M, Eichhorn ME, Schmid G, Ischenko I, Papyan A, Graeb C, Seeliger H, Geissler EK, Jauch KW, Bruns CJ (2005) Rapamycin induces tumor-specific thrombosis via tissue factor in the presence of VEGF. Blood 105:4463–4469

Gurm HS, Boyden T, Welch KB (2008) Comparative safety and efficacy of a sirolimus-eluting versus paclitaxel-eluting stent: a meta-analysis. Am Heart J 155:630–639

Hackstein H, Taner T, Logar AJ, Thomson AW (2002) Rapamycin inhibits macropinocytosis and mannose receptor-mediated endocytosis by bone marrow-derived dendritic cells. Blood 100:1084–1087

Hackstein H, Taner T, Zahorchak AF, Morelli AE, Logar AJ, Gessner A, Thomson AW (2003) Rapamycin inhibits IL-4-induced dendritic cell maturation in vitro and dendritic cell mobilization and function in vivo. Blood 101:4457–4463

Hartford CM, Ratain MJ (2007) Rapamycin: something old, something new, sometimes borrowed and now renewed. Clin Pharmacol Ther 82:381–388

Hay N, Sonenberg N (2004) Upstream and downstream of mTOR. Genes Dev 18:1926–1945

Horibe EK, Sacks J, Unadkat J, Raimondi G, Wang Z, Ikeguchi R, Marsteller D, Ferreira LM, Thomson AW, Lee WP, Feili-Hariri M (2008) Rapamycin-conditioned, alloantigen-pulsed dendritic cells promote indefinite survival of vascularized skin allografts in association with T regulatory cell expansion. Transplant Immunol 18:307–318

Ikeguchi R, Sacks JM, Unadkat JV, Solari M, Horibe EK, Thomson AW, Lee AW, Feili-Hariri M (2008) Long-term survival of limb allografts induced by pharmacologically conditioned, donor alloantigen-pulsed dendritic cells without maintenance immunosuppression. Transplantation 85:237–246

Ikonen TS, Gummert JF, Hayase M, Honda Y, Hausen B, Christians U, Berry GJ, Yock PG, Morris RE (2000) Sirolimus (rapamycin) halts and reverses progression of allograft vascular disease in non-human primates. Transplantation 70:969–975

Jensen PE (2007) Recent advances in antigen processing and presentation. Nature Immunol 8:1041–1048

Kahan BD, Camardo JS (2001) Rapamycin: clinical results and future opportunities. Transplantation 72:1181–1193

Kahan BD, Julian BA, Pescovitz MD, Vanrenterghem Y, Neylan J (1999) Sirolimus reduces the incidence of acute rejection episodes despite lower cyclosporine doses in caucasian recipients of mismatched primary renal allografts: a phase II trial. Rapamune Study Group. Transplantation 68:1526–1532

Kenna TJ, Thomas R, Steptoe RJ (2008) Steady-state dendritic cells expressing cognate antigen terminate memory CD8+ T-cell responses. Blood 111:2091–2100

Kim HS, Raskova J, Degiannis D, Raska K, Jr. (1994) Effects of cyclosporine and rapamycin on immunoglobulin production by preactivated human B cells. Clin Exp Immunol 96:508–512

Lai JH, Tan TH (1994) CD28 signaling causes a sustained down-regulation of I kappa B alpha which can be prevented by the immunosuppressant rapamycin. J Biol Chem 269:30077–30080

Larsen CP, Ritchie SC, Hendrix R, Linsley PS, Hathcock KS, Hodes RJ, Lowry RP, Pearson TC (1994) Regulation of immunostimulatory function and costimulatory molecule (B7–1 and B7–2) expression on murine dendritic cells. J Immunol 152:5208–5219

Lechler RI, Batchelor JR (1982) Restoration of immunogenicity to passenger cell-depleted kidney allografts by the addition of donor strain dendritic cells. J Exp Med 155:31–41

Lechler RI, Ng WF, Steinman RM (2001) Dendritic cells in transplantation – friend or foe? Immunity 14:357–368

Lee YR, Yang IH, Lee YH, Im SA, Song S, Li H, Han K, Kim K, Eo SK, Lee CK (2005) Cyclosporin A and tacrolimus, but not rapamycin, inhibit MHC-restricted antigen presentation pathways in dendritic cells. Blood 105:3951–3955

Levings MK, Gregori S, Tresoldi E, Cazzaniga S, Bonini C, Roncarolo MG (2005) Differentiation of Tr1 cells by immature dendritic cells requires IL-10 but not CD25 + CD4 + Tr cells. Blood 105:1162–1169

Li Y, Li XC, Zheng XX, Wells AD, Turka LA, Strom TB (1999) Blocking both signal 1 and signal 2 of T-cell activation prevents apoptosis of alloreactive T cells and induction of peripheral allograft tolerance. Nat Med 5:1298–1302

Lotze MT, Thomson AW (eds) (2001) Dendritic cells: biology and clinical applications, 2nd edn. Academic Press, London, San Diego, pp. 1–794

Lotze MT, Zeh HJ, Rubartelli A, Sparvero LJ, Amoscato AA, Washburn NR, Devera ME, Liang X, T√∂r M, Billiar T (2007) The grateful dead: damage-associated molecular pattern molecules and reduction/oxidation regulate immunity. Immunol Rev 220:60–81

Lu L, Thomson AW (2001) Dendritic cell tolerogenicity and prospects for dendritic cell-based therapy of allograft rejection and autoimmune disease. In: Lotze MT, Thomson AW (eds) Dendritic cells, 2nd edn. Academic Press, San Diego, pp 587–607

Lui S, Yung S, Tsang R, Zhang F, Chan K, Tam S, Chan T (2008) Rapamycin prevents the development of nephritis in lupus-prone NZB/W F1 mice. Lupus 17:305–313

Luo H, Chen H, Daloze P, Chang JY, St-Louis G, Wu J (1992) Inhibition of in vitro immunoglobulin production by rapamycin. Transplantation 53:1071–1076

MacDonald AS (2001) A worldwide, phase III, randomized, controlled, safety and efficacy study of a sirolimus/cyclosporine regimen for prevention of acute rejection in recipients of primary mismatched renal allografts. Transplantation 71:271–280

Mancini D, Pinney S, Burkhoff D, LaManca J, Itescu S, Burke E, Edwards N, Oz M, Marks AR (2003) Use of rapamycin slows progression of cardiac transplantation vasculopathy. Circulation 108:48–53

Meikle L, Pollizzi K, Egnor A, Kramvis I, Lane H, Sahin M, Kwiatkowski DJ (2008) Response of a neuronal model of tuberous sclerosis to mammalian target of rapamycin (mTOR) inhibitors: effects on mTORC1 and Akt signaling lead to improved survival and function. J Neurosci 28:5422–5432

Mondino A, Mueller DL (2007) mTOR at the crossroads of T cell proliferation and tolerance. Semin Immunol 19:162–172

Montaner S (2007) Akt/TSC/mTOR activation by the KSHV G protein-coupled receptor: emerging insights into the molecular oncogenesis and treatment of Kaposi's sarcoma. Cell Cycle (Georgetown, Tex) 6:438–443

Monti P, Mercalli A, Leone BE, Valerio DC, Allavena P, Piemonti L (2003) Rapamycin impairs antigen uptake of human dendritic cells. Transplantation 75:137–145

Morelli AE, Hackstein H, Thomson AW (2001) Potential of tolerogenic dendritic cells for transplantation. Semin Immunol 13:323–335

Morelli AE, Thomson AW (2003) Dendritic cells: regulators of alloimmunity and opportunities for tolerance induction. Immunol Rev 196:125–146

Morelli AE, Thomson AW (2007) Tolerogenic dendritic cells and the quest for transplant tolerance. Nat Rev Immunol 7:610–621

Obar H, Nagasaki K, Hsieh CL, Ogura Y, Esquivel CO, Martinez OM, Krams SM (2005) IFN-gamma, produced by NK cells that infiltrate liver allografts early after transplantation, links the innate and adaptive immune responses. Am J Transplant 5:2094–2103

Ohtani M, Nagai S, Kondo S, Mizuno S, Nakamura K, Tanabe M, Takeuchi T, Matsuda S, Koyasu S (2008) mTOR and GSK3 differentially regulate LPS-induced IL-12 production in dendritic cells. Blood:43

Pearl JP, Parris J, Hale DA, Hoffmann SC, Bernstein WB, McCoy KL, Swanson SJ, Mannon RB, Roederer M, Kirk AD (2005) Immunocompetent T-cells with a memory-like phenotype are the dominant cell type following antibody-mediated T-cell depletion. Am J Transplant 5:465–474

Raught B, Gingras AC, Sonenberg N (2001) The target of rapamycin (TOR) proteins. Proc Natl Acad Sci USA 98:7037–7044

Rigol M, Solanes N, Sionis A, Galvez C, Martorell J, Rojo I, Brunet M, Ramirez J, Roque M, Roig E, Perez-Villa F, Barquin L, Pomar JL, Sanz G, Heras M (2008) Effects of cyclosporine, tacrolimus and sirolimus on vascular changes related to immune response. J Heart Lung Transplant 27:416–422

Ruggenenti P, Perico N, Gotti E, Cravedi P, D'Agati V, Gagliardini E, Abbate M, Gaspari F, Cattaneo D, Noris M, Casiraghi F, Todeschini M, Cugini D, Conti S, Remuzzi G (2007) Sirolimus versus cyclosporine therapy increases circulating regulatory T cells, but does not protect renal transplant patients given alemtuzumab induction from chronic allograft injury. Transplantation 84:956–964

Sallusto F, Schaerli P, Loetscher P, Schaniel C, Lenig D, Mackay CR, Qin S, Lanzavecchia A (1998) Rapid and coordinated switch in chemokine receptor expression during dendritic cell maturation. Eur J Immunol 28:2760–2769

Saunders RN, Metcalfe MS, Nicholson ML (2001) Rapamycin in transplantation: a review of the evidence. Kidney Int 59:3–16

Sehgal SN (1998) Rapamune (RAPA, rapamycin, sirolimus): mechanism of action immunosuppressive effect results from blockade of signal transduction and inhibition of cell cycle progression. Clin Biochem 31:335–340

Sehgal SN (2003) Sirolimus: its discovery, biological properties, and mechanism of action. Transplant Proc 35:7S–14S

Sordi V, Bianchi G, Buracchi C, Mercalli A, Marchesi F, D'Amico G, Yang CH, Luini W, Vecchi A, Mantovani A, Allavena P, Piemonti L (2006) Differential effects of immunosuppressive drugs on chemokine receptor CCR7 in human monocyte-derived dendritic cells: selective upregulation by rapamycin. Transplantation 82:826–834

Steinman RM, Hawiger D, Nussenzweig MC (2003) Tolerogenic dendritic cells. Annu Rev Immunol 21:685–711

Taner T, Hackstein H, Wang Z, Morelli AE, Thomson AW (2005) Rapamycin-treated, alloantigen-pulsed host dendritic cells induce Ag-specific T cell regulation and prolong graft survival. Am J Transplant 5:228–236

Thomson AW, Lu L (1999) Are dendritic cells the key to liver transplant tolerance? Immunol Today 20:27–32

Turnquist HR, Raimondi G, Zahorchak AF, Fischer RT, Wang Z, Thomson AW (2007) Rapamycin-conditioned dendritic cells are poor stimulators of allogeneic $CD4^+$ T cells, but enrich for antigen-specific $Foxp3^+$ T regulatory cells and promote organ transplant tolerance. J Immunol 178:7018–7031

Turnquist H, Sumpter T, Tsung A, Zahorchak Z, Nakao A, Nau J, Liew F, Geller D, Thomson A (2008) IL-1beta-driven ST2L expression promotes maturation resistance in rapamycin-conditioned dendritic cells. J Immunol 181:62–72

Ueno H, Klechevsky E, Morita R, Aspord C, Cao T, Matsui T, Di Pucchio T, Connolly J, Fay JW, Pascual V, Palucka AK, Banchereau J (2007) Dendritic cell subsets in health and disease. Immunolo Rev 219:118–142

Uss E, Yong SL, Hooibrink B, van Lier RA, ten Berge IJ (2007) Rapamycin enhances the number of alloantigen-induced human CD103 + CD8+ regulatory T cells in vitro. Transplantation 83:1098–1106

Vogelsang GB, Hess AD (1993) Rapamycin effects on immunologic reconstitution. Transplant Proc 25:727–728

Wai LE, Fujiki M, Takeda S, Martinez OM, Krams SM (2008) Rapamycin, but not cyclosporine or FK506, alters natural killer cell function. Transplantation 85:145–149

Walsh PT, Taylor DK, Turka LA (2004) Tregs and transplantation tolerance. J Clin Invest 114:1398–1403

Wasowska B, Wieder KJ, Hancock WW, Zheng XX, Berse B, Binder J, Strom TB, Kupiec-Weglinski JW (1996) Cytokine and alloantibody networks in long term cardiac allografts in rat recipients treated with rapamycin. J Immunol 156:395–404

Wells AD, Li XC, Li Y, Walsh MC, Zheng XX, Wu Z, Nunez G, Tang A, Sayegh M, Hancock WW, Strom TB, Turka LA (1999) Requirement for T-cell apoptosis in the induction of peripheral transplantation tolerance. Nat Med 5:1303–1307

Woltman AM, van der Kooij SW, Coffer PJ, Offringa R, Daha MR, van Kooten C (2003) Rapamycin specifically interferes with GM-CSF signaling in human dendritic cells, leading to apoptosis via increased $p27^{KIP1}$ expression. Blood 101:1439–1445

Woo J, Lu L, Rao AS, Li Y, Subbotin V, Starzl TE, Thomson AW (1994) Isolation, phenotype, and allostimulatory activity of mouse liver dendritic cells. Transplantation 58:484–491

Wullschleger S, Loewith R, Hall MN (2006) TOR signaling in growth and metabolism. Cell 124:471–484

Zahorchak AF, Kean LS, Tokita D, Turnquist HR, Abe M, Finke J, Hamby K, Rigby MR, Larsen CP, Thomson AW (2007) Infusion of stably immature monocyte-derived dendritic cells plus CTLA4Ig modulates alloimmune reactivity in rhesus macaques. Transplantation 84:196–206

Zeng LH, Xu L, Gutmann DH, Wong M (2008) Rapamycin prevents epilepsy in a mouse model of tuberous sclerosis complex. Ann Neurol 63:444–453

Zheng Y, Zha Y, Gajewski T (2008) Molecular regulation of T-cell anergy. EMBO reports 9:50–55

Handbook of Experimental Pharmacology "Dendritic Cells"

The Use of Dexamethasone in the Induction of Tolerogenic DCs

Cees van Kooten, Annelein S. Stax, Andrea M. Woltman, and Kyra A. Gelderman

Contents

Abstract Dendritic cells (DCs) have a central role in immune regulation, ranging from tolerance induction to the induction of specific immune responses. DCs serve as an essential link between innate and adaptive immunity. This broad range of powerful immune stimulatory as well as regulatory functions has made DCs as targets for vaccine development strategies. One approach to promote the tolerogenicity of

---

C. van Kooten (✉)
Leiden University Medical Center, Department of Nephrology, C3P, Albinusdreef 2, P.O. Box 9600, NL-2300RC Leiden, The Netherlands
C.van_Kooten@lumc.nl

G. Lombardi, Y. Riffo-Vasquez (eds.), *Dendritic Cells,* Handbook of Experimental Pharmacology 188,

DCs is to suppress their maturation by pharmacological agents, including glucocorticoids (GCs). In the present chapter we will review GCs used in vitro with cultured DCs, applied in vivo, or used to generate tolerogenic DCs for cellular therapy.

1 Introduction

Dendritic cells (DCs) are bone marrow-derived cells that populate all lymphoid and nonlymphoid organs. They have a central role in immune regulation, ranging from tolerance induction and the prevention of autoimmunity to the induction of antitumor immunity and the protection against infectious agents. Although DCs are a heterogeneous group of cells that represent differences in origin, anatomic location, cell surface phenotype, and function, they all have potent antigen presenting capacity for stimulating naive, memory, effector and/or regulatory T cells. Therefore, DCs serve as an essential link between innate and adaptive immune responses (Banchereau and Steinman 1998; Steinman and Banchereau 2007).

This broad range of powerful immune stimulatory and regulatory functions has made DCs targets for vaccine development strategies. This includes cellular vaccination for treatment of cancer or infectious diseases, as well as "negative vaccination" for the treatment of autoimmune diseases and prevention of allograft rejections. The latter can be accomplished by inhibiting the immunostimulatory capacity of DCs, or more importantly, exploiting tolerogenic DCs to specifically silence immune responses. One approach to promote the tolerogenicity of DCs is to suppress their maturation using antiinflammatory cytokines or pharmacological agents or genetically engineered DCs expressing immunosuppressive molecules, as recently reviewed by several groups (Hackstein and Thomson 2004; Woltman and van Kooten 2003; Adorini et al. 2004; Morelli and Thomson 2007). One class of agents that have shown promising effects on prevention of DC maturation, and widely applicable are glucocorticoids (GC). In the present chapter we will specifically focus on the use of GC, either in vitro in cell cultures or applied in vivo, or used to generate tolerogenic DCs for cellular therapy.

2 Glucocorticoids

Glucocorticoids (GC) are among the most potent immunosuppressive and anti inflammatory drugs currently available and are efficacious in the treatment of both Th-1 and Th-2 associated inflammatory diseases, including allograft rejection, rheumatoid arthritis and asthma (Wilckens and De Rijk 1997). The therapeutic effects of GC were initially ascribed to the strong inhibitory effect on T cells. At the moment, however, it is obvious that also antigen presenting cells (APC) are strongly affected by GC. It has been demonstrated that GC downregulates the production of proinflammatory cytokines by monocytes and macrophages and also affect DC function; the subject of the present review. Various derivatives of GC are used in clinical practice and, as far as we know, there are no differences in the functional effects on DCs between the different compounds, although their in vivo efficacy might be different. Most experimental studies have used dexamethasone (Dex), but other GC have shown similar effects.

Next to exogenously administered GC, endogenous GC also plays an important physiological role. It is recognized that GC are an essential link between the central nervous system and regulation of the innate immune system (Sternberg 2006). Endogenous GC exist in two different forms, being either the active 11-hydroxy (cortisol) or the inactive 11-keto (cortisone) form. Regulation of endogenous GC activity is fine-tuned by an intracellular conversion through the enzyme 11β-hydroxysteroid dehydrogenase (11β-HSD) whereas the type-2 form of this enzyme (highly expressed in kidney and fetus) can inactivate cortisol via dehydrogenation. The type-1 enzyme has reductase activity and generates cortisol from cortisone. This process is also known as the cortisol-cortisone shuttle. Both cortisol and cortisone are normally present in serum in concentrations ranging from 10^{-7}–10^{-9} M, mostly with an excess of inactive cortisone (Sternberg et al. 1992).

Recently, it was shown that immature DCs start to express functional 11β-HSD1 when developing in vitro from human monocytes or from mouse bone marrow cells (Zhang et al. 2005; Freeman et al. 2005). When physiological concentrations of inactive cortisone are added to DC cultures, this inhibits DC activation through local generation of cortisol, an effect which could be prevented by an 11β-HSD inhibitor. This suggests that immature monocyte-derived DCs are biased towards maintenance of the immature state. Maturation induced by CD40L activation, as a mimic of T cell-mediated signals, resulted in a strong decrease in 11β-HSD activity. In contrast, 'innate maturation' induced by TNF-α or a panel of different TLR ligands showed no effect or negligible enhancement of 11β-HSD activity (Freeman et al. 2005). This suggests that especially CD40L-matured DC actively prevents the generation of endogenous GC. This adds important information to recent findings that different modes of DC activation result in different stages of maturation (Reis E Sousa 2006).

3 Immunoregulatory Effects of Dexamethasone

3.1 In Vitro Analysis of Dex-Mediated Effects

Dexamethasone and other GC have been widely investigated for their immune modulatory effects on dendritic cells. Results described in the literature have been obtained with dendritic cells from different origins, directly isolated or generated in vitro mostly from either peripheral monocytes (in the case of humans) or from bone marrow precursors (for mice and rats). Although there are many similarities between the modulating activities on these different DC subsets, we will indicate where specific effects have been observed. Furthermore, the modulating effects of Dex and other GC have demonstrated large resemblance to agents like Vitamin D3 or IL-10. These factors will be discussed in separate chapters and are therefore outside the scope of this present review. However, where relevant, we will indicate specific differences between these modulating agents.

3.2 Morphological and Phenotypic Characteristics

A consistent finding has been the inhibitory effect of GC on the development of immature DCs from monocytes or bone marrow precursors. The GC-treated human monocytes retain a monocyte/macrophage phenotype with high CD14 expression and no expression of CD1a, as a typical DC marker, but also lack expression of CD68, as one of the typical macrophage markers (Piemonti et al. 1999b; Canning et al. 2000; Woltman et al. 2000). However, these cells do express the DC marker DC-SIGN (Woltman et al. 2006). Treatment of monocyte-derived DC (moDC) with Dex decreased DC-SIGN expression, whereas it dose-dependently increases MGL/ASGPR (recognizing terminal GalNAc) expression. This effect was not seen with IL-10 treated DC (van Vliet et al. 2006a, b).

We have shown that addition of GC to monocyte cultures for a minimum of 48 h completely prevented normal DC development upon a 7-day culture period in GM-CSF and IL-4 (Woltman et al. 2000). A similar durable immature state was shown by others and suggested to be the result of high endogenous IL-10 production (Xia et al. 2005).

Glucocorticoids also inhibited various aspects of maturation of DCs, when applied to already differentiated immature DCs. However, the strength of inhibition seemed to be dependent on the type of maturation signal, ranging from strong inhibition of LPS- or cytokine-induced maturation (Piemonti et al. 1999b; de Jong et al. 1999; Vieira et al. 1998; Vanderheyde et al. 1999; Manome et al. 2000; Matasic et al. 1999) to variable inhibition of CD40L-induced maturation (Piemonti et al. 1999b; de Jong et al. 1999; Vanderheyde et al. 1999; Rea et al. 2000).

Glucocorticoids have similar effects on different types of DC. Addition of GC also prevented the development of interstitial DCs from human $CD34^+$ precursors by specific induction of apoptosis in $CD14^+$-DC precursors and blocked differentiation of $CD14^+$-DC precursors into fully differentiated $CD1a^+$ interstitial DCs (Woltman et al. 2002). In a slightly different culture system, also starting with cord blood precursors, a similar dramatic effect on DC development and induction of apoptosis was observed (Mainali and Tew 2004). In contrast, in the described culture system starting with $CD34^+$ cells, Langerhans cells (LC) developed normally and showed comparable functional activities (IL-12 production and T cell stimulation), even when exposed to GC for the whole 12-day culture period (Woltman et al. 2002). This shows that not all DC subsets are equally sensitive for GC treatment.

3.3 Apoptosis Induction by Glucocorticoids

Contradictory results exist on the effect of glucocorticoids on the survival of human DCs in vitro. Glucocorticoids were shown to induce caspase-independent apoptosis in immature moDCs (Kim et al. 2001), although several other studies did not find any apparent apoptosis in moDCs (Woltman et al. 2000; Matasic et al. 1999; Vanderheyde et al. 1999). However, strong indications for GC-induced apoptosis in vivo were found in rats treated with Dex. These animals showed decreased numbers of airway DCs preceded and accompanied by an increase in apoptotic cells (Brokaw et al. 1998). Moreover, in mice, epicutaneous application of CS resulted in decreased numbers of LC in the skin and a reduced MHC class II expression on these cells. Although a direct in situ induction of apoptosis in the skin was demonstrated, it may have been an indirect effect via inhibition of GM-CSF production by keratinocytes (Hoetzenecker et al. 2004). More convincing results for a proapoptotic action of GC have been obtained with DC precursors (see Sect. 3.2) and with plasmacytoid DC (see Sect. 4.2) (Boor et al. 2006).

3.4 Antigen Uptake Machinery

Glucocorticoid treatment of DCs increased the endocytic and pinocytic activity of these cells, partially because of an up-regulation of mannose receptors (Piemonti et al. 1999a). Also in macrophages, it was shown that GC increased phagocytosis of apoptotic cells, which was associated with cytoskeletal changes including absence of phosphorylation of paxillin/pyk2 and an increased Rac activation (Giles et al. 2001).

3.5 Costimulatory Molecules and T Cell Stimulation

Upon stimulation of Dex-treated DCs, these cells were strongly hampered in their up-regulation of costimulatory and MHC molecules (Piemonti et al. 1999b; Woltman et al. 2000). This reduced expression was observed with different modes of activation, including proinflammatory cytokines, LPS or CD40L and cannot be explained by a reduced receptor expression. In fact, TLR2, TLR3, and TLR4 (the LPS receptor) are even expressed at a higher level on GC-treated dendritic cells (Duperrier et al. 2005; Rozkova et al. 2006). Although Dex DCs express lower levels of the costimulatory molecules CD80 and CD86, compared to control DC these cells express higher levels of the B7 family member, B7-H1 (Duperrier et al. 2005; Woltman et al. 2006). As a consequence, Dex DCs become poor stimulators of allogeneic T cells (Piemonti et al. 1999b; Woltman et al. 2000). Moreover, T cells recovered from this primary stimulation showed a hyporesponsiveness upon secondary challenge. This poor stimulatory capacity of dexDCs could be restored either by applying activating signals (antiCD28 and supernatant of activated control DCs) or by blocking the immune regulatory molecules B7-H1 and IL-10 (Woltman et al. 2006). Importantly, induction of hyporesponsiveness was observed both in naive and memory T cells and was operational in the absence of natural regulatory T cells. Hyporesponsiveness was observed for proliferative responses, especially when IFN-γ production was strongly suppressed. This points towards a role for cytokines produced by activated DCs, since these are a determining factor for the development of different functional T cell subsets.

3.6 Cytokines

Activation of Dex-treated DCs results in a reduced production of proinflammatory cytokines, including IL-6, TNF-α, IL-1β, and IL-12 (Piemonti et al. 1999b; Woltman et al. 2000; Vieira et al. 1998; Rea et al. 2000). Importantly, the same conditions result in an increased production of the antiinflammatory cytokine IL-10. It is thought that the balance between IL-10 and IL-12 is important for the outcome of T cell activation. Dex-treated DC showed high expression of the phosphorylated form of the ERK kinase and IL-10 production was inhibited by the ERK inhibitor PD98059 (Xia et al. 2005). An increased IL-10 production after treatment with Dex has been observed in other cells, including monocytes (Mozo et al. 2004; Visser et al. 1998).

Also the production of other cytokines and chemokines is affected by treatment with GC. CCL18 is a chemokine which has been associated with alternatively activated macrophages. Along with this, IL-10 and VitD3 were shown to increase CCL18 expression by human immature moDC. Surprisingly, under similar conditions, Dex inhibited the production of CCL18 by DCs (Vulcano et al. 2003). Using murine DC, Dex was shown to inhibit MIP-1α and MCP-1 production (protein and mRNA), whereas production of both chemokines was stimulated by VitD3 (Xing et al. 2002).

3.7 Interaction between T Cells and DC

Although control DC showed an upregulation of costimulatory molecules upon contact with allogeneic T cells, this was not observed for Dex-DC, confirming that they were resistant to maturation signals and "frozen" in an immature state (Woltman et al. 2006). When various drugs were investigated for their capacity to interfere with functional DC–T cell interactions, Dex was found to be most efficient (Matsue et al. 2002). Interestingly, coculture of APC with regulatory T cells was shown to directly affect the APC function, with decreased MHC class II and CD80/CD86 expression on murine BM-DC (Vendetti et al. 2000) and generation of alternatively activated human monocytes/macrophages with increased expression of CD206/MR, CD163, CCL18 and phagocytic capacity (Tiemessen et al. 2007).

3.8 Molecular Effects of Dex – Signaling and Other Gene Products

Both for Dex and IL10, GILZ (glucocorticoid induced leucine zipper) was identified as a gene induced in DCs, which was both necessary and sufficient to mediate Dex effects including increased expression of B7H1 and ILT3. (Cohen et al. 2006). Various studies have shown that also in DCs, Dex can inhibit NF-kB activation, and down stream signals like NO and ROS (Tan et al. 2005; Vital et al.

2003). The NF-kB transcription factor has been used as a specific target for the generation of tolerogenic DCs (Li et al. 2007). Similar, NF-kB directed mechanisms have been proposed as effector pathways upon treatment with IL-10 and VitD3, although subtle biological differences with different agents have been observed. One explanation might be that the NF-kB pathway consists of different family members, which might not be equally affected by these agents and which have been shown to regulate different biological functions of DCs (Ouaaz et al. 2002).

Dex treatment in vivo was shown to induce GITR on CD4 T cells and GITRL on pDC, and interaction between these members of the TNF-TNFR family drive the generation of IDO as an important immunosuppressive mechanism (Grohmann et al. 2007). This action of Dex seems to be mediated through inhibition of the noncanonical NF-kB pathway.

Recently, there has been an interest in linking between dendritic cells and the production of components of the Complement system (Castellano et al. 2004). It was shown that Dex increased expression of two described receptors for C1q (gC1qR and cC1qR)(Vegh et al. 2003) and moderately increased mRNA levels of C3 (Reis et al. 2006). Moreover, mDC (but not pDC) are a source of the long pentraxin PTX3 after activation with LPS or CD40L. This production is inhibited by addition of Dex and VitD3 but enhanced by IL10 (Doni et al. 2006). The relevance of complement components for the antiinflammatory functions of dexDC is at present unclear.

3.9 Molecular Effects of Dex – Gene Arrays

To achieve a genome wide view on the effects of Dex on gene expression profiles, microarray analysis has been applied to LPS and Dex-treated murine D1 cells (Vizzardelli et al. 2006). Apart from clustering of differentially expressed genes, two issues obtained specific attention. Dex inhibited induction of CCR7 expression, and as a functional consequence interfered with the DC migratory capacity in vivo. Moreover, combinations of LPS and Dex resulted in a synergistic induction of lipocalin 24p3, a gene previously implicated in the induction of T cell apoptosis. However, the role of this protein in the tolerogenic function of dex-treated DCs remains to be determined.

3.10 The Use of Dendritic Cell Lines

For some type of investigations, such as transfection studies, and biochemistry with a large number of cells and reproducibility between different labs – the use of cell lines of DC origin have been an attractive option. Using a mouse epidermal derived cell line XS52, the first modulating effects of glucocorticoids have been described (Kitajima et al. 1996). The mouse cell line D1, derived from growth factor dependent long-term cultures, has been widely used, and has been instrumental in showing the modulating effects of Dex (Matyszak et al. 2000). They have also been used for molecular profiling (Vizzardelli et al. 2006). Recently a new murine cell line was described resembling DCs (SP37A3), and treatment of these cells with Dex, induced tolerogenic characteristics with strongly reduced T cell proliferation and IFN-γ production, but an intact IL-10 and IL-4 response (Bros et al. 2007). At the mRNA level, Dex treatment reduced IL-12 and Ox40L, but increased FcγRIIB and IL1RA expression.

For the human, KG-1 cells have been used as a model (Bharadwaj et al. 2005). Also the human $CD34^{+}$AML cell line (MUTZ-3) has been demonstrated to have the potential to differentiate into interstitial DC and Langerhans cells, characterized by DC-SIGN vs Langerin and Birbeck granules, respectively (Santegoets et al. 2006). For these human cell lines, there is no information on the modulating effects of GC.

4 Effects of In Vivo Glucocorticoid Treatment on DC

The strong effects of GC on DC biology and the widely used clinical application of this drug make it tempting to speculate the therapeutic use of GC, not to mention that its important antiinflammatory actions might also be partially mediated by effects on DC. The characterization of specific markers on DC populations in blood and specific staining strategies using multicolor FACS analysis have made it possible to directly investigate this question.

4.1 In Vivo Effects of GC in Inflammatory Disorders

High dose GC treatment is a first line therapy in several autoimmune and inflammatory disorders. A very dramatic decrease of mDC and pDC numbers was observed at day 4, after a 3-day course of intraveneous GC (1 g/day) in 20 patients with various inflammatory diseases (Suda et al. 2003). Interestingly, 4 days later, most of the circulating mDC pool had been reconstituted, whereas pDC numbers were still strongly reduced. On one hand, high dose GC treatment in patients with Immune Thrombocytopenic Purpura (ITP), administered with oral dexamethasone 40 mg[1] per day for 4 days, also show a reduction in pDC numbers, but an increase in mDC numbers at the end of therapy (Ling et al. 2007). On the other hand, others found that ITP patients treated with prednisone showed reduced numbers of mDC and pDC (Hsu et al. 2004). Finally, high dose CS Solu Medrol resulted in decreased mDC and strongly reduced pDC in circulation of 5 patients who had systemic onset, juvenile idiopathic arthritis (Rozkova et al. 2006).

4.2 In Vivo Effects of GC in Transplantation

Also in transplantation, several groups have monitored DC subsets in blood and have tried to correlate this to the applied immunosuppressive regimen. In these cases interpretation is complicated by the fact that different combinations of drugs are commonly used. Moreover, the surgical procedure might also have an impact and results in decreased DC numbers in circulation, as shown in donors of living organ donation (Hesselink et al. 2005). Finally, it cannot be excluded that transplantation of different organs might have different impact on the pool of circulating DC.

In a large study, comparing 87 renal transplant recipients with 87 matched controls, it was clearly demonstrated that long term IS showed a negative impact on the number of circulating DCs (Hackstein et al. 2005). This was observed both for myeloid and plasmacytoid DC, although strongest effects were seen on pDC numbers. When the relative contribution of individual drugs was analyzed (with 53% of patients using GC), a strong relation between GC use and reduced pDC numbers was observed.

In a group of kidney/pancreas recipients, no difference in mDC numbers was observed when compared to controls. However, circulating cells did show reduced expression of costimulatory molecules but a normal responsiveness upon activation (Sebelin et al. 2006). In addition, the development of MoDC occurred was comparable to controls. Circulating mDC numbers were found to be lower in 12 transplant recipients after more than 3 years of prednisone + tacrolimus therapy (Macedo et al. 2005). In this case, DC generated from monocytes of these patients showed less maturation upon activation.

Several groups have investigated pDC and mDC numbers in cadaver-liver transplant recipients. Initially it was shown that successful weaning of IS was associated with a high DC2/DC1 ratio (Mazariegos et al. 2003). When the effect of prednisone dose was investigated, this was associated with a nonsignificant decrease in absolute DC numbers, and has no effect on the DC2/DC1 ratio (Mazariegos et al. 2005). However, both mDC and pDC were reduced in liver transplant recipients, which seemed to normalize with GC withdrawal, but not with calcineurin inhibitor withdrawal (Bosma et al. 2007). In vitro, there was no indication of apoptosis of mDC, whereas this was observed with pDC. Circulating mDC in patients showed reduced expression of costimulatory molecules, however, they showed a normal responsiveness and maturation upon ex vivo activation.

4.3 In Vivo Effects of GC on Tissue Distribution of DC

Although at first glance, there might still be some controversy, it is safe to conclude that GC treatment certainly affects the pool of circulating DCs, with especially very prominent effects on the pDC population. However, a potential drawback of the presented analysis is the fact that mostly blood has been used for monitoring. This leaves the option that treatment interferes with migration and retention of the cells in lymphoid or nonlymphoid organs. Therefore, these results should be combined with analysis at the tissue level. Recently it was shown that Dex administration in mouse also resulted in reduced pDC levels in spleen, liver and LN (Abe and Thomson 2006). Similarly, mice treated with Dex demonstrated relatively decreased splenic DC numbers and increased splenic macrophage numbers (Moser et al. 1995). This shift in the myeloid cellular compartment of the spleen upon Dex-treatment might be caused by an altered differentiation process of myeloid progenitor cells. In addition, GC administration to *Rhesus macaques* also changed DC subsets in lymph nodes (Koopman et al. 2001). Recently, we were able to characterize and quantify both mDC and pDC in human renal tissue (Woltman et al. 2007). These methods will allow the investigation of changes in composition of DC subsets in transplanted organs upon different immunosuppressive strategies.

5 In Vivo Use of Dex-DC

In view of the critical role of DC in immune regulation, these cells hold a great potential for cellular immunotherapy. This can work in the directions of powerful stimulation of the immune response, as desired in tumor therapy or in vaccination strategies against infectious agents. However, also for negative vaccination, i.e. suppression of specific immune responses, DC might be useful in situations of autoimmunity or transplantation. In the latter case, controlling the maturation stage of the DC is of critical importance. Based on the in vitro findings, Dex has been used to freeze DC in an immature state and investigate their tolerogenicity in vivo.

5.1 In Vivo Use of Dex-DC in Autoimmunity

Evidence that DCs can be used or manipulated to combat autoimmune diseases has come initially from studies in experimental models of type 1 diabetes and multiple sclerosis (Ludewig et al. 2001; Feili-Hariri et al. 1999). Prevention of experimental autoimmune diseases can be achieved by transferring manipulated syngeneic DCs, such as semimature tumor necrosis factor α (TNF-α)-treated DCs, interferon γ (IFN-γ)-treated DCs, and CTLA4Ig-treated DCs. (Shinomiya et al. 1999; Link et al. 2001; Menges et al. 2002). More recently, a side-by-side comparison has been made for the use of Dex-DC, IL-10-DC, and TNF-DC, in the prevention of collagen induced arthritis (van Duivenvoorde et al. 2007). Interestingly, all the three cell types were able to interfere with disease induction, but their molecular mechanisms appeared to be different, as shown by differential regulation of the notch family members delta 4 and jagged1, difference in the control of antibody responses against collagen and the induction of cytokine response (especially IL-10 and IL-5) by antigen specific T cells. In these experiments, Dex treatment was combined with LPS activation, a concept also used in the context of transplantation and referred to as “alternatively activated” DC.

5.2 *In Vivo Use of Dex-DC in Transplantation*

In transplantation, DCs have been used for cell-based therapies to prolong allograft survival or even more importantly to induce donor-specific tolerance. Mice pretreated with donor-derived immature DCs showed prolonged allograft survival in models of pancreatic islet and heart transplantation (Rastellini et al. 1995; Lutz et al. 2000; Fu et al. 1996). Similarly, the regulatory role of DCs was shown by adoptive transfer of allopeptide-loaded recipient-derived lymphoid and myeloid DCs, which were able to prolong cardiac and islet allograft survival in rat transplantation models (Garrovillo et al. 2001; Oluwole et al. 2001).

In view of the need to control DC maturation, and the fear that use of immature DC could result in further maturation after administration, these cells have been treated with several of the modulating agents as described above. Several studies have used the fully mismatched combination of C57BL/6 to Balb/c transplantation in mice. Pretreatment with 10E6 Dex-treated D1 cells (a DC cell line of BL/6 origin) resulted in prolonged skin graft survival from 17 to 35 days, whereas third party skins were rejected with the same speed (Roelen et al. 2003). DCs used for treatment were treated with Dex from day 6 onwards, whereas LPS in addition was included from day 7 for the last 48 h. A similar model and approach was used in a heart transplantation model. Pretreatment with alternatively activated LPS-Dex DC generated from donor bone marrow prolonged heart allograft survival from 10 to 20 days (Emmer et al. 2006). This prolongation was not observed when Dex-DCs were used without LPS activation. The requirement for activation of the tolerogenic DC to obtain optimal effects was also demonstrated with other modes of DC modulation (IL-10 + TGF-β) (Lan et al. 2006). Interestingly, heart allograft prolongation was also obtained when immDC were combined with Dex treatment in vivo, however, this was successful only when Dex was added after, but not before, the transplantation procedure (Emmer et al. 2006). In contrast, administration of LPS-Dex-DC of donor origin was not able to prevent rejection of fully mismatched or haploidentical stem cells (Vanclee et al. 2006).

We have recently investigated the ability of tolerogenic donor DC to prolong renal allograft survival in two fully mismatched rat models (BN to LEW and DA to LEW). Using LPS activated Dex-treated donor DC, which displayed tolerogenic properties in vitro, we were able to induce donor specific unresponsiveness in the recipient; however, this did not result in prolonged graft survival (Stax, manuscript in preparation). Nevertheless, indefinite renal graft survival has been induced in rats using a DC vaccination strategy. In this case, F1 DC (LEW x AUG) were administered to LEW recipients in combination with CTLA4-Ig treatment 10 days before transplantation and recipients were treated with CsA (10 mg kg^{1} per day) for the first 10 days after transplantation (Mirenda et al. 2004). This conditioning resulted in the development of T cell anergy and induction of allo-specific, self-restricted regulatory T cells and a completely normal histology at day 100. Importantly, these results could not be observed when donor DC, treated and applied in the same way, or when mature nonDex-treated F1 DCs were used (Mirenda et al. 2004). Therefore, this study has important implications: (1) a cotreatment with CTLA4-Ig together with cellular therapy might be important to prevent an immunogenic re presentation of injected cells by APC of the recipient. (2) cotreatment at the time of transplantation might be required to suppress immunity and inflammation at the time of transplantation. (3) the superior effect of F1 DC points to the importance of controlling both direct and indirect pathway of antigen presentation (4) the induction of a regulatory network is compatible with a short term treatment of CsA.

6 Concluding Remarks

For ethical reasons, cellular therapy in a clinical setting has to be applied in combination with standard immunosuppressive strategies. Although it has been suggested that calcineurin inhibitors are detrimental for tolerance induction, results described above suggest that this will not always be the case. However, rapamycin which is often considered a protolerogenic drug, was shown to prevent graft prolongation induced by immature bone marrow derived DC (Peche et al. 2005). Similarly, dexamethasone treatment in vivo was shown to inhibit the induction of oral tolerance (Stock et al. 2005). Therefore, despite the overwhelming information of protolerogenic effects of Dex as discussed in this review, more detailed information on the regulation and fine tuning of immune responses is required before tolerogenic cell therapy can be reliably and safely introduced into clinical practice.

References

Abe M, Thomson AW (2006) Dexamethasone preferentially suppresses plasmacytoid dendritic cell differentiation and enhances their apoptotic death. Clin Immunol 118:300–306

Adorini L, Giarratana N, Penna G (2004) Pharmacological induction of tolerogenic dendritic cells and regulatory T cells. Semin Immunol 16:127–134

Banchereau J, Steinman RM (1998) Dendritic cells and the control of immunity. Nature 392: 245–252

Bharadwaj U, Zhang R, Yang H, Li M, Doan LX, Chen C, Yao Q (2005) Effects of cyclophilin A on myeloblastic cell line KG-1 derived dendritic like cells (DLC) through p38 MAP kinase activation. J Surg Res 127:29–38

Boor PP, Metselaar HJ, Mancham S, Tilanus HW, Kusters JG, Kwekkeboom J (2006) Prednisolone suppresses the function and promotes apoptosis of plasmacytoid dendritic cells. Am J Transplant 6:2332–2341

Bosma BM, Metselaar HJ, Tra WM, Mancham S, Kuipers EJ, Tilanus HW, Kwekkeboom J (2007) Impairment of circulating myeloid dendritic cells in immunosuppressed liver transplant recipients. Clin Exp Immunol 149:525–534

Brokaw JJ, White GW, Baluk P, Anderson GP, Umemoto EY, McDonald DM (1998) Glucocorticoid-induced apoptosis of dendritic cells in the rat tracheal mucosa. Am J Respir Cell Mol Biol 19:598–605

Bros M, Jahrling F, Renzing A, Wiechmann N, Dang NA, Sutter A, Ross R, Knop J, Sudowe S, Reske-Kunz AB (2007) A newly established murine immature dendritic cell line can be differentiated into a mature state, but exerts tolerogenic function upon maturation in the presence of glucocorticoid. Blood 109:3820–3829

Canning MO, Grotenhuis K, De Wit HJ, Drexhage HA (2000) Opposing effects of dehydroepiandrosterone and dexamethasone on the generation of monocyte-derived dendritic cells. Eur J Endocrinol 143:687–695

Castellano G, Woltman AM, Nauta AJ, Roos A, Trouw LA, Seelen MA, Schena FP, Daha MR, van Kooten C (2004) Maturation of dendritic cells abrogates C1q production in vivo and in vitro. Blood 103:3813–3820

Cohen N, Mouly E, Hamdi H, Maillot MC, Pallardy M, Godot V, Capel F, Balian A, Naveau S, Galanaud P, Lemoine FM, Emilie D (2006) GILZ expression in human dendritic cells redirects their maturation and prevents antigen-specific T lymphocyte response. Blood 107:2037–2044

de Jong EC, Vieira PL, Kalinski P, Kapsenberg ML (1999) Corticosteroids inhibit the production of inflammatory mediators in immature monocyte-derived DC and induce the development of tolerogenic DC3. J Leukoc Biol 66:201–204

Doni A, Michela M, Bottazzi B, Peri G, Valentino S, Polentarutti N, Garlanda C, Mantovani A (2006) Regulation of PTX3, a key component of humoral innate immunity in human dendritic cells: stimulation by IL-10 and inhibition by IFN-gamma. J Leukoc Biol 79:797–802

Duperrier K, Velten FW, Bohlender J, Demory A, Metharom P, Goerdt S (2005) Immunosuppressive agents mediate reduced allostimulatory properties of myeloid-derived dendritic cells despite induction of divergent molecular phenotypes. Mol Immunol 42:1531–1540

Emmer PM, van d, V, Adema GJ, Hilbrands LB (2006) Dendritic cells activated by lipopolysaccharide after dexamethasone treatment induce donor-specific allograft hyporesponsiveness. Transplantation 81:1451–1459

Feili-Hariri M, Dong X, Alber SM, Watkins SC, Salter RD, Morel PA (1999) Immunotherapy of NOD mice with bone marrow-derived dendritic cells. Diabetes 48:2300–2308

Freeman L, Hewison M, Hughes SV, Evans KN, Hardie D, Means TK, Chakraverty R (2005) Expression of 11beta-hydroxysteroid dehydrogenase type 1 permits regulation of glucocorticoid bioavailability by human dendritic cells. Blood 106:2042–2049

Fu F, Li Y, Qian S, Lu L, Chambers F, Starzl TE, Fung JJ, Thomson AW (1996) Costimulatory molecule-deficient dendritic cell progenitors (MHC class II+, CD80dim, CD86−) prolong cardiac allograft survival in nonimmunosuppressed recipients. Transplantation 62:659–665

Garrovillo M, Ali A, Depaz HA, Gopinathan R, Oluwole OO, Hardy MA, Oluwole SF (2001) Induction of transplant tolerance with immunodominant allopeptide-pulsed host lymphoid and myeloid dendritic cells. Am J Transplant 1:129–137

Giles KM, Ross K, Rossi AG, Hotchin NA, Haslett C, Dransfield I (2001) Glucocorticoid augmentation of macrophage capacity for phagocytosis of apoptotic cells is associated with reduced p130Cas expression, loss of paxillin/pyk2 phosphorylation, and high levels of active Rac. J Immunol 167:976–986

Grohmann U, Volpi C, Fallarino F, Bozza S, Bianchi R, Vacca C, Orabona C, Belladonna ML, Ayroldi E, Nocentini G, Boon L, Bistoni F, Fioretti MC, Romani L, Riccardi C, Puccetti P (2007) Reverse signaling through GITR ligand enables dexamethasone to activate IDO in allergy. Nat Med 13:579–586

Hackstein H, Renner FC, Bohnert A, Nockher A, Frommer T, Bein G, Weimer R (2005) Dendritic cell deficiency in the blood of kidney transplant patients on long-term immunosuppression: results of a prospective matched-cohort study. Am J Transplant 5:2945–2953

Hackstein H, Thomson AW (2004) Dendritic cells: emerging pharmacological targets of immunosuppressive drugs. Nat Rev Immunol 4:24–35

Hesselink DA, Vaessen LM, Hop WC, Schoordijk W, Ijzermans JN, Baan CC, Weimar W (2005) The effects of renal transplantation on circulating dendritic cells. Clin Exp Immunol 140: 384–393

Hoetzenecker W, Meingassner JG, Ecker R, Stingl G, Stuetz A, Elbe-Burger A (2004) Corticosteroids but not pimecrolimus affect viability, maturation and immune function of murine epidermal Langerhans cells. J Invest Dermatol 122:673–684

Hsu NC, Chung CY, Horng HC, Chang CS (2004) Corticosteroid administration depresses circulating dendritic cells in ITP patients. Platelets 15:451–454

Kim KD, Choe YK, Choe IS, Lim JS (2001) Inhibition of glucocorticoid-mediated, caspase-independent dendritic cell death by CD40 activation. J Leukoc Biol 69:426–434
Kitajima T, Ariizumi K, Bergstresser PR, Takashima A (1996) A novel mechanism of glucocorticoid-induced immune suppression: the inhibiton of T cell-mediated terminal maturation of a murine dendritic cell line. J Clin Invest 98:142–147
Koopman G, Dalgleish AG, Bhogal BS, Haaksma AG, Heeney JL (2001) Changes in dendritic cell subsets in the lymph nodes of rhesus macaques after application of glucocorticoids. Hum Immunol 62:208–214
Lan YY, Wang Z, Raimondi G, Wu W, Colvin BL, de CA, Thomson AW (2006) "Alternatively activated" dendritic cells preferentially secrete IL-10, expand Foxp3 + CD4+ T cells, and induce long-term organ allograft survival in combination with CTLA4-Ig. J Immunol 177:5868–5877
Li M, Zhang X, Zheng X, Lian D, Zhang ZX, Ge W, Yang J, Vladau C, Suzuki M, Chen D, Zhong R, Garcia B, Jevnikar AM, Min WP (2007) Immune modulation and tolerance induction by RelB-silenced dendritic cells through RNA interference. J Immunol 178:5480–5487
Ling Y, Cao X, Yu Z, Ruan C (2007) Circulating dendritic cells subsets and CD4 + Foxp3+ regulatory T cells in adult patients with chronic ITP before and after treatment with high-dose dexamethasome. Eur J Haematol 79:310–316
Link H, Huang YM, Masterman T, Xiao BG (2001) Vaccination with autologous dendritic cells: from experimental autoimmune encephalomyelitis to multiple sclerosis. J Neuroimmunol 114:1–7
Ludewig B, Junt T, Hengartner H, Zinkernagel RM (2001) Dendritic cells in autoimmune diseases. Curr Opin Immunol 13:657–662
Lutz MB, Suri RM, Niimi M, Ogilvie AL, Kukutsch NA, Rossner S, Schuler G, Austyn JM (2000) Immature dendritic cells generated with low doses of GM-CSF in the absence of IL-4 are maturation resistant and prolong allograft survival in vivo. Eur J Immunol 30:1813–1822
Macedo C, Popescu I, bu-Elmagd K, Reyes J, Shapiro R, Zeevi A, Berghaus JM, Wang LF, Lu L, Thomson AW, Storkus WJ, Fung JJ, Metes D (2005) Augmentation of type-1 polarizing ability of monocyte-derived dendritic cells from chronically immunosuppressed organ-transplant recipients. Transplantation 79:451–459
Mainali ES, Tew JG (2004) Dexamethasone selectively inhibits differentiation of cord blood stem cell derived-dendritic cell (DC) precursors into immature DCs. Cell Immunol 232:127–136
Manome H, Aiba S, Singh S, Yoshino Y, Tagami H (2000) Dexamethasone and cyclosporin A affect the maturation of monocyte-derived dendritic cells differently. Int Arch Allergy Immunol 122:76–84
Matasic R, Dietz AB, Vuk-Pavlovic S (1999) Dexamethasone inhibits dendritic cell maturation by redirecting differentiation of a subset of cells. J Leukoc Biol 66:909–914
Matsue H, Yang C, Matsue K, Edelbaum D, Mummert M, Takashima A (2002) Contrasting impacts of immunosuppressive agents (rapamycin, FK506, cyclosporin A, and dexamethasone) on bidirectional dendritic cell-T cell interaction during antigen presentation. J Immunol 169:3555–3564
Matyszak MK, Citterio S, Rescigno M, Ricciardi-Castagnoli P (2000) Differential effects of corticosteroids during different stages of dendritic cell maturation. Eur J Immunol 30:1233–1242
Mazariegos GV, Zahorchak AF, Reyes J, Chapman H, Zeevi A, Thomson AW (2005) Dendritic cell subset ratio in tolerant, weaning and non-tolerant liver recipients is not affected by extent of immunosuppression. Am J Transplant 5:314–322
Mazariegos GV, Zahorchak AF, Reyes J, Ostrowski L, Flynn B, Zeevi A, Thomson AW (2003) Dendritic cell subset ratio in peripheral blood correlates with successful withdrawal of immunosuppression in liver transplant patients. Am J Transplant 3:689–696
Menges M, Rossner S, Voigtlander C, Schindler H, Kukutsch NA, Bogdan C, Erb K, Schuler G, Lutz MB (2002) Repetitive injections of dendritic cells matured with tumor necrosis factor alpha induce antigen-specific protection of mice from autoimmunity. J Exp Med 195:15–21
Mirenda V, Berton I, Read J, Cook T, Smith J, Dorling A, Lechler RI (2004) Modified dendritic cells coexpressing self and allogeneic major histocompatability complex molecules: an efficient way to induce indirect pathway regulation. J Am Soc Nephrol 15:987–997

Morelli AE, Thomson AW (2007) Tolerogenic dendritic cells and the quest for transplant tolerance. Nat Rev Immunol 7:610–621

Moser M, De Smedt T, Sornasse T, Tielemans F, Chentoufi AA, Muraille E, Van Mechelen M, Urbain J, Leo O (1995) Glucocorticoids down-regulate dendritic cell function in vitro and in vivo. Eur J Immunol 25:2818–2824

Mozo L, Suarez A, Gutierrez C (2004) Glucocorticoids up-regulate constitutive interleukin-10 production by human monocytes. Clin Exp Allergy 34:406–412

Oluwole OO, Depaz HA, Gopinathan R, Ali A, Garrovillo M, Jin MX, Hardy MA, Oluwole SF (2001) Indirect allorecognition in acquired thymic tolerance: induction of donor-specific permanent acceptance of rat islets by adoptive transfer of allopeptide-pulsed host myeloid and thymic dendritic cells. Diabetes 50:1546–1552

Ouaaz F, Arron J, Zheng Y, Choi Y, Beg AA (2002) Dendritic cell development and survival require distinct NF-kappaB subunits. Immunity 16:257–270

Peche H, Trinite B, Martinet B, Cuturi MC (2005) Prolongation of heart allograft survival by immature dendritic cells generated from recipient type bone marrow progenitors. Am J Transplant 5:255–267

Piemonti L, Monti P, Allavena P, Leone BE, Caputo A, Di C, V (1999a) Glucocorticoids increase the endocytic activity of human dendritic cells. Int Immunol 11:1519–1526

Piemonti L, Monti P, Allavena P, Sironi M, Soldini L, Leone BE, Socci C, Di C, V (1999b) Glucocorticoids affect human dendritic cell differentiation and maturation. J Immunol 162:6473–6481

Rastellini C, Lu L, Ricordi C, Starzl TE, Rao AS, Thomson AW (1995) Granulocyte/macrophage colony-stimulating factor-stimulated hepatic dendritic cell progenitors prolong pancreatic islet allograft survival. Transplantation 60:1366–1370

Rea D, van Kooten C, Van Meijgaarden KE, Melief CJM, Offringa R (2000) Glucocorticoids transform CD40-triggering of dendritic cells into an alternative activation pathway resulting in antigen presenting cells that secrete IL-10. Blood 95:3162–3167

Reis E, Sousa C (2006) Dendritic cells in a mature age. Nat Rev Immunol 6:476–483

Reis ES, Barbuto JA, Isaac L (2006) Human monocyte-derived dendritic cells are a source of several complement proteins. Inflamm Res 55:179–184

Roelen DL, Schuurhuis DH, van den Boogaardt DE, Koekkoek K, van Miert PP, van Schip JJ, Laban S, Rea D, Melief CJ, Offringa R, Ossendorp F, Claas FH (2003) Prolongation of skin graft survival by modulation of the alloimmune response with alternatively activated dendritic cells. Transplantation 76:1608–1615

Rozkova D, Horvath R, Bartunkova J, Spisek R (2006) Glucocorticoids severely impair differentiation and antigen presenting function of dendritic cells despite upregulation of Toll-like receptors. Clin Immunol 120:260–271

Santegoets SJ, Masterson AJ, van der Sluis PC, Lougheed SM, Fluitsma DM, Van den Eertwegh AJ, Pinedo HM, Scheper RJ, de Gruijl TD (2006) A CD34(+) human cell line model of myeloid dendritic cell differentiation: evidence for a CD14(+)CD11b(+) Langerhans cell precursor. J Leukoc Biol 80:1337–1344

Sebelin K, Schulzki A, Kloetzel PM, Dorken B, Pezzutto A, Subklewe M (2006) Impairment of circulating myeloid dendritic cells in immunosuppressed renal/pancreas transplant recipients. Transplantation 82:779–787

Shinomiya M, Fazle Akbar SM, Shinomiya H, Onji M (1999) Transfer of dendritic cells (DC) ex vivo stimulated with interferon-gamma (IFN-gamma) down-modulates autoimmune diabetes in non-obese diabetic (NOD) mice. Clin Exp Immunol 117:38–43

Steinman RM, Banchereau J (2007) Taking dendritic cells into medicine. Nature 449:419–426

Sternberg EM (2006) Neural regulation of innate immunity: a coordinated nonspecific host response to pathogens. Nat Rev Immunol 6:318–328

Sternberg EM, Chrousos GP, Wilder RL, Gold PW (1992) The stress response and the regulation of inflammatory disease. Ann Intern Med 117:854–866

Stock P, Akbari O, DeKruyff RH, Umetsu DT (2005) Respiratory tolerance is inhibited by the administration of corticosteroids. J Immunol 175:7380–7387

Suda T, Chida K, Matsuda H, Hashizume H, Ide K, Yokomura K, Suzuki K, Kuwata H, Miwa S, Nakano H, Fujisawa T, Enomoto N, Matsushita A, Nakamura H (2003) High-dose intravenous glucocorticoid therapy abrogates circulating dendritic cells. J Allergy Clin Immunol 112:1237–1239

Tan PH, Sagoo P, Chan C, Yates JB, Campbell J, Beutelspacher SC, Foxwell BM, Lombardi G, George AJ (2005) Inhibition of NF-kappa B and oxidative pathways in human dendritic cells by antioxidative vitamins generates regulatory T cells. J Immunol 174:7633–7644

Tiemessen MM, Jagger AL, Evans HG, van Herwijnen MJ, John S, Taams LS (2007) CD4 + CD25 + Foxp3+ regulatory T cells induce alternative activation of human monocytes/macrophages. Proc Natl Acad Sci U S A 104:19446–19451

van Duivenvoorde LM, Han WG, Bakker AM, Louis-Plence P, Charbonnier LM, Apparailly F, van der Voort EI, Jorgensen C, Huizinga TW, Toes RE (2007) Immunomodulatory dendritic cells inhibit Th1 responses and arthritis via different mechanisms. J Immunol 179:1506–1515

van Vliet SJ, Gringhuis SI, Geijtenbeek TB, van Kooyk Y (2006a) Regulation of effector T cells by antigen-presenting cells via interaction of the C-type lectin MGL with CD45. Nat Immunol 7:1200–1208

van Vliet SJ, van Liempt E, Geijtenbeek TB, van Kooyk Y (2006b) Differential regulation of C-type lectin expression on tolerogenic dendritic cell subsets. Immunobiology 211:577–585

Vanclee A, Schouten HC, Bos GM (2006) Murine dendritic cells that are resistant to maturation are unable to induce tolerance to allogeneic stem cells. Transpl Immunol 16:8–13

Vanderheyde N, Verhasselt V, Goldman M, Willems F (1999) Inhibition of human dendritic cell functions by methylprednisolone. Transplantation 67:1342–1347

Vegh Z, Goyarts EC, Rozengarten K, Mazumder A, Ghebrehiwet B (2003) Maturation-dependent expression of C1q-binding proteins on the cell surface of human monocyte-derived dendritic cells. Int Immunopharmacol 3:345–357

Vendetti S, Chai JG, Dyson J, Simpson E, Lombardi G, Lechler R (2000) Anergic T cells inhibit the antigen-presenting function of dendritic cells. J Immunol 165:1175–1181

Vieira PL, Kalinski P, Wierenga EA, Kapsenberg ML, de Jong EC (1998) Glucocorticoids inhibit bioactive IL-12p70 production by in vitro-generated human dendritic cells without affecting their T cell stimulatory potential. J Immunol 161:5245–5251

Visser J, van Boxel-Dezaire A, Methorst D, Brunt T, De Kloet ER, Nagelkerken L (1998) Differential regulation of interleukin-10 (IL-10) and IL-12 by glucocorticoids in vitro. Blood 91:4255–4264

Vital AL, Goncalo M, Cruz MT, Figueiredo A, Duarte CB, Lopes MC (2003) Dexamethasone prevents granulocyte-macrophage colony-stimulating factor-induced nuclear factor-kappaB activation, inducible nitric oxide synthase expression and nitric oxide production in a skin dendritic cell line. Mediators Inflamm 12:71–78

Vizzardelli C, Pavelka N, Luchini A, Zanoni I, Bendickson L, Pelizzola M, Beretta O, Foti M, Granucci F, Nilsen-Hamilton M, Ricciardi-Castagnoli P (2006) Effects of dexamethazone on LPS-induced activationand migration of mouse dendritic cells revealed by a genome-wide transcriptional analysis. Eur J Immunol 36:1504–1515

Vulcano M, Struyf S, Scapini P, Cassatella M, Bernasconi S, Bonecchi R, Calleri A, Penna G, Adorini L, Luini W, Mantovani A, Van DJ, Sozzani S (2003) Unique regulation of CCL18 production by maturing dendritic cells. J Immunol 170:3843–3849

Wilckens T, De Rijk R (1997) Glucocorticoids and immune function: unknown dimensions and new frontiers. Immunol Today 18:418–424

Woltman AM, De Fijter JW, Kamerling SW, Paul LC, Daha MR, van Kooten C (2000) The effect of calcineurin inhibitors and corticosteroids on the differentiation of human dendritic cells. Eur J Immunol 30:1807–1812

Woltman AM, De Fijter JW, Zuidwijk K, Vlug AG, Bajema IM, Van der Kooij SW, van Ham V, van Kooten C (2007) Quantification of dendritic cell subsets in human renal tissue under normal and pathological conditions. Kidney Int 71:1001–1008

Woltman AM, Massacrier C, De Fijter JW, Caux C, van Kooten C (2002) Corticosteroids prevent generation of CD34+-derived dermal dendritic cells but do not inhibit Langerhans cell development. J Immunol 168:6181–6188

Woltman AM, Van der Kooij SW, De Fijter JW, van Kooten C (2006) Maturation-resistant dendritic cells induce hyporesponsiveness in alloreactive CD45RA+ and CD45RO+ T-cell populations. Am J Transplant 6:2580–2591

Woltman AM, van Kooten C (2003) Functional modulation of dendritic cells to suppress adaptive immune responses. J Leukoc Biol 73:428–441

Xia CQ, Peng R, Beato F, Clare-Salzler MJ (2005) Dexamethasone induces IL-10-producing monocyte-derived dendritic cells with durable immaturity. Scand J Immunol 62:45–54

Xing N, L Maldonado ML, Bachman LA, McKean DJ, Kumar R, Griffin MD (2002) Distinctive dendritic cell modulation by vitamin D(3) and glucocorticoid pathways. Biochem Biophys Res Commun 297:645–652

Zhang TY, Ding X, Daynes RA (2005) The expression of 11 beta-hydroxysteroid dehydrogenase type I by lymphocytes provides a novel means for intracrine regulation of glucocorticoid activities. J Immunol 174:879–889

Induction of Tolerogenic Dendritic Cells by Vitamin D Receptor Agonists

Luciano Adorini and Giuseppe Penna

Contents

Abstract Dendritic cells induce and regulate T cell responses, and tolerogenic dendritic cells (DCs) can promote the development of regulatory T cells with suppressive activity. Thus, the possibility to manipulate DCs using different pharmacological or biological agents enables them to exert tolerogenic activities, could be exploited to better control a variety of chronic inflammatory conditions, from autoimmune diseases to allograft rejection. A variety of both biological and pharmacological agents can induce tolerogenic DCs, and several in vitro studies have demonstrated that human regulatory T cells can be induced by DCs manipulated to acquire and/or enhance tolerogenic properties, with in vivo data also accumulating. Within this context, we have explored the immunoregulatory activities of vitamin

L. Adorini (✉)
Intercept Pharma, Via Togliatti 22 bis, 06073 Corciano (Perugia), Italy
LAdorini@interceptpharma.com

G. Lombardi, Y. Riffo-Vasquez (eds.), *Dendritic Cells,* Handbook of Experimental Pharmacology 188,

D receptor (VDR) agonists, secosteroid hormones able to induce tolerogenic DCs and regulatory T cells. Tolerogenic DCs induced by a short treatment with VDR agonists promote $CD4^+$ $CD25^+$ $Foxp3^+$ suppressor T cells that are able to mediate transplantation tolerance and to arrest the development of autoimmune diseases. VDR agonists not only favour the induction of $CD4^+$ $CD25^+$ regulatory T cells, but can also enhance their recruitment to inflammatory sites. VDR agonists have been proven effective and safe drugs in a variety of autoimmune disease and graft rejection models, highlighting their potential applicability to chronic inflammatory conditions sustained by autoreactive or alloreactive immune responses. In addition to the topical treatment of psoriasis, a Th1-mediated autoimmune disease of the skin where VDR agonists are the most used topical drugs; these agents might eventually find a broader application in the treatment of inflammatory conditions, where their modulatory effects on DCs enhancing T cells with regulatory functions could turn out to be quite beneficial.

1 Introduction

Dendritic cells (DCs), a highly specialized antigen-presenting cell (APC) system critical for the initiation of $CD4^+$ T cell responses are present, in different stages of maturation, in the circulation as well as in lymphoid and non-lymphoid organs, where they exert a sentinel function. After antigen uptake, DCs migrate through the afferent lymph to T-dependent areas of secondary lymphoid organs where they can prime naive T cells. During migration to lymphoid organs, DCs mature into potent APCs by increasing their immunostimulatory properties, while decreasing antigen-capturing capacity (Steinman and Banchereau 2007).

DCs are heterogeneous not only in terms of maturation state, but also of origin, morphology, phenotype and function. Two distinct DC subpopulations were originally defined in the human blood based on the expression of CD11c, and they have been subsequently characterized as belonging to the myeloid or lymphoid lineage, and defined as myeloid (M-DCs) and plasmacytoid (P-DCs) DCs (Shortman and Liu 2002; Colonna et al. 2004). M-DCs are characterized by a monocytic morphology; express myeloid markers like CD13 and CD33, the β2 integrin CD11c, the activatory receptor (immunoglobulin-like transcripts, ILT1) and low levels of the IL-3 receptor α chain CD123. Conversely, P-DCs have a morphology resembling plasma cells, are devoid of myeloid markers, express high levels of CD4, CD62L and CD123. M-DCs produce high levels of IL-12, while P-DCs high levels of IFN-α. (Colonna et al. 2004), cytokines with clearly distinct effects on T cell activation and differentiation.

It is now clear that DCs can be not only immunogenic but also tolerogenic, both intrathymically and in the periphery, and they can modulate T cell development (Steinman and Banchereau 2007). In particular, immature DCs have been found to have tolerogenic properties, and to induce T cells with suppressive activity. However, the simplistic concept that immature DCs are intrinsically and uniquely able to induce regulatory/suppressor T cells (Treg) has been dispelled by the observation that mature DCs can also be very efficient inducers of Treg cells (Yamazaki et al. 2003), a property already noted for semi-mature DCs (Lutz and Schuler 2002).

Among the various populations of regulatory and suppressor T cells described, naturally occurring thymic and peripheral $CD4^+$ T cells that co-express CD25 are currently most actively investigated (Shevach et al. 2006). $CD4^+$ $CD25^+$ Treg cells prevent the activation and proliferation of potentially autoreactive T cells that have escaped thymic deletion. They fail to proliferate and secrete cytokines in response to polyclonal or antigen-specific stimulation, and are not only anergic but also inhibit the activation of responsive T cells. Although CD25, CD152, and glucocorticoid-induced TNF-related protein (GITR) are markers of $CD4^+$ $CD25^+$ Treg cells, they are also expressed by activated T cells (Shevach et al. 2006). A more faithful marker distinguishing $CD4^+$ $CD25^+$ Treg cells from recently activated $CD4^+$ T cells is Foxp3, a member forkhead family of transcription factors that is required for $CD25^+$ Treg development and is sufficient for their suppressive function (Miyara and Sakaguchi 2007). $Foxp3^+$ $CD4^+$ $CD25^+$ Treg cells play an important role in preventing the induction of several autoimmune diseases, such as the autoimmune syndrome induced by day 3 thymectomy in genetically susceptible mice, inflammatory bowel disease, type 1 diabetes (T1D) in thymectomized rats and in NOD mice. A defect in peripheral regulatory cells affecting both $CD25^+$ Treg and NK cells has been described also in T1D patients, and autoreactive T cells in diabetics are skewed to a proinflammatory Th1 phenotype lacking the IL-10-secreting T cells found in non-diabetic, HLA-matched controls. The clinical relevance of $CD4^+$ $CD25^+$ Treg cells has also been shown in patients affected by rheumatoid arthritis and multiple sclerosis (Baecher-Allan and Hafler 2006).

Because DCs are pleiotropic modulators of T-cell activity, manipulation of DC function, to favour the induction of DCs with tolerogenic properties leading to the development of Treg cells, could be exploited to modulate immune responses. Considerable efforts are ongoing to translate this concept into clinical practice, also by rationalizing the tolerogenic effects exerted by immunosuppressive and immunomodulatory drugs currently used to control autoimmune diseases and graft rejection (Adorini et al. 2004; Hackstein and Thomson 2004).

2 Tolerogenic Dendritic Cells: Mechanistic Insights

Tolerogenic DCs are characterized by reduced expression of costimulatory molecules, in particular CD40, CD80, CD86, although this is not an absolute requirement. In addition, they usually show reduced IL-12 and increased IL-10 production, and often an early stage of maturation (Steinman et al. 2003). While these well-established phenotypic and functional properties of tolerogenic DCs can easily explain their propensity to induce regulatory rather than effector T cells, several other mechanisms may play a role in favouring Treg cell induction by tolerogenic DCs.

2.1 Indoleamine 2,3-Dioxygenase

One mechanism by which DCs can regulate T cell responses is via expression of indoleamine 2,3-dioxygenase (IDO), the rate-limiting enzyme of tryptophan catabolism. IDO-transgenic DCs decrease the concentration of tryptophan, increase the concentration of kynurenine, the main tryptophan metabolite, and suppress allogeneic T cell proliferation in vitro due to T cell death, because suppressive tryptophan catabolites exert a cytotoxic action preferentially on activated T cells (Terness et al. 2002). Although the concept that cells expressing IDO can suppress T-cell responses and promote tolerance is a relatively new paradigm in immunology, accumulating evidence supports this possibility, including studies on maternal tolerance to the fetus, tumour resistance, chronic infections and autoimmune diseases (Mellor and Munn 2004). In particular, IDO-expressing DCs contribute to the generation and maintenance of peripheral tolerance by depleting autoreactive T cells (Mellor and Munn 2004). Interestingly, $CD4^+$ $CD25^+$ Treg cells can condition DCs to express IDO suppressive properties, indicating that IDO could act as a bridge between DCs and Tregs (Puccetti and Grohmann 2007). Mouse P-DCs can also initiate the immunosuppressive pathway of tryptophan catabolism, suggesting an important role for IDO-expressing P-DCs in controlling the balance between inflammation and tolerance (Fallarino et al. 2007), and further supporting the view that inducible IDO expression plays an important role in rendering DC tolerogenic.

2.2 Inhibitory Receptors

Most cell types involved in innate or acquired immune responses including myeloid, lymphoid and dendritic cells, express at least one member of the ILTs family receptors structurally and functionally related to killer cell inhibitory receptors (Yokoyama 1997) that have been shown to be involved in immunoregulation (Colonna et al. 1999). ILT family members can be subdivided into two main types. One, comprising ILT1, ILT7, ILT8, and leukocyte Ig-like receptor 6, is characterized by a short cytoplasmic tail delivering an activating signal through the immunoreceptor tyrosine-based activatory motif (ITAM) of the associated common γ chain of the Fc receptor. Members of the second type, including ILT2, ILT3, ILT4, and ILT5, contain a cytoplasmic immunoreceptor tyrosine-based inhibitory motif (ITIM) transducing a negative signal (Colonna et al. 2000). When inhibitory ILTs are activated, their ITIM domains become phosphorylated, and recruit $p56^{lck}$ and SH2-containing protein-tyrosine-phosphatase 1 (SHP-1), leading to downstream events and gene modulation (Ravetch and Lanier 2000). For example, the inhibitory receptor ILT3 has been shown to negatively regulate activation of antigen-presenting cells (Cella et al. 1997).

A connection between ILTs and tolerance induction has been established by the observation that $CD8^+$ $CD28^-$ suppressor T cells upregulate ILT3 and ILT4 expression on DCs, rendering them tolerogenic (Chang et al. 2002). Such tolerogenic

DCs have been reported to anergize alloreactive $CD4^+$ $CD45RO^+$ $CD25^+$ T cells converting them into regulatory T cells which, in turn, continue the cascade of suppression by tolerizing other DCs (Suciu-Foca and Cortesini 2007). Alloantigen specific $CD8^+$ $CD28^-Foxp3^+$ T suppressor cells have also been shown to induce $ILT3^+$ $ILT4^+$ tolerogenic endothelial cells, inhibiting alloreactivity (Manavalan et al. 2004). Consistent with these results, rat $CD8^+$ $Foxp3^+$ Treg cells have been shown to induce PIR-B, an hortologue of inhibitory ILTs (Takai and Ono 2001), in DCs and heart endothelial cells, and to mediate tolerance to allogeneic heart transplants (Liu et al. 2004). ILT3 appears to be responsible for induction of $CD8^+$ suppressor T cells in cancer patients, suggesting that depletion and/or blockade of soluble ILT3 may be crucial to the success of anti-tumor immunotherapy (Cortesini 2007).

2.3 Cytokines

Cytokines represent the best known class of biological agents currently used to favour the induction of tolerogenic DCs. In particular, DCs differentiated in the presence of IL-10, TGF-β, TNF-α, or Granulocyte colony-stimulating factor (G-CSF) can acquire phenotypic and functional properties, characteristic of tolerogenic DCs.

The intrinsically strong anti-inflammatory properties of IL-10 are further enhanced by its capacity to induce Treg cells. In particular, the presence of IL-10 during differentiation of $CD4^+$ T cells results in the development of a defined subset of regulatory T cells (Tr1 cells) characterized by low proliferation, absence of IL-2 production, and a specific cytokine profile with IL-10 and IFN-γ but neither IL-4 nor IL-5 production (Groux et al. 1997). In vivo, the differentiation of Tr1 cells is likely controlled by DCs which promote IL-10 production and may express tolerogenic co-stimulatory molecules (Roncarolo et al. 2006).

Several studies have shown that TGF-β1 inhibits in vitro activation and maturation of DCs, preventing the upregulation of critical T-cell co-stimulatory molecules on DC surface, inhibiting IL-12 production, and reducing their antigen-presenting capacity (Lyakh et al. 2005; Fogel-Petrovic et al. 2007). Thus, in addition to direct inhibitory effects of TGF-β1 on effector T lymphocytes, and to induction of the Treg transcription factor Foxp3 (Yamazaki et al. 2007), its modulatory effects at the DC level may critically contribute to the development of tolerogenic DCs leading to Treg induction.

Tumor necrosis factor (TNF)-α is a proinflammatory cytokine with interesting immunoregulatory properties which can modulate DC development, phenotype and function (Lutz and Schuler 2002). Maturation by TNF-α induce high levels of MHC class II and co-stimulatory molecules on DCs, but they remain weak producers of proinflammatory cytokines, in particular IL-12 (Lutz and Schuler 2002). These incompletely matured DCs (semi-mature DCs) induce peptide-specific IL-10-producing T cells in vivo and prevent EAE (Menges et al. 2002). DCs with a similar phenotype were previously found to inhibit, when injected 1 week before transplantation, haplotype-specific cardiac allograft rejection, with a marked increase in median graft survival time from 8 to > 100 days (Lutz et al. 2000). Injection of semi-mature DCs could also protect mice from GVHD and induce the expansion of IL-10-producing $CD4^+$ $CD25^+$ Treg cells (Sato et al. 2003), suggesting that semi-mature DCs may be beneficial in the treatment of several immune-mediated diseases.

G-CSF, the key hematopoietic growth factor of the myeloid lineage, has also been found to possess marked immunoregulatory properties (Franzke et al. 2003; Rutella and Lemoli 2004). $CD4^+$ T cells exposed in vivo to G-CSF acquire Tr1-type properties once triggered in vitro through the T-cell receptor, with an IL-10-dominated cytokine production profile, low intrinsic proliferation, and contact-independent suppression of antigen-driven proliferation (Rutella et al. 2002). The immunomodulatory effects of G-CSF might be mediated by DCs expressing high levels of co-stimulatory molecules and HLA-DR, but decreased IL-12p70 secretion and poor allostimulatory capacity (Rutella et al. 2004), reminiscent of semi-mature DCs (Lutz and Schuler 2002). The ability of G-CSF to promote key tolerogenic interactions between DCs and Treg cells has been demonstrated by the enhanced recruitment of TGF-β1-expressing $CD4^+$ $CD25^+$ Treg cells after adoptive transfer of DCs isolated from G-CSF- compared to vehicle-treated mice into naive NOD recipients (Kared et al. 2005).

3 Induction of Tolerogenic Dendritic Cells by VDR Agonists

The activated form of vitamin D, $1,25(OH)_2D_3$, is a secosteroid hormone which has, in addition to its central function in calcium and bone metabolism, important effects on the growth and differentiation of many cell types, and pronounced immunoregulatory properties (Deluca and Cantorna 2001; Adorini 2002a, b; Mathieu and Adorini 2002; Griffin et al. 2003). The biological effects of $1,25(OH)_2D_3$ are mediated by the vitamin D receptor (VDR), a member of the superfamily of nuclear hormone receptors functioning as a agonist-activated transcription factor which binds to specific DNA sequence elements in vitamin D responsive genes, and influences their rate of RNA polymerase II-mediated transcription (Carlberg 2003).

APCs, and notably DCs, express the VDR and are key targets of VDR agonists, both in vitro and in vivo (Adorini and Penna 2008). A number of studies, summarized in Table 1, has clearly demonstrated that $1,25(OH)_2D_3$ and its analogues markedly modulate DC phenotype and function (Berer et al. 2000; Griffin et al. 2000; Penna and Adorini 2000; Piemonti et al. 2000; Canning et al. 2001; van Halteren et al. 2002). These studies, performed either on monocyte-derived DCs from human peripheral blood or on bone-marrow derived mouse DCs, have consistenly shown that in vitro treatment of DCs with VDR agonists leads to down-regulated expression of the co-stimulatory molecules CD40, CD80, CD86, and to decreased IL-12 and enhanced IL-10 production, resulting in decreased T-cell activation (Fig. 1). The block of maturation, coupled with abrogation of IL-12 and strongly enhanced production of IL-10, highlight the important functional effects of VDR agonists on DCs and are, at least in part, responsible for the induction of

Table 1 Phenotypic and functional modifications induced by VDR ligands in human myeloid dendritic cells

Phenotypic marker	Effect
Maturation marker expression	
CD83	Decreased
DC-LAMP	Decreased
Antigen uptake	
Mannose receptor expression	Increased
Costimulatory molecule expression	
CD40	Decreased
CD80	Decreased
CD86	Decreased
Inhibitory molecule expression	
ILT3	Increased
ILT4	Unmodified
B7-H1	Unmodified
Chemokine receptor expression	
CCR7	Decreased
Function	**Effect**
Cytokine production	
IL-1	Decreased
IL-6	Decreased
IL-10	Increased
IL-12/23p40	Decreased
IL-12p75	Decreased
IL-23	Decreased
Chemokine production	
CCL2	Increased
CCL17	Decreased
CCL18	Increased
CCL20	Decreased
CCL22	Increased
CXCL10	Decreased
Apoptosis	
Maturation-induced	Increased
Transcription factors	
NF-κBp65 nuclear translocation	Decreased
IRF-4 expression	Decreased
T-cell activation	
Response to alloantigens	Decreased
Response to autoantigens	Decreased

Compiled from Penna and Adorini (2000), Vulcano et al. (2003), Penna et al. (2005, 2007) and from the author's unpublished data

DCs with tolerogenic properties. The combination of these effects can explain the capacity of VDR agonists to induce DCs with tolerogenic properties which favor Treg cell enhancement.

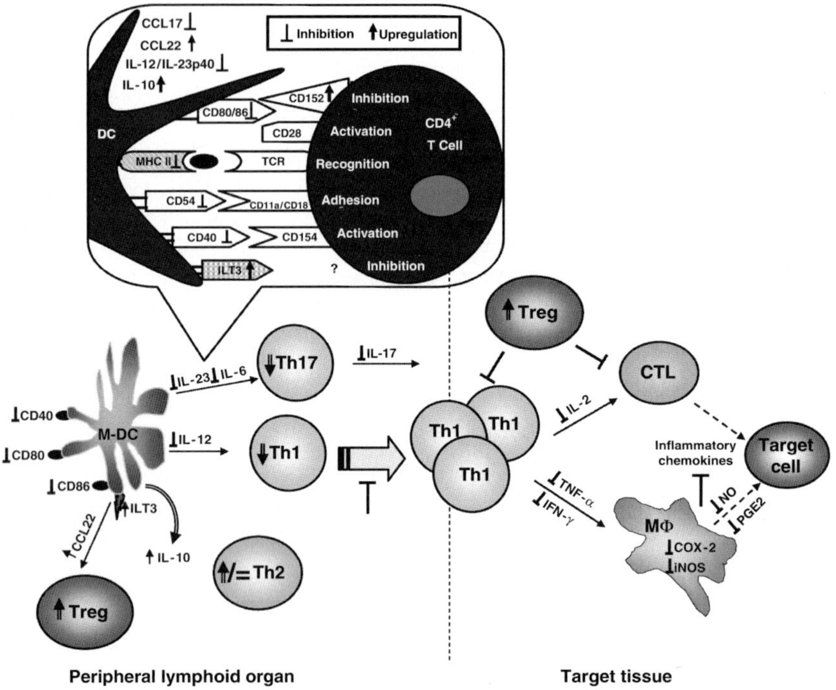

Fig. 1 Immunomodulatory effects of VDR agonists on myeloid dendritic cells and CD4$^+$ T cells. VDR agonists inhibit in myeloid dendritic cells (M-DC), but not in plasmacytoid DCs, expression of surface costimulatory molecules, e.g. CD40, CD80, CD86, as well as MHC class II and CD54 molecules. Production of cytokines affecting T cell differentiation into Th1 and Th17, IL-12 and IL-23, respectively, are also inhibited in M-DCs. Conversely, expression of surface inhibitory molecules like ILT3, and of secreted inhibitory cytokines like IL-10 are markedly upregulated. Chemokines potentially able to recruit CCR4$^+$ regulatory T cells like CCL22 are also upregulated, whereas the CCR4 ligand CCL17 is downregulated. Upon interaction with M-DCs, CD4$^+$ T cells upregulate expression of the inhibitory molecule CD152 (CTLA-4). DCs expressing low levels of costimulatory molecules, secreting IL-10, and expressing high levels of inhibitory molecules (e.g. ILT3) favour the induction and/or the enhancement of regulatory/suppressor T cells.

VDR agonists can modulate the inflammatory response via several mechanisms in secondary lymphoid organs and in target tissues. In secondary lymphoid organs, VDR agonists inhibit IL-12 and IL-23 production and down-regulate costimulatory molecule expression (CD40, CD80, CD86) expressed by myeloid DCs (M-DCs), while upregulating their IL-10 production and ILT3 expression. M-DC modulation by VDR agonists inhibits development of Th1 and Th17 cells whilst inducing CD4$^+$ CD25$^+$ Foxp3$^+$ regulatory T cells and, under certain conditions, Th2 cells. VDR agonists can also inhibit the migration of Th1 cells, and they upregulate CCL22 production by M-DC, enhancing the recruitment of CD4$^+$ CD25$^+$ regulatory T cells and of Th2 cells. In addition, VDR agonists exert direct effects on T cells by inhibiting IL-2 and IFN-γ production. In target tissues, pathogenic Th1 cells, that can damage target cells via induction of cytotoxic T cells (CTL) and activated macrophages (MΦ), are reduced in number and their activity is further inhibited by CD4$^+$ CD25$^+$ regulatory T cells and by Th2 cells induced by VDR agonists. IL-17 production by Th17 cells is also inhibited. In MΦ, important inflammatory molecules like cyclo-oxygenase 2 (COX-2) and inducible nitric oxide synthase (iNOS) are inhibited by VDR agonists, leading to decreased production of nitric oxide (NO) and prostaglandin E2 (PGE2). MΦs, as well as DCs and T cells, can synthesize $1{,}25(OH)_2D_3$ and this may also contribute to the regulation of the local immune response. Blunted arrows indicate inhibition, and broken arrows cytotoxicity

DCs are able to synthesize 1,25$(OH)_2D_3$ in vitro as a consequence of increased 1α-hydroxylase expression (Hewison et al. 2003), and this could also contribute to promote regulatory T cell induction. It is also possible that 1,25$(OH)_2D_3$ may contribute to the physiological control of immune responses, and possibly be also involved in maintaining tolerance to self antigens, as suggested by the enlarged lymph nodes containing a higher frequency of mature DCs in VDR-deficient mice (Griffin et al. 2001). This appealing concept has been recently highlighted by the observation that vitamin D_3 induced by sunlight in the skin is hydroxylated by local DCs into the active hormone, which in turn upregulates on activated T cells expression of the epidermiotropic chemokine receptor CCR10, a primary VDR-responsive gene, enabling them to migrate in response to the epidermal chemokine CCL27 (Sigmundsdottir et al. 2007). Thus, the autocrine production of 1,25$(OH)_2D_3$ by DCs can program the homing of skin-associated T cells, which could include regulatory T cells able to counteract the pro-inflammatory effects induced in the skin by sun exposure. Interestingly, B cells can also synthesize 1,25$(OH)_2D_3$ (Chen et al. 2007) and can preferentially expand Foxp3$^+$ Treg cells (Chen and Jensen 2007), suggesting that the tolerogenic potential of B cells could perhaps be associated with their capacity to produce 1,25$(OH)_2D_3$.

3.1 Tolerogenic Dendritic Cells Induced by VDR Agonists Lead to Enhancement of Regulatory T Cells

The prevention of DC differentiation and maturation as well as the modulation of their activation and survival leading to DCs with tolerogenic phenotype and function (Table 1) play an important role in the immunoregulatory activity of VDR agonists, and appear to be critical for the capacity of this hormones to induce CD4$^+$ CD25$^+$ Treg cells that are able to control autoimmune responses and allograft rejection (Table 2).

VDR agonists enhance CD4$^+$ CD25$^+$ Treg cells and promote tolerance induction in transplantation and autoimmune disease models. A short treatment with 1,25$(OH)_2D_3$ and mycophenolate mofetil (MMF), a selective inhibitor of T and B cell proliferation that also modulates APCs, induces tolerance to islet allografts associated with an increased frequency of CD4$^+$ CD25$^+$ Treg cells able to adoptively transfer transplantation tolerance (Gregori et al. 2001). The induction of tolerogenic DCs could indeed represent a therapeutic strategy promoting tolerance to allografts (Adorini 2002) and the observation that immature myeloid DCs can induce T cell tolerance to specific antigens in human volunteers represents an important proof of concept for this approach (Dhodapkar et al. 2001).

CD4$^+$ CD25$^+$ Treg cells able to inhibit the T cell response to a pancreatic autoantigen and to significantly delay disease transfer by pathogenic CD4$^+$ CD25$^-$ T cells are also induced by treatment of adult nonobese diabetic (NOD) mice with the VDR agonist BXL-219 (Gregori et al. 2002). This treatment arrests insulitis, blocks the progression of Th1 cell infiltration into the pancreatic islets, and inhibits

Table 2 VDR agonists foster the induction of regulatory T cells

In dendritic cells
Inhibit IL-12
Enhance IL-10
Down-regulate CD40, CD80, CD86
Block maturation
Upregulate ILT3 expression
Leading to T cells characterized by
Reduced Th1 development
Hyporesponsiveness to auto and alloantigens
Increased CTLA-4 expression
Decreased CD40L expression
Enhanced $CD4^+CD25^+$ suppressor T cells

Compiled from references Berer et al. (2000), Griffin et al. (2000), Penna and Adorini (2000), Piemonti et al. (2000), Canning et al. (2001), Penna et al. (2002), van Halteren et al. (2002), Penna et al. (2005) and from the author unpublished results

type 1 diabetes development at non-hypercalcemic doses (Gregori et al. 2002). Although the type 1 diabetes and islet transplantation models are quite different, in both cases administration of VDR agonists doubles the number of $CD4^+$ $CD25^+$ Treg cells, in the spleen and pancreatic lymph nodes, respectively (Gregori et al. 2001, 2002). $1,25(OH)_2D_3$ has also been shown to prevent and treat TNBS-induced colitis, by reducing Th1 and Th17 cells while upregulating $Foxp3^+$ Treg cells, associated with significant reduction of IL-12p75, IL-23p19, and IL-6 production by DCs (Daniel et al. 2007).

However, tolerogenic DCs may not always be necessarily involved in the generation of Treg cells by VDR agonists. A combination of $1,25(OH)_2D_3$ and dexamethasone has been shown to induce human and mouse naive $CD4^+$ T cells to differentiate in vitro into Treg cells, even in the absence of APCs (Barrat et al. 2002). These Treg cells produced IL-10, but neither IL-5 nor IFN-γ, thus distinguishing them from the previously described Tr1 cells (Groux et al. 1997). Upon transfer, the IL-10-producing Treg cells could prevent central nervous system inflammation, indicating their capacity to exert a suppressive function in vivo (Barrat et al. 2002). Thus, although DCs appear to be primary targets for the immunomodulatory activities of VDR agonists, they can also act directly on T cells, as expected by VDR expression in both cell types and by the presence of common targets in their signal transduction pathways, such as the nuclear factor NF-κB that is down-regulated in both APCs and T cells.

Interestingly, agonists of the peroxisome proliferator-activated receptor γ (PPARγ), another member of the steroid hormone receptor superfamily, also inhibit DC maturation and Ag-presenting capacity in a NF-κB-dependent fashion (Klotz et al. 2007). Unlike its down-regulatory effect on other cells of the immune system, the PPARγ agonist ciglitazone has been found to exert an enhancing effect on both inducible and natural Tregs (Wohlfert et al. 2007), similarly to VDR agonists. In addition, using PPARγ-deficient $CD4^+$ T cells obtained from tissue-specific PPARγ null mice it has been suggested that endogenous PPARγ activation represents a Treg intrinsic mechanism for down-regulation of effector $CD4^+$ T cell function and prevention of colitis (Hontecillas and Bassaganya-Riera 2007). Thus, PPARγ as well as VDR agonists can promote Treg activity, likely involving in both cases induction of tolerogenic DCs.

3.2 Upregulation of Inibitory Receptor Expression in Dendritic Cells by VDR Agonists

To further characterize mechanisms accounting for the induction of DCs with tolerogenic properties by VDR agonists, we have examined the ILT expression by $1,25(OH)_2D_3$-treated DCs. We have found that incubation of monocyte-derived human DCs, either immature or during maturation, with $1,25(OH)_2D_3$ leads to a selective upregulation of ILT3 (Adorini et al. 2004). Analysis of DC subsets revealed a higher ILT3 expression on P-DCs compared to M-DCs (Cella et al. 1999; Penna et al. 2001). CD40 ligation reduced ILT3 expression on M-DCs but had little effect on P-DCs (Penna et al. 2005). Maintaining high ILT3 expression on P-DCs matured via CD40 ligation is of interest, because this cell population has been shown to induce $CD8^+$ regulatory T cells able to suppress the proliferation of naïve $CD8^+$ cells through an IL-10-dependent pathway (Gilliet and Liu 2002). While incubation with $1,25(OH)_2D_3$ did not affect the already high ILT3 expression by P-DCs, it increased ILT3 expression on M-DCs considerably (Penna et al. 2005). The down-regulation of ILT3 on M-DCs by T cell-dependent signals, and the up-regulation of this inhibitory receptor by $1,25(OH)_2D_3$ in DCs suggests a novel mechanism for the immunomodulatory properties of this hormone that could play a role in the control of T cell responses.

As tolerogenic DCs induced by different pharmacological agents share several properties, we have analyzed upregulation of ILT3 expression in immature and mature DCs by selected immunomodulatory agents. $1,25(OH)_2D_3$ markedly upregulates ILT3 expression on both immature and mature DCs, whereas IL-10 has a much less pronounced effect, and dexamethasone no observable activity. In the same experiment, all the three agents inhibited DC maturation, as shown by decreased CD83 expression (Adorini et al. 2004). An in vivo correlate could be established by the marked upregulation of ILT3 expression in DCs of psoriatic lesions treated with the VDR agonist calcipotriol, whereas no ILT3 expression was induced by topical treatment of psoriatic plaques with the glucocorticoid mometazone (Penna et al. 2005). These results indicate that drug-induced ILT3 upregulation is not a general feature of tolerogenic DCs, as proposed (Manavalan et al. 2003), and are consistent with the view that VDR agonists and glucocorticoids modulate DCs using distinctive pathways (Xing et al. 2002). Analysis of DC subsets revealed a differential regulation of ILT3 expression by $1,25(OH)_2D_3$, with a marked up-regulation in M-DCs but no effect on its expression by P-DCs. A regulatory role for ILT3 expressed on DCs was shown by the increased IFN-γ secretion promoted by anti-ILT3 addition to cultures of DCs and T cells, which was blunted in $1,25(OH)_2D_3$-treated DCs, suggesting ILT3-independent mechanisms able to regulate T-cell activation. Although ILT3 expression by DCs is required for induction of regulatory T cells, DC pretreatment with $1,25(OH)_2D_3$ leads to induction of $CD4^+$ $Foxp3^+$ T cells with suppressive activity irrespective of the presence of neutralizing anti-ILT3 mAb, indicating that ILT3 expression is dispensable for the capacity of $1,25(OH)_2D_3$-treated DCs to induce regulatory T cells (Penna et al. 2005).

3.3 Modulation of Chemokine Production by VDR Agonists Can Affect Recruitment of Effector T Cells and $CD4^+$ $CD25^+$ Treg Cells to Inflammatory Sites

In both islet transplantation and type 1 diabetes models, treatment with VDR agonists has a profound effect on the migration of effector T cells, preventing their entry into the pancreatic islets (Gregori et al. 2001, 2002). The VDR agonist BXL-219 significantly downregulates in vitro and in vivo proinflammatory chemokine production by islet cells, inhibiting T cell recruitment into the pancreatic islets and T1D development (Giarratana et al. 2004). The inhibition of CXCL10 is particularly relevant, consistent with the decreased recruitment of Th1 cells into sites of inflammation by treatment with an anti-CXCR3 antibody (Xie et al. 2003), and with the substantial delay of T1D development observed in CXCR3-deficient mice (Frigerio et al. 2002). The inhibition of islet chemokine production by BXL-219 treatment in vivo is associated with upregulation of IκBα transcription, an inhibitor of nuclear factor κB (NF-κB), and with arrest of NF-κBp65 nuclear translocation (Giarratana et al. 2004), highlighting a novel mechanism of action exerted by VDR agonists potentially relevant for the treatment of T1D and other autoimmune diseases. These observations expand the known mechanisms of action exerted by vitamin D analogs in the treatment of T1D and other experimental autoimmune diseases, that include arrest of DC maturation, inhibition of Th1 cell responsiveness, and enhancement of regulatory T cells (Adorini 2002; Mathieu and Adorini 2002; Griffin et al. 2003). In addition to modulating chemokine production in target tissues such as pancreatic islets, it is also possible that VDR agonists can affect the migration of $CD25^+$ Treg cells by regulating their chemokine receptor expression, a hypothesis that we are currently testing.

Both human (D'Ambrosio et al. 2003) and mouse (Giarratana et al. 2007) $CD4^+$ $CD25^+$ Treg cells express CCR4, and selectively migrate in response to CCR4 agonists like CCL22. An interesting confirmation to this finding is provided by the observation that human ovarian tumors produce CCL22, the cognate ligand of the CCR4 receptor, promoting the recruitment of $CCR4^+$ $CD4^+$ $CD25^+$ Treg cells that act as a tumor-protective mechanism (Curiel et al. 2004).

We have found that, in contrast to the high production by circulating human M-DCs, the CCR4 agonists CCL17 and CCL22 are poorly produced by P-DCs

(Penna et al. 2002). It is noteworthy that blood-borne M-DCs, in contrast to P-DCs, constitutively produce CCL17 and CCL22 ex vivo (Penna et al. 2002). This selective constitutive production of CCR4 agonists by immature M-DCs could lead to the preferential attraction of $CD4^+$ $CD25^+$ Treg cells, a mechanism expected to favor tolerance induction. This has been observed in ovarian carcinoma patients, in which $Foxp3^+$ $CCR4^+$ $CD25^+$ Treg cells are selectively recruited by tumor-produced CCL22, and suppress anti-tumor responses leading to reduced patient survival (Curiel et al. 2004). Intriguingly, the production of CCL22 is markedly enhanced by $1{,}25(OH)_2D_3$ in blood M-DCs but not P-DCs (Penna et al. 2007). Besides maintaining peripheral immunological tolerance in homeostatic conditions, $CD4^+$ $CD25^+$ Treg cells could turn-off and limit ongoing inflammatory responses. Inflammatory signals strongly induce maturation and influx of both M-DCs and P-DCs to secondary lymphoid tissues (Shortman and Liu 2002), and maturation of M-DCs and P-DCs enhances their production of several proinflammatory chemokines that can potentially attract different T-cell subsets. Interestingly, maturing P-DCs, similarly to activated B cells, produce large quantities of the CCR5 agonist CCL4 (Penna et al. 2002). Thus, in analogy with the proposed role for CCL4 in $CD4^+$ $CD25^+$ Treg cells attraction by activated B cells, mature P-DCs could recruit these cells to limit ongoing inflammatory responses.

3.4 *VDR Agonists Selectively Modulates Tolerogenic Properties in Myeloid but Not Plasmacytoid Dendritic Cells*

Although the immunomodulatory effects of VDR agonists on DCs are well established, the capacity of this hormone to modulate DC subsets has only recently been addressed. Myeloid (M-DCs) and plasmacytoid (P-DCs) DC subsets play complementary roles in the induction and regulation of innate and adaptive immune responses (Colonna et al. 2004). M-DCs are the most efficient APCs directly able to prime naïve T cells and can become, under different conditions, immunogenic or tolerogenic (Steinman and Hemmi 2006), whereas P-DCs, under steady-state conditions, appear to play a key role in maintaing peripheral immune tolerance, and can be considered naturally occurring tolerogenic DCs (Liu 2005).

Analysis of immunomodulatory effects exerted by $1{,}25(OH)_2D_3$ on human blood M-DCs and P-DCs demonstrates a differential capacity of this hormone to modulate cytokine and chemokine production in DC subsets, showing marked effects in M-DCs and negligible ones in P-DCs (Penna et al. 2007). In addition to CCL22 and CCL17, neither IFN-α, the signature cytokine produced by P-DCs (Liu 2005), nor expression of MHC class II molecules or CCR7, a key regulator of DC migration to secondary lymphoid organs, are affected in P-DCs by $1{,}25(OH)_2D_3$ treatment (Penna et al. 2007). Conversely, production of IL-12, the M-DC signature cytokine, as well as MHC class II and CCR7 expression are markedly inhibited by $1{,}25(OH)_2D_3$ in M-DCs (Penna et al. 2007). All these molecules are controlled by NF-κB, a signal transduction pathway crucially involved in the inflammatory response (Li and Verma 2002). Our data showing inhibition of RelA nuclear translocation by $1,25(OH)_2D_3$ in M-DCs but not P-DCs demonstrate a mechanism of action selectively targeting NF-κB in DC subpopulations (Penna et al. 2007). The selective targeting of NF-κB components by VDR agonists in M-DCs could thus contribute to explain the lack of activity of these agents on cytokine and chemokine production by P-DCs. These cells however respond to $1,25(OH)_2D_3$, as shown by CYP24 upregulation, although less markedly than M-DCs, as indicated by the three fold reduction in the number of modulated genes by microarray analysis. Also inhibition of Th1 development and enhancement of $CD4^+$ suppressor T cell activity are selectively induced by $1,25(OH)_2D_3$ in M-DCs but not P-DCs. This differential capacity of DC subsets to respond to $1,25(OH)_2D_3$ is not due to a diverse VDR expression or VDR-dependent signal transduction, as shown (Fig. 2a) by the marked

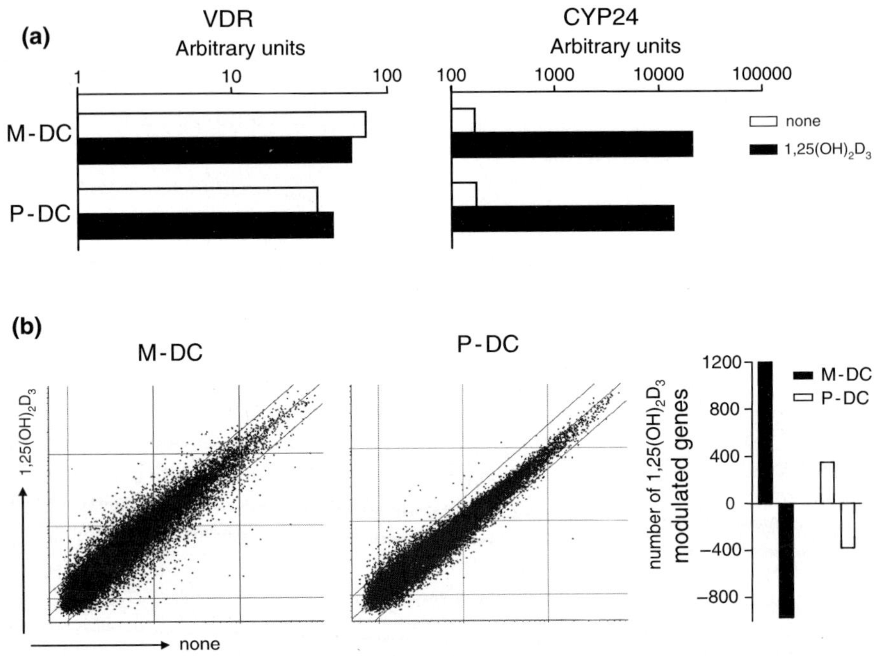

Fig. 2 Gene modulation induced by $1,25(OH)_2D_3$ in M-DCs and P-DCs. **(a)** M-DCs and P-DCs express similar levels of VDR and upregulate equally well primary VDR response genes following stimulation with $1,25(OH)_2D_3$. Magnetically purified blood M-DCs and P-DCs (2×10^4 cells/well) were cultured with or without 10 nM $1,25(OH)_2D_3$. After 2 h, RNA was extracted and expression of VDR and CYP24 transcripts evaluated by real time RT-PCR. Bars represents arbitrary units (A.U.) normalized to GAPDH signals and are from one representative experiment out of 5 performed. **(b)** Microarray analysis of ex-vivo purified DC subpopulations incubated with $1,25(OH)_2D_3$. Magnetically purified blood M-DCs and P-DCs were cultured in GM-CSF or IL-3, with or without 100 nM $1.25(OH)_2D_3$. After 24 h, cDNA was generated from pools of 5 donors and microarray gene expression profiles were obtained using GE Healthcare Human 40 k BioArrays, and analyzed using GeneSpring software. The outer diagonal lines in the scatter plots represent the two-fold cut-off for upregulated or downregulated genes. Bars represents the number of genes upregulated or downregulated at least 2-fold by $1,25(OH)_2D_3$ treatment in M-DCs (filled bars) and P-DCs (open bars)

up-regulation of CYP24 a primary VDR response gene rapidly induced following exposure to $1,25(OH)_2D_3$ (Carlberg 2003). Thus, both M-DCs and P-DCs express similar VDR levels and respond equally well to VDR ligation.

To further assess responsiveness of DC subsets to $1,25(OH)_2D_3$, we determined its effects at the genome level. Microarray analysis of ex-vivo purified DC subpopulations incubated for 24 h with or without 100 nM $1,25(OH)_2D_3$ revealed a three fold lower number of modulated genes in P-DCs compared to M-DCs (Fig. 2b). The cut-off for gene modulation was a two-fold difference, marked by the outer diagonal lines in the scatter plots (Fig. 2b). P-DCs can therefore respond to VDR agonists, which however do not appear to modify their tolerogenic potential.

Thus, $1,25(OH)_2D_3$ appears to upregulate tolerogenic properties, selectively in M-DCs, downregulating IL-12 and Th1 cell development, while promoting $CD4^+$ suppressor T cell activity and enhancing the production of CCL22, a chemokine able to recruit regulatory T cells. In contrast, no immunomodulatory effects appear to be induced by $1,25(OH)_2D_3$ in P-DCs, a DC subset prone to favour tolerance (Liu 2005). P-DCs, characterized by an intrinsic ability to prime naïve $CD4^+$ T cells to differentiate into IL-10-producing T cells and $CD4^+$ $CD25^+$ regulatory T cells, and to suppress immune responses, may represent naturally occurring regulatory DCs (Liu 2005; Puccetti and Fallarino 2007), and the lack of P-DC modulation by $1,25(OH)_2D_3$ would thus leave this tolerogenic potential unmodified.

4 Common Features of Agents Leading to Induction of Tolerogenic DCs

A variety of immunosuppressive agents are currently used to inhibit transplantation rejection and to treat autoimmune diseases. Interestingly, the mechanism of action of major immunosuppressive drugs, like the calcineurin inhibitors cyclosporine A and tacrolimus, has been only understood after almost 20 years of clinical use (Allison 2000). Thus, it is perhaps not surprising that a novel mechanism of action shared by many immunosuppressive and anti-inflammatory drugs, based on the induction of DCs with tolerogenic properties, has only recently emerged (Lagaraine and Lebranchu 2003; Woltman and van Kooten 2003; Adorini et al. 2004; Hackstein and Thomson 2004).

Indeed, several immunosuppressive agents currently used to treat allograft rejection and autoimmune diseases have been shown to induce DCs with tolerogenic phenotype and function. Notable examples are glucocorticoids (Vieira et al. 1998; Matasic et al. 1999; Piemonti et al. 1999; Woltman et al. 2000), MMF (Mehling et al. 2000; Colic et al. 2003), and sirolimus (Woltman et al. 2001; Hackstein et al. 2003). These agents impair DC maturation and inhibit upregulation of co-stimulatory molecules, secretion of proinflammatory cytokines, in particular IL-12, and allostimulatory capacity. Sirolimus appears to be a very interesting agent, because it induces tolerogenic DCs (Hackstein et al. 2003), and sirolimus-treated alloantigen-pulsed DCs infused one week before transplantation inhibit antigen-specific T cell responsiveness and prolong graft survival (Taner et al. 2005).

Conversely, controversial effects of calcineurin inhibitors, like cyclosporine A and tacrolimus, have been reported on DC maturation, although these drugs have a clear inhibitory effect on DC, decreasing their cytokine production and allostimulatory capacity (Lee et al. 1999; Woltman et al. 2000; Szabo et al. 2001). Other immunosuppressive agents, like desoxyspergualin, also inhibit the allostimulatory capacity of DCs, impairing their maturation and IL-12 production as well (Contreras et al. 1998; Thomas et al. 1999, 2001). Similar effects are exerted on DCs by anti-inflammatory agents, such as acetylsalicylic acid (Matasic et al. 2000; Hackstein et al. 2001; Buckland et al. 2006a, b), Butyric acid (Millard et al. 2002) and N-acetyl-L-cysteine (Verhasselt et al. 1999). Interestingly, Aspirin-modified DCs, expressing a tolerogenic phenotype and high levels of ILT3 (Buckland et al. 2006a), are potent inducers of allo-specific regulatory T-cells (Buckland et al. 2006b).

Although the pro-tolerogenic effects of several pharmacological agents on DCs are well established, little is known about their capacity to induce regulatory T cells promoting transplantation tolerance. MMF was able, as a monotherapy, to induce some limited levels of transplantation tolerance even if no induction of tolerogenic DCs was observed in vivo (Gregori et al. 2001). Conversely, calcineurin inhibitors have been reported to prevent transplantation tolerance induced by co-stimulation blockers, although the issue is still unresolved (Izawa et al. 2004), but successful establishment of alloantigen-specific hyporesponsiveness by NF-κB inhibitor-treated DCs was not inhibited by concomitant calcineurin inhibition (Saemann et al. 2004). In addition, the sirolimus derivative everolimus did not hamper in vitro the suppressive activity of $CD4^+$ $CD25^+$ Treg cells, suggesting that these cells may still exert suppressive activity in transplant recipients treated with drugs interfering with IL-2 signaling (Game et al. 2005). Finally, as discussed in detail above, $1,25(OH)_2D_3$ and its analogues have also been found to inhibit DC maturation, leading to reduced expression of costimulatory molecules and IL-12 production. These tolerogenic DCs show decreased capacity to stimulate alloreactive T cells, and promote the differentiation of $CD4^+$ $CD25^+$ Treg cells.

Common features shared by biological and pharmacological agents favoring the induction of tolerogenic DCs are their capacity to inhibit differentiation, maturation, co-stimulatory molecule expression, and IL-12 production, leading to decreased allostimulatory capacity (Adorini et al. 2004). Co-stimulatory molecule expression is almost invariably reduced in tolerogenic DCs, with the exception of exposure to agents inducing semi-mature DCs (Lutz and Schuler 2002). In any case, all the tolerogenic agents tested inhibit DC maturation and reduce their capacity to stimulate alloreactive T cells in a mixed leukocyte reaction assay. Another common feature of DC-targeting drugs is the inhibition of IL-12, a cytokine critically involved in the development of Th1-dependent diseases. In contrast, only VDR agonists, among the agents tested, are able to enhance the secretion by DCs of IL-10, a cytokine favoring the induction of regulatory T cells (Adorini et al. 2004).

Several of these effects could be mediated by NF-κB, a signal transduction pathway crucially involved in the inflammatory response (Bonizzi and Karin 2004). The NF-κB family member RelB is required for myeloid DC differentiation, and antigen-pulsed DCs in which RelB function is inhibited can induce regulatory $CD4^+$

T cells able to transfer tolerance to primed recipients in an IL-10-dependent fashion (Martin et al. 2003). Our data showing upregulation of transcripts encoding IκBα and inhibition of RelA nuclear translocation by BXL-219 in pancreatic islet cells (Giarratana et al. 2004) demonstrate a novel mechanism of action in the targeting NF-κB by VDR ligands, in addition to inhibition of NF-κB1 and c-Rel (Yu et al. 1995), as well as RelB (Dong et al. 2003) expression. Interestingly, this mechanism of action has been previously demonstrated for glucorticoids, anti-inflammatory drugs that binds to a nuclear receptor in the same superfamily as the VDR, by showing that dexamethasone upregulates the transcription of *Nfkbia*, which results in increased rate of IκBα synthesis and in reduced NF-κB translocation to the nucleus (Auphan et al. 1995; Scheinman et al. 1995). The promoter of the *Nfkbia* gene encoding IκBα contains, as the *Relb* gene (Dong et al. 2003), several vitamin D responsive elements, some of which are highly conserved between human and mouse homologs, suggesting a direct transcriptional regulation of IκBα by BXL-219 (Giarratana et al. 2004). The direct targeting of NF-κB components by VDR agonists exemplified by arrest of NF-κBp65 nuclear translocation in M-DCs (Penna et al. 2007) could thus contribute to explain their capacity to induce tolerogenic DCs, as well as their inhibitory effects on proinflammatory cytokine and chemokine production by DCs.

5 Conclusions

VDR agonists share with several immunomodulatory agents, the capacity to target DCs, rendering them tolerogenic and fostering the induction of regulatory rather than effector T cells. Multiple mechanisms contribute to induction of DC tolerogenicity by VDR agonists, from downregulation of co-stimulatory molecules, both membrane-bound as CD40, CD80, CD86 and secreted as IL-12, to upregulation of inhibitory molecules like ILT3 and IL-10, to modulation of chemokine secretion, enhancing the production of chemokines able to recruit regulatory and suppressor T cells, and inhibiting production of chemokines recruiting inflammatory cells by the target organ in inflammatory conditions.

In principle, these VDR agonist-induced mechanisms favoring DC tolerogenicity could be exploited in two ways. The first could rely on the in vitro manipulation of DCs to promote tolerogenic properties, followed by reinfusion into the patient. However, this, as any cell-based therapy, poses tremendous hurdles to clinical applicability. The standardization of effective and reproducible protocols would be very difficult, but even more problematic will be to ensure the capacity of the reinfused DCs to maintain a tolerogenic function in vivo, under inflammatory conditions. In contrast to therapies based on ex-vivo manipulation of DCs, treatments with immunosuppressive and anti-inflammatory drugs able to promote tolerogenic DCs have been in clinical use for decades to control allograft rejection and autoimmune diseases. Administration of these agents can directly target both DCs and T cells, leading to the inhibition of pathogenic effector T cells and enhancing the frequency of T cells with suppressive properties, effects that appear to be largely mediated via induction of tolerogenic DCs. Thus, direct treatment of patients with DC-tolerizing agents appears to represent a preferable therapeutic option. In addition to low molecular weight drugs like VDR agonists, biological agents, in particular cytokines, could be directly administered in vivo to promote induction of tolerogenic DCs. However, issues related to immunogenicity, short and long-term adverse events, and high cost are likely to place important limitations on their clinical applicability.

References

Adorini L (2002a) Immunomodulatory effects of vitamin D receptor ligands in autoimmune diseases. Int Immunopharmacol 2:1017–1028

Adorini L (2002b) 1,25-Dihydroxyvitamin D3 analogs as potential therapies in transplantation. Curr Opin Invest Drugs 3:1458–1463

Adorini L, Giarratana N, Penna G (2004) Pharmacological induction of tolerogenic dendritic cells and regulatory T cells. Semin Immunol 16:127–134

Adorini L and Penna G (2008) Control of autoimmune disease by the vitamin D endocrine system. Nat Clin Pract Rheumatol 4(8):404–412

Allison AC (2000) Immunosuppressive drugs: the first 50 years and a glance forward. Immunopharmacology 47:63–83

Auphan N, DiDonato JA, Rosette C, Helmberg A, Karin M (1995) Immunosuppression by glucocorticoids: inhibition of NF-kappa B activity through induction of I kappa B synthesis. Science 270:286–290

Baecher-Allan C, Hafler DA (2006) Human regulatory T cells and their role in autoimmune disease. Immunol Rev 212:203–216

Barrat FJ, Cua DJ, Boonstra A, Richards DF, Crain C, Savelkoul HF, de Waal-Malefyt R, Coffman RL, Hawrylowicz CM, O'Garra A (2002) In vitro generation of interleukin 10-producing regulatory CD4(+) T cells is induced by immunosuppressive drugs and inhibited by T helper type 1 (Th1)- and Th2-inducing cytokines. J Exp Med 195:603–616

Berer A, Stockl J, Majdic O, Wagner T, Kollars M, Lechner K, Geissler K, Oehler L (2000) 1,25-Dihydroxyvitamin D(3) inhibits dendritic cell differentiation and maturation in vitro. Exp Hematol 28:575–583

Bonizzi G, Karin M (2004) The two NF-kappaB activation pathways and their role in innate and adaptive immunity. Trends Immunol 25:280–288

Buckland M, Jago C, Fazekesova H, George A, Lechler R, Lombardi G (2006a) Aspirin modified dendritic cells are potent inducers of allo-specific regulatory T-cells. Int Immunopharmacol 6:1895–1901

Buckland M, Jago CB, Fazekasova H, Scott K, Tan PH, George AJ, Lechler R, Lombardi G (2006b) Aspirin-treated human DCs up-regulate ILT-3 and induce hyporesponsiveness and regulatory activity in responder T cells. Am J Transplant 6:2046–2059

Canning MO, Grotenhuis K, de Wit H, Ruwhof C, Drexhage HA (2001) 1-alpha,25-Dihydroxyvitamin D3 (1,25(OH)(2)D(3)) hampers the maturation of fully active immature dendritic cells from monocytes. Eur J Endocrinol 145:351–357

Carlberg C (2003) Current understanding of the function of the nuclear vitamin D receptor in response to its natural and synthetic ligands. Recent Results Cancer Res 164:29–42

Cella M, Dohring C, Samaridis J, Dessing M, Brockhaus M, Lanzavecchia A, Colonna M (1997) A novel inhibitory receptor (ILT3) expressed on monocytes, macrophages, and dendritic cells involved in antigen processing. J Exp Med 185:1743–1751

Cella M, Jarrossay D, Facchetti F, Alebardi O, Nakajima H, Lanzavecchia A, Colonna M (1999) Plasmacytoid monocytes migrate to inflamed lymph nodes and produce large amounts of type I interferon. Nat Med 5:919–923

Chang CC, Ciubotariu R, Manavalan JS, Yuan J, Colovai AI, Piazza F, Lederman S, Colonna M, Cortesini R, Dalla-Favera R, Suciu-Foca N (2002) Tolerization of dendritic cells by T(S) cells: the crucial role of inhibitory receptors ILT3 and ILT4. Nat Immunol 3:237–243

Chen X, Jensen PE (2007) Cutting edge: primary B lymphocytes preferentially expand allogeneic FoxP3 + CD4 T cells. J Immunol 179:2046–2050

Chen S, Sims GP, Chen XX, Gu YY, Lipsky PE (2007) Modulatory effects of 1,25-dihydroxyvitamin D3 on human B cell differentiation. J Immunol 179:1634–1647

Colic M, Stojic-Vukanic Z, Pavlovic B, Jandric D, Stefanoska I (2003) Mycophenolate mofetil inhibits differentiation, maturation and allostimulatory function of human monocyte-derived dendritic cells. Clin Exp Immunol 134:63–69

Colonna M, Nakajima H, Navarro F, Lopez-Botet M (1999) A novel family of Ig-like receptors for HLA class I molecules that modulate function of lymphoid and myeloid cells. J Leukoc Biol 66:375–381

Colonna M, Nakajima H, Cella M (2000) A family of inhibitory and activating Ig-like receptors that modulate function of lymphoid and myeloid cells. Semin Immunol 12:121–127

Colonna M, Trinchieri G, Liu YJ (2004) Plasmacytoid dendritic cells in immunity. Nat Immunol 5:1219–1226

Contreras JL, Wang PX, Eckhoff DE, Lobashevsky AL, Asiedu C, Frenette L, Robbin ML, Hubbard WJ, Cartner S, Nadler S, Cook WJ, Sharff J, Shiloach J, Thomas FT, Neville DM, Jr., Thomas JM (1998) Peritransplant tolerance induction with anti-CD3-immunotoxin: a matter of proinflammatory cytokine control. Transplantation 65:1159–1169

Cortesini R (2007) Pancreas cancer and the role of soluble immunoglobulin-like transcript 3 (ILT3). Jop 8:697–703

Curiel TJ, Coukos G, Zou L, Alvarez X, Cheng P, Mottram P, Evdemon-Hogan M, Conejo-Garcia JR, Zhang L, Burow M, Zhu Y, Wei S, Kryczek I, Daniel B, Gordon A, Myers L, Lackner A, Disis ML, Knutson KL, Chen L, Zou W (2004) Specific recruitment of regulatory T cells in ovarian carcinoma fosters immune privilege and predicts reduced survival. Nat Med 10: 942–949

D'Ambrosio D, Sinigaglia F, Adorini L (2003) Special attractions for suppressor T cells. Trends Immunol 24:122–126

Daniel C, Sartory NA, Zahn N, Radeke HH, Stein JM (2007) Immune modulatory treatment of TNBS colitis with calcitriol is associated with a change of a Th1/Th17 to a Th2 and regulatory T cell profile. J Pharmacol Exp Ther 324:23–33

Deluca HF, Cantorna MT (2001) Vitamin D: its role and uses in immunology. Faseb J 15:2579–2585

Dhodapkar MV, Steinman RM, Krasovsky J, Munz C, Bhardwaj N (2001) Antigen-specific inhibition of effector T cell function in humans after injection of immature dendritic cells. J Exp Med 193:233–238

Dong X, Craig TA, Xing N, Bachman LA, Paya CV, Weih F, McKean DJ, Kumar R, Griffin MD (2003) Direct transcriptional regulation of RelB by 1alpha,25-dihydroxyvitamin D3 and its analogs: physiologic and therapeutic implications for dendritic cell function. J Biol Chem 278:49378–49385

Fallarino F, Gizzi S, Mosci P, Grohmann U, Puccetti P (2007) Tryptophan catabolism in IDO + plasmacytoid dendritic cells. Curr Drug Metab 8:209–216

Fogel-Petrovic M, Long JA, Misso NL, Foster PS, Bhoola KD, Thompson PJ (2007) Physiological concentrations of transforming growth factor beta1 selectively inhibit human dendritic cell function. Int Immunopharmacol 7:1924–1933

Franzke A, Piao W, Lauber J, Gatzlaff P, Konecke C, Hansen W, Schmitt-Thomsen A, Hertenstein B, Buer J, Ganser A (2003) G-CSF as immune regulator in T cells expressing the G-CSF receptor: implications for transplantation and autoimmune diseases. Blood 102:734–739

Frigerio S, Junt T, Lu B, Gerard C, Zumsteg U, Hollander GA, Piali L (2002) Beta cells are responsible for CXCR3-mediated T-cell infiltration in insulitis. Nat Med 8:1414–1420

Game DS, Hernandez-Fuentes MP, Lechler RI (2005) Everolimus and Basiliximab Permit Suppression by Human CD4CD25 Cells in vitro. Am J Transplant 5:454–464

Giarratana N, Penna G, Amuchastegui S, Mariani R, Daniel KC, Adorini L (2004) A vitamin D analog downregulates proinflammatory chemokine production by pancreatic islets inhibiting T cell recruitment and type 1 diabetes development. J Immunol 173:2280–2287

Giarratana N, Penna G, Adorini L (2007) Animal models of spontaneous autoimmune disease: type 1 diabetes in the nonobese diabetic mouse. Methods Mol Biol 380:285–312

Gilliet M, Liu YJ (2002) Generation of human CD8 T regulatory cells by CD40 ligand-activated plasmacytoid dendritic cells. J Exp Med 195:695–704

Gregori S, Casorati M, Amuchastegui S, Smiroldo S, Davalli AM, Adorini L (2001) Regulatory T cells induced by 1α, 25-Dihydroxyvitamin D_3 and mycophenolate mofetil treatment mediate transplantation tolerance. J Immunol 167:1945–1953

Gregori G, Giarratana N, Smiroldo S, Uskokovic M, Adorini L (2002) A 1(,25-Dihydroxyvitamin D_3 analog enhances regulatory T cells and arrests autoimmune diabetes in NOD mice. Diabetes 51:1367–1374

Griffin MD, Lutz WH, Phan VA, Bachman LA, McKean DJ, Kumar R (2000) Potent inhibition of dendritic cell differentiation and maturation by vitamin D analogs. Biochem Biophys Res Commun 270:701–708

Griffin MD, Lutz W, Phan VA, Bachman LA, McKean DJ, Kumar R (2001) Dendritic cell modulation by 1alpha,25 dihydroxyvitamin D3 and its analogs: a vitamin D receptor-dependent pathway that promotes a persistent state of immaturity in vitro and in vivo. Proc Natl Acad Sci USA 22:22

Griffin MD, Xing N, Kumar R (2003) Vitamin D and its analogs as regulators of immune activation and antigen presentation. Annu Rev Nutr 23:117–145

Groux H, O'Garra A, Bigler M, Rouleau M, Antonenko S, de Vries JE, Roncarolo MG (1997) A CD4+ T-cell subset inhibits antigen-specific T-cell responses and prevents colitis. Nature 389:737–742

Hackstein H, Thomson AW (2004) Dendritic cells: emerging pharmacological targets of immunosuppressive drugs. Nat Rev Immunol 4:24–34

Hackstein H, Morelli AE, Larregina AT, Ganster RW, Papworth GD, Logar AJ, Watkins SC, Falo LD, Thomson AW (2001) Aspirin inhibits in vitro maturation and in vivo immunostimulatory function of murine myeloid dendritic cells. J Immunol 166:7053–7062

Hackstein H, Taner T, Zahorchak AF, Morelli AE, Logar AJ, Gessner A, Thomson AW (2003) Rapamycin inhibits IL-4 – induced dendritic cell maturation in vitro and dendritic cell mobilization and function in vivo. Blood 101:4457–4463

Hewison M, Freeman L, Hughes SV, Evans KN, Bland R, Eliopoulos AG, Kilby MD, Moss PA, Chakraverty R (2003) Differential regulation of vitamin D receptor and its ligand in human monocyte-derived dendritic cells. J Immunol 170:5382–5390

Hontecillas R, Bassaganya-Riera J (2007) Peroxisome proliferator-activated receptor gamma is required for regulatory CD4+ T cell-mediated protection against colitis. J Immunol 178:2940–2949

Izawa A, Sayegh MH, Chandraker A (2004) The antagonism of calcineurin inhibitors and costimulatory blockers: fact or fiction? Transplant Proc 36:570S–573S

Kared H, Masson A, Adle-Biassette H, Bach JF, Chatenoud L, Zavala F (2005) Treatment with granulocyte colony-stimulating factor prevents diabetes in NOD mice by recruiting plasmacytoid dendritic cells and functional CD4(+)CD25(+) regulatory T-cells. Diabetes 54:78–84

Klotz L, Dani I, Edenhofer F, Nolden L, Evert B, Paul B, Kolanus W, Klockgether T, Knolle P, Diehl L (2007) Peroxisome proliferator-activated receptor gamma control of dendritic cell function contributes to development of CD4+ T cell anergy. J Immunol 178:2122–2131

Lagaraine C, Lebranchu Y (2003) Effects of immunosuppressive drugs on dendritic cells and tolerance induction. Transplantation 75:37S–42S

Lee JI, Ganster RW, Geller DA, Burckart GJ, Thomson AW, Lu L (1999) Cyclosporine A inhibits the expression of costimulatory molecules on in vitro-generated dendritic cells: association with reduced nuclear translocation of nuclear factor kappa B. Transplantation 68:1255–1263

Li Q, Verma IM (2002) NF-kappaB regulation in the immune system. Nat Rev Immunol 2:725–734

Liu YJ (2005) IPC: professional type 1 interferon-producing cells and plasmacytoid dendritic cell precursors. Annu Rev Immunol 23:275–306

Liu J, Liu Z, Witkowski P, Vlad G, Manavalan JS, Scotto L, Kim-Schulze S, Cortesini R, Hardy MA, Suciu-Foca N (2004) Rat CD8 + FOXP3 + T suppressor cells mediate tolerance to allogeneic heart transplants, inducing PIR-B in APC and rendering the graft invulnerable to rejection. Transpl Immunol 13:239–247

Lutz MB, Schuler G (2002) Immature, semi-mature and fully mature dendritic cells: which signals induce tolerance or immunity? Trends Immunol 23:445–449

Lutz MB, Suri RM, Niimi M, Ogilvie AL, Kukutsch NA, Rossner S, Schuler G, Austyn JM (2000) Immature dendritic cells generated with low doses of GM-CSF in the absence of IL-4 are maturation resistant and prolong allograft survival in vivo. Eur J Immunol 30:1813–1822

Lyakh LA, Sanford M, Chekol S, Young HA, Roberts AB (2005) TGF-{beta} and Vitamin D3 Utilize Distinct Pathways to Suppress IL-12 Production and Modulate Rapid Differentiation of Human Monocytes into CD83+ Dendritic Cells. J Immunol 174:2061–2070

Manavalan JS, Rossi PC, Vlad G, Piazza F, Yarilina A, Cortesini R, Mancini D, Suciu-Foca N (2003) High expression of ILT3 and ILT4 is a general feature of tolerogenic dendritic cells. Transpl Immunol 11:245–258

Manavalan JS, Kim-Schulze S, Scotto L, Naiyer AJ, Vlad G, Colombo PC, Marboe C, Mancini D, Cortesini R, Suciu-Foca N (2004) Alloantigen specific CD8 + CD28 − FOXP3 + T suppressor cells induce ILT3 + ILT4+ tolerogenic endothelial cells, inhibiting alloreactivity. Int Immunol 16:1055–1068

Martin E, O'Sullivan B, Low P, Thomas R (2003) Antigen-specific suppression of a primed immune response by dendritic cells mediated by regulatory T cells secreting interleukin-10. Immunity 18:155–167

Matasic R, Dietz AB, Vuk-Pavlovic S (1999) Dexamethasone inhibits dendritic cell maturation by redirecting differentiation of a subset of cells. J Leukoc Biol 66:909–914

Matasic R, Dietz AB, Vuk-Pavlovic S (2000) Cyclooxygenase-independent inhibition of dendritic cell maturation by aspirin. Immunology 101:53–60

Mathieu C, Adorini L (2002) The coming of age of 1,25-dihydroxyvitamin D(3) analogs as immunomodulatory agents. Trends Mol Med 8:174–179.

Mehling A, Grabbe S, Voskort M, Schwarz T, Luger TA, Beissert S (2000) Mycophenolate mofetil impairs the maturation and function of murine dendritic cells. J Immunol 165:2374–2381.

Mellor AL, Munn DH (2004) IDO expression by dendritic cells: tolerance and tryptophan catabolism. Nat Rev Immunol 4:762–774

Menges M, Rossner S, Voigtlander C, Schindler H, Kukutsch NA, Bogdan C, Erb K, Schuler G, Lutz MB (2002) Repetitive injections of dendritic cells matured with tumor necrosis factor alpha induce antigen-specific protection of mice from autoimmunity. J Exp Med 195:15–21

Millard AL, Mertes PM, Ittelet D, Villard F, Jeannesson P, Bernard J (2002) Butyrate affects differentiation, maturation and function of human monocyte-derived dendritic cells and macrophages. Clin Exp Immunol 130:245–255

Miyara M, Sakaguchi S (2007) Natural regulatory T cells: mechanisms of suppression. Trends Mol Med 13:108–116

Penna G, Adorini L (2000) 1,25-dihydroxyvitamin D3 inhibits differentiation, maturation, activation and survival of dendritic cells leading to impaired alloreactive T cell activation. J Immunol 164:2405–2411

Penna G, Sozzani S, Adorini L (2001) Cutting edge: selective usage of chemokine receptors by plasmacytoid dendritic cells. J Immunol 167:1862–1866

Penna G, Vulcano M, Roncari A, Facchetti F, Sozzani S, Adorini L (2002) Differential chemokine production by myeloid and plasmacytoid dendritic cells. J Immunol 169:6673–6676

Penna G, Roncari A, Amuchastegui S, Daniel KC, Berti E, Colonna M, Adorini L (2005) Expression of the inhibitory receptor ILT3 on dendritic cells is dispensable for induction of CD4 + Foxp3+ regulatory T cells by 1,25-dihydroxyvitamin D3. Blood 106:3490–3497

Penna G, Amuchastegui S, Giarratana N, Daniel KC, Vulcano M, Sozzani S, Adorini L (2007) 1,25-Dihydroxyvitamin D3 selectively modulates tolerogenic properties in myeloid but not plasmacytoid dendritic cells. J Immunol 178:145–153

Piemonti L, Monti P, Allavena P, Sironi M, Soldini L, Leone BE, Socci C, Di Carlo V (1999) Glucocorticoids affect human dendritic cell differentiation and maturation. J Immunol 162:6473–6481

Piemonti L, Monti P, Sironi M, Fraticelli P, Leone BE, Dal Cin E, Allavena P, Di Carlo V (2000) Vitamin D3 affects differentiation, maturation, and function of human monocyte-derived dendritic cells. J Immunol 164:4443–4451

Puccetti P, Fallarino F (2007) Generation of T cell regulatory activity by plasmacytoid dendritic cells and tryptophan catabolism. Blood Cells Mol Dis 40:101–105

Puccetti P, Grohmann U (2007) IDO and regulatory T cells: a role for reverse signalling and non-canonical NF-kappaB activation. Nat Rev Immunol 7:817–823

Ravetch JV, Lanier LL (2000) Immune inhibitory receptors. Science 290:84–89

Roncarolo MG, Gregori S, Battaglia M, Bacchetta R, Fleischhauer K, Levings MK (2006) Interleukin-10-secreting type 1 regulatory T cells in rodents and humans. Immunol Rev 212:28–50

Rutella S, Lemoli RM (2004) Regulatory T cells and tolerogenic dendritic cells: from basic biology to clinical applications. Immunol Lett 94:11–26

Rutella S, Pierelli L, Bonanno G, Sica S, Ameglio F, Capoluongo E, Mariotti A, Scambia G, d'Onofrio G, Leone G (2002) Role for granulocyte colony-stimulating factor in the generation of human T regulatory type 1 cells. Blood 100:2562–2571

Rutella S, Bonanno G, Pierelli L, Mariotti A, Capoluongo E, Contemi AM, Ameglio F, Curti A, De Ritis DG, Voso MT, Perillo A, Mancuso S, Scambia G, Lemoli RM, Leone G (2004) Granulocyte colony-stimulating factor promotes the generation of regulatory DC through induction of IL-10 and IFN-alpha. Eur J Immunol 34:1291–1302

Saemann MD, Kelemen P, Bohmig GA, Horl WH, Zlabinger GJ (2004) Hyporesponsiveness in alloreactive T-cells by NF-kappaB inhibitor-treated dendritic cells: resistance to calcineurin inhibition. Am J Transplant 4:1448–1458

Sato K, Yamashita N, Baba M, Matsuyama T (2003) Regulatory dendritic cells protect mice from murine acute graft-versus-host disease and leukemia relapse. Immunity 18:367–379

Scheinman RI, Cogswell PC, Lofquist AK, Baldwin AS, Jr. (1995) Role of transcriptional activation of I kappa B alpha in mediation of immunosuppression by glucocorticoids. Science 270:283–286

Shevach EM, DiPaolo RA, Andersson J, Zhao DM, Stephens GL, Thornton AM (2006) The lifestyle of naturally occurring CD4 + CD25 + Foxp3 + regulatory T cells. Immunol Rev 212:60–73

Shortman K, Liu YJ (2002) Mouse and human dendritic cell subtypes. Nat Rev Immunol 2: 151–161.

Sigmundsdottir H, Pan J, Debes GF, Alt C, Habtezion A, Soler D, Butcher EC (2007) DCs metabolize sunlight-induced vitamin D3 to 'program' T cell attraction to the epidermal chemokine CCL27. Nat Immunol 8:285–293

Steinman RM, Banchereau J (2007) Taking dendritic cells into medicine. Nature 449:419–426

Steinman RM, Hemmi H (2006) Dendritic cells: translating innate to adaptive immunity. Curr Top Microbiol Immunol 311:17–58

Steinman RM, Hawiger D, Nussenzweig MC (2003) Tolerogenic dendritic cells. Annu Rev Immunol 21:685–711

Suciu-Foca N, Cortesini R (2007) Central role of ILT3 in the T suppressor cell cascade. Cell Immunol 248:59–67

Szabo G, Gavala C, Mandrekar P (2001) Tacrolimus and cyclosporine A inhibit allostimulatory capacity and cytokine production of human myeloid dendritic cells. J Invest Med 49:442–449

Takai T, Ono M (2001) Activating and inhibitory nature of the murine paired immunoglobulin-like receptor family. Immunol Rev 181:215–222

Taner T, Hackstein H, Wang Z, Morelli AE, Thomson AW (2005) Rapamycin-treated, alloantigen-pulsed host dendritic cells induce ag-specific T cell regulation and prolong graft survival. Am J Transplant 5:228–236

Terness P, Bauer TM, Rose L, Dufter C, Watzlik A, Simon H, Opelz G (2002) Inhibition of allogeneic T cell proliferation by indoleamine 2,3-dioxygenase-expressing dendritic cells: mediation of suppression by tryptophan metabolites. J Exp Med 196:447–457

Thomas JM, Contreras JL, Jiang XL, Eckhoff DE, Wang PX, Hubbard WJ, Lobashevsky AL, Wang W, Asiedu C, Stavrou S, Cook WJ, Robbin ML, Thomas FT, Neville DM, Jr. (1999) Peritransplant tolerance induction in macaques: early events reflecting the unique synergy between immunotoxin and deoxyspergualin. Transplantation 68:1660–1673

Thomas JM, Hubbard WJ, Sooudi SK, Thomas FT (2001) STEALTH matters: a novel paradigm of durable primate allograft tolerance. Immunol Rev 183:223–233

van Halteren AG, van Etten E, de Jong EC, Bouillon R, Roep BO, Mathieu C (2002) Redirection of human autoreactive T-cells upon interaction with dendritic cells modulated by TX527, an analog of 1,25 dihydroxyvitamin D(3). Diabetes 51:2119–2125

Verhasselt V, Vanden Berghe W, Vanderheyde N, Willems F, Haegeman G, Goldman M (1999) N-acetyl-L-cysteine inhibits primary human T cell responses at the dendritic cell level: association with NF-kappaB inhibition. J Immunol 162:2569–2574

Vieira PL, Kalinski P, Wierenga EA, Kapsenberg ML, de Jong EC (1998) Glucocorticoids inhibit bioactive IL-12p70 production by in vitro-generated human dendritic cells without affecting their T cell stimulatory potential. J Immunol 161:5245–5251

Vulcano M, Struyf S, Scapini P, Cassatella M, Bernasconi S, Bonecchi R, Calleri A, Penna G, Adorini L, Luini W, Mantovani A, Van Damme J, Sozzani S (2003) Unique regulation of CCL18 production by maturing dendritic cells. J Immunol 170:3843–3849

Wohlfert EA, Nichols FC, Nevius E, Clark RB (2007) Peroxisome proliferator-activated receptor gamma (PPARgamma) and immunoregulation: enhancement of regulatory T cells through PPARgamma-dependent and -independent mechanisms. J Immunol 178:4129–4135

Woltman AM, van Kooten C (2003) Functional modulation of dendritic cells to suppress adaptive immune responses. J Leukoc Biol 73:428–441

Woltman AM, de Fijter JW, Kamerling SW, Paul LC, Daha MR, van Kooten C (2000) The effect of calcineurin inhibitors and corticosteroids on the differentiation of human dendritic cells. Eur J Immunol 30:1807–1812

Woltman AM, de Fijter JW, Kamerling SW, van Der Kooij SW, Paul LC, Daha MR, van Kooten C (2001) Rapamycin induces apoptosis in monocyte- and CD34-derived dendritic cells but not in monocytes and macrophages. Blood 98:174–180

Xie JH, Nomura N, Lu M, Chen SL, Koch GE, Weng Y, Rosa R, Di Salvo J, Mudgett J, Peterson LB, Wicker LS, DeMartino JA (2003) Antibody-mediated blockade of the CXCR3 chemokine receptor results in diminished recruitment of T helper 1 cells into sites of inflammation. J Leukoc Biol 73:771–780

Xing N, ML LM, Bachman LA, McKean DJ, Kumar R, Griffin MD (2002) Distinctive dendritic cell modulation by vitamin D(3) and glucocorticoid pathways. Biochem Biophys Res Commun 297:645–652

Yamazaki S, Iyoda T, Tarbell K, Olson K, Velinzon K, Inaba K, Steinman RM (2003) Direct expansion of functional CD25+CD4+ regulatory T cells by antigen-processing dendritic cells. J Exp Med 198:235–247

Yamazaki S, Bonito AJ, Spisek R, Dhodapkar M, Inaba K, Steinman RM (2007) Dendritic cells are specialized accessory cells along with TGF-{beta} for the differentiation of Foxp3+ CD4+ regulatory T cells from peripheral Foxp3- precursors. Blood 110:4293–4302

Yokoyama WM (1997) What goes up must come down: the emerging spectrum of inhibitory receptors. J Exp Med 186:1803–1808

Yu XP, Bellido T, Manolagas SC (1995) Down-regulation of NF-kappa B protein levels in activated human lymphocytes by 1,25-dihydroxyvitamin D3. Proc Natl Acad Sci USA 92:10990–10994

Use of Adenovirus in Vaccines for HIV

Steven Patterson, Timos Papagatsias, and Adel Benlahrech

Contents

Abstract The best hope of controlling the HIV pandemic is the development of an effective vaccine. In addition to the stimulation of virus neutralising antibodies, a vaccine will need an effective T-cell response against the virus. Vaccines based on recombinant adenoviruses (rAd) are promising candidates to stimulate anti-HIV T-cell responses. This review discusses the different rAd vector types, problems raised by host immune responses against them and strategies that are being adopted to overcome this problem. Vaccines need to target and stimulate dendritic cells and thus the tropism and interaction of rAd-based vaccines with these cells is covered. Different rAd vaccination regimes and the need to stimulate mucosal responses are discussed together with data from animal studies on immunogenicity and virus challenge experiments. The review ends with a discussion of the recent disappointing Merck HIV vaccine trial.

S. Patterson (✉)
Department of Immunology, Imperial College, Chelsea and Westminster Hospital, London, UK
s.patterson@imperial.ac.uk

G. Lombardi, Y. Riffo-Vasquez (eds.), *Dendritic Cells,* Handbook of Experimental Pharmacology 188,

Today according to the World Health Organisation (WHO) statistics, there are 33.2 million people infected with the human immunodeficiency virus-1 (HIV-1), with two thirds of these cases occurring in sub-Saharan Africa. Over the last 20 years HIV-1 has caused 20 million deaths and currently there are some 2.5 million new infections and 2.1 million deaths per year. Effective combination anti-retroviral drug therapy was introduced in the mid-1990s and has greatly reduced the death rate caused by the virus in the developed world. However, infected individuals require expensive life long treatment which causes significant side effects. Furthermore, treatment reaches only a minority of infected individuals in the underdeveloped world where the problem is greatest. Additionally, drug-resistant virus can be generated due to the high mutation rate of HIV-1. The most effective solution to the Acquired Immunodeficiency Syndrome (AIDS) pandemic is an effective vaccine but despite 20 years of research there are no prospects of such a vaccine in the near future.

Most successful antiviral vaccines mediate protection by inducing neutralising antibodies (NAbs) but the consensus view is that protection from disease caused by HIV-1 will require stimulation of both humoral and T-cell responses. Vaccination that induces sterilising immunity may not be achieved but it is hoped that vaccination will result in control of virus replication and prevent progression to AIDS. The perceived importance of the T-cell response, particularly of CD8 T cells, is based on a number of observations; virus load reduction shortly after infection correlates with the appearance of HIV-specific CD8 T cells (Borrow et al. 1994; Koup et al. 1994); depletion of CD8 T cells from macaques infected with the related simian immunodeficiency virus (SIV) results in an increase in virus load (Matano et al. 1998; Schmitz et al. 1999); soon after infection and the appearance of HIV-specific CD8 T cells, virus CD8 escape mutants appear (Phillips et al. 1991; Borrow et al. 1997). Thus strategies to induce antiviral CD8 responses have been at the forefront of HIV-1 vaccine research.

1 Adenoviruses as Vectors

Many different viruses have been engineered to carry foreign genes that can be targeted by humoral and cellular immune responses (Liniger et al. 2007). The most widely tested vectors for HIV-1 vaccines to date are pox- and adenovirus-based vectors. This review will focus on the latter.

There are 51 known strains of adenovirus which are divided into seven (A–F) sera groups (group B is further divided into subgroups B1 and B2) and most are associated with mild respiratory and gastrointestinal infections. The properties of the virus important for vector construction include infection of dividing and non-dividing cells, ease of molecular manipulation and growth to high titre. An added advantage of the replication defective vectors that are most widely used is that, there is limited synthesis of adenovirus genes that may compete with the transgene product for presentation on major histocompatibility (MHC) molecules.

Adenoviruses are icosahedral non-enveloped viruses with a diameter of approximately 90–100 nm. The viral capsid is made up of three major proteins, the hexon, penton base and fibre. The hexon units form the icosahedral capsid surface with the penton base proteins forming the 12 capsid vertices. The fibre protein, an antenna-like structure, is attached to the penton base and protrudes outwards from the capsid. At the end of the fibre is a globular "knob" domain responsible for attachment to primary receptors. The fibre proteins of the majority of viruses, including adenovirus type 5 (Ad5) most widely employed as a vector, use the coxsackie virus and adenovirus receptor (CAR) for cellular attachment (Bergelson et al. 1997). CAR is expressed by many cell types including epithelial, endothelial, muscle, and hepatocytes but is not expressed by most cells of the immune system including dendritic cells (DC). Group B2 adenoviruses, including Ad11 and Ad35, use a complement regulatory protein, CD46, as a cellular attachment receptor (Gaggar et al. 2003). This receptor is expressed by DC and other immune system cells but, surprisingly, vaccine vectors based on these viruses seem to be less immunogenic than Ad5-based vectors.

On virus uptake at coated pits into early endosomes, there is interaction with cellular integrins via an arginyl-glycyl-aspartic acid (RGD) motif in the penton base of the viral capsid which, together with the acidification of the endosome facilitates endosome disruption and release of the virus into the cytoplasm (Wickham et al. 1993). The viral capsid is partially disrupted during transit into the cytoplasm and subsequently with the aid of microtubules and dynein migrates towards the nucleus and enters via a nuclear pore to initiate the replication cycle (Leopold et al. 2000).

1.1 Vector Construction

A description of the different replication defective vector constructs and their manufacture is given by He and colleagues (He et al. 1998). The genome of adenoviruses is 34–43 kb in length and so-called first generation vectors, the most widely used, are made by replacing either the E1 and/or E3 genes with the transgene. E3 is not required for virus replication but plays a role in virus escape of immune recognition (Burgert et al. 2002) and thus E3-deleted viruses only can be used for the construction of replication competent vectors (Peng et al. 2005). The adenovirus E1 gene is synthesised early in infection and mediates activation of other viral genes. First generation vectors, deleted in E1, cannot replicate and are grown in packaging cell lines, such as 293 human embryonic kidney (HEK) or 911 human embryonic retinoblastoma (HER), that supply E1 *in trans*. Removal of E1 enables accommodation of up to 5 kb of foreign genetic material and to further increase capacity to 7.5 kb, E1/E3 deleted vectors have been developed. To counter problems of anti-vector immunity and destruction of transgene-expressing cells caused by low level leaky expression of adenovirus genes, the virus has additionally been depleted in the E2 and E4 genes (Gorziglia et al. 1999). So called "gutless" vectors have also been engineered in which the final vector lacks any adenovirus genes (Mitani et al. 1995; Parks et al. 1996). The E1 gene in the 293HEK and 911HER packaging cell lines has flanking sequences complementary to the E1 flanking sequences in the adenoviral genome. Homologous recombination can lead to the generation of replication competent adenovirus (RCA) by replacement of the transgene with E1 from the packaging cell line. To overcome this problem the PER.C6 cell line, a 911 derivative, has been developed in which the E1 gene is controlled by the human phosphoglycerate kinase (PGK) promoter with no overlap with the adenovirus backbone (Fallaux et al. 1998).

2 Blunting of Immunogenicity by Pre-Existing Immunity to Vectors

Infection with adenovirus is widespread but there are marked differences in seroprevalence to different strains of the virus. A study of seropositivity to all 51 known types in a Belgium population found that 60–80% of individuals had NAbs to serotype C viruses, the group to which Ad5 belongs. By contrast the serogroup B viruses, which includes Ad11 and Ad35, had a seroprevalence of less than 10% (Vogels et al. 2003). To date most recombinant Ad (rAd) vector vaccine studies have used an Ad5 vector and, in view of the widespread seropositivity to Ad5, a perceived problem is that NAb will blunt the effectiveness of vaccination. This could be a particular problem in sub-Saharan Africa where NAb titres against Ad5 are fivefold higher than in the USA (Sumida et al. 2005). This fear is borne out by studies in the mouse and rhesus macaque (Sumida et al. 2004;Yang et al. 2003; Barouch et al. 2003; Casimiro et al. 2003). A single vaccination in non-Ad immune animals induces humoral and cellular immunity to the vector (Juillard et al. 1995; Yang et al. 1995) thus anti-Ad immunity is likely to be a problem even in those individuals that are Ad seronegative since vaccination regimes may involve repeated boosting vaccinations. Many approaches have been adopted to overcome this problem. Priming with DNA followed by boosting with the adenovector is more effective than prime and boost with rAd vector alone (Santra et al. 2005). Following this principle, prime and boost vaccinations have been performed with pox and rAd vectors or with two different serotypes of rAd vector (Barratt-Boyes et al. 2006). Significant effort has been made to develop vectors from adenoviruses that are serologically less prevalent, notably the B type viruses Ad11 and Ad35, and there is also interest in developing vectors from other primates such as chimpanzee (Farina et al. 2001; Fitzgerald et al. 2003; Reyes-Sandoval et al. 2004).

Neutralising antibodies may be directed against penton, hexon, or fibre components of the virus, however, the most potent neutralising activity is against the hexon (Sumida et al. 2005; Youil et al. 2002). The hexon has 7 hypervariable loops that can bind NAbs, and to overcome NAb immunity these determinants have been replaced in rAd5 with those of a rare serotype, Ad48 (Roberts et al. 2006). The resulting chimeric viruses were used to construct vectors carrying a SIV *gag* gene and were found to be as immunogenic as unmodified rAd5 vectors even in the presence of NAbs.

A novel approach to overcome blunting by NAbs is to coat the virions with a polymer to block antibody binding. Two polymers have been used, polyethylene glycol (PEG) and a multivalent hydrophilic polymer based on poly-[N-(2-hydroxy-propyl)methacrylamide (pHPMA) (O'Riordan et al. 1999; Fisher et al. 2001). PEG coating maintains biological activity of the vector including infection, pHPMA, on the other hand, blocks infection. Conjugation of cellular ligands onto pHPMA-coated vectors has overcome this problem. Fibroblast growth factor (FGF) and vascular endothelial growth factor (VEGF) molecules were attached to the polymer coating and shown to mediate vector cellular entry. In addition to overcoming NAb, this system allows vector retargeting to different cell types by selecting appropriate cellular ligands.

In gene therapy applications where transgene expression is required for a longer period, anti-Ad CD8 responses destroy infected cells (Yang et al. 1994, 1995). Vaccines require shorter transgene expression, but despite this, adoptive transfer of CD8 cells from Ad5 seropositive mice caused a 50% reduction in CD8 responses against the transgene in mice vaccinated with a rAd5 vaccine (Sumida et al. 2004). Pre-existing NAbs to Ad5 can reduce the generation of CD8 responses against the transgene by 90% or more but can be overcome by vaccinating with a vector based on a serologically distinct strain of adenovirus. However, anti-Ad CD8 T cells that are cross-reactive between different serotypes have been reported and could potentially blunt vaccination with rAd vectors from rarer serotypes (Smith et al. 1998). This possibility is supported by studies in mice exposed to Ad5 and then immunised with a rAd vector derived from chimpanzee, Ad68, coding for HIV-1 Gag. Anti-Gag CD8 responses were reduced by approximately 30% in animals initially exposed to Ad5 and shown to be due to cross reactive CD8 T cells (Fitzgerald et al. 2003).

3 Immunogenicity of rAd Vectors

3.1 Tropism

Dendritic cells (DC) initiate immune responses by processing foreign antigen into short peptides which bind to MHC class I and II molecules and stimulate antigen-specific CD8 and CD4 T cells. To initiate an effector immune response DC require a maturation stimulus which induces up-regulation of co-stimulatory molecules and expression of the chemokine receptor CCR7 to mediate migration to the draining lymph node (Banchereau and Steinman 1998). This stimulus is usually delivered by pathogen associated molecules recognised by pattern recognition receptors (PRRs) such as toll-like receptors (TLRs) or through inflammatory cytokines. Thus vaccine-derived antigens must reach DC and induce their maturation to initiate immune responses. As mentioned previously, group C adenoviruses utilise CAR which is not expressed by DC, nevertheless, rAd5 vectors can infect these cells. Recent data suggests the DC infection is not mediated by the penton RGD motif that binds cellular integrins but through a region of the fibre shaft that recognises and binds to a heparin-sensitive receptor on DC (Cheng et al. 2007). Unsurprisingly, vectors based on group B2 viruses, such as Ad11 or Ad35, or chimeric viruses that comprise of the icosahedral core of Ad5 and group B virus fibre that recognises CD46, transduce DC more efficiently (Rozis et al. 2005). To more efficiently target DC, the RGD sequence has been engineered into the fibre knob in order to enhance binding to cellular integrins and shown to increase transduction of a murine DC line and human DC (Okada et al. 2001). Similarly, in a mouse bone marrow-derived DC model, 8-fold higher transduction was observed by a rAd with an RGD-modified fibre knob than with an unmodified vector (Worgall et al. 2004). Vaccination of mice with such fibre knob-modified vectors expressing β-galactosidase significantly enhanced CD4 and CD8 responses to the transgene (Worgall et al. 2004).

3.2 Immunogenicity of Type B Viruses

Although, viruses utilising the CD46 receptor for cellular entry may be expected to be more antigenic than group C vectors that use CAR, because they infect DC more efficiently, several reports have surprisingly reported otherwise. Rhesus macaques vaccinated with HIV-1 Gag-expressing group B vectors, rAd35 and rAd34, and group C rAd5, found higher levels of responses to the transgene stimulated by Ad5 (Shiver and Emini 2004). These studies have been extended by Barouch and colleagues, who confirmed that Ad35 was less immunogenic than Ad5 in macaques but found that the immunogenicity of Ad35 was similar to that of Ad5 in chimeric 35/5 viruses expressing the CAR binding fibre knob of Ad5 (Nanda et al. 2005). This work is supported by studies in which Ad5 was shown to be more immunogenic in monkeys than chimeric Ad5 with the fibre of Ad35 (Ophorst et al. 2004). The more potent immunogenicity of Ad5 may reflect more rapid escape from the endosome and efficient trafficking to the nucleus whereas group B viruses are retained for longer in endosome (Shayakhmetov et al. 2003; Miyazawa et al. 2001).

Cellular entry mediated by CD46 may be associated with reduced immunogenicity of serogroup B rAd vectors since other immunosuppressive viruses, such as measles and HHV6 (McChesney and Oldstone 1989; Smith et al. 2003) both use CD46 as a receptor (Dorig et al. 1993; Santoro et al. 1999). Furthermore there is evidence that cross-linking CD46 can induce regulatory cells that suppress T-cell responses (Barchet et al. 2006). However, studies in CD46 transgenic mice found that a chimeric rAd5/35 vector that had the CD46-binding fibre protein of Ad35 was not associated with immunosuppression (DiPaolo et al. 2006).

3.3 Dendritic Cell Activation

To induce an effector immune response DC need to be activated to mature as presentation of antigen by immature DC can induce tolerance (Dhodapkar et al. 2001). Numerous studies in the mouse and rhesus macaque models describe intramuscular vaccination with rAd vectors expressing HIV-1 genes leading to the generation of T-cell and antibody responses. For this to be achieved there must be activation of DC but whether this is due to a direct effect of the virus on DC, or due to tissue injury-induced inflammation caused by the injection or both is not clear. Some studies found that adenovirus infection of human DC does not induce maturation (Rozis et al. 2005; Zhong et al. 1999; Smith et al. 2001; Ranieri et al. 1999) whilst other investigators observed DC maturation (Rea et al. 1999; Schumacher et al. 2004). One possible explanation for these discrepancies is that those investigations in which DC activation was observed used up to tenfold more virus. Mice are frequently used as vaccination models for HIV-1 vaccines, however, there may be differences between murine and human DC with respect to Ad-induced maturation. For example, mouse myeloid DC express the TLR9 receptor that may be activated through CpG motifs in adenovirus DNA whereas human myeloid DC do not express TLR9 (Krug et al. 2001; Kadowaki et al. 2001; Jarrossay et al. 2001; Edwards et al. 2003). The knob component of Ad5 is reported to be required for induction of maturation of bone marrow-derived DC (Molinier-Frenkel et al. 2003) whilst it was shown that molecular events involved activation of the nuclear factor-kappa B (NF-κB) pathway (Morelli et al. 2000). By contrast, mutation of the RGD motif in the Ad penton base was found to suppress vector-induced maturation. Evidence was presented to suggest that the vector induces DC to secrete tumour necrosis factor alpha (TNFα) through a phosphoinositide-3 (PI-3) kinase pathway and that TNFα acts in an autocrine manner to induce maturation (Philpott et al. 2004). Differential sensitivity to Ad-mediated activation of mouse and human DC may thus influence the outcome of Ad vaccination.

4 Vaccination with rAd Vectors

4.1 Animal Models

Vaccination protocols using rAd vectors have either focussed on immunogenicity alone or vaccination followed by virus challenge. Immunogenicity has been studied in mice, rhesus macaques and chimpanzees. HIV-1 infects chimpanzees but not macaques, thus challenge studies in these species have been conducted with HIV-1 and SIV respectively. The current view is that T-cell immunity alone is unlikely to induce sterilising immunity but may prevent disease progression. The drawback of the chimpanzee model is that chimpanzees do not develop an AIDS-like disease and thus assessing the effectiveness of preventing disease progression is difficult. An optimal HIV-1 vaccine is likely to require both T cells and envelope NAbs. Although SIV-infected macaques develop an AIDS-like disease, differences have been noted in the immunogenicity of SIV and HIV-1 envelopes (Weiss et al. 1986). To overcome this problem chimeric SIVs have been constructed in which the SIV *env* gene has been replaced by that of HIV-1 (Kuwata et al. 1995). These constructs are termed, simian-human immunodeficiency viruses (SHIVs), have been extensively used in challenge studies.

4.2 Replication Competent and Defective Vectors

Vaccination studies with rAd vectors have used either replication-competent, E3-deleted virus, or E1a replication-defective virus. A possible concern with using replication competent virus is that, there will be synthesis of adenovirus proteins in the antigen presenting cell which may compete with the transgene protein for binding to the MHC molecules resulting in a reduced immune response to the transgene. Most of the available evidence suggests that this is not a major concern and may reflect synthesis of larger amounts of transgene antigen over a longer period of time. However, in this context it is interesting to note that a recent study has shown that when replication defective rAd vector is given by the intramuscular route, transgene expression could be detected at the site of injection 5 weeks later and low levels of vector DNA sequences could be detected in a number of tissues after one year (Tatsis et al. 2007). It was suggested that prolonged low level transgene expression facilitated the observed generation of a mix of effector, effector memory and central memory CD8 T cell populations. This combination of cells may be optimal for controlling HIV-1 infection since effectors would be expected to be active in peripheral tissues at the site of infection whilst the higher proliferative capacity of central memory cells would be important in the generation of more HIV-specific effectors and control virus that spreads from the infection site.

Vaccination of chimpanzees, rhesus macaques or mice with replication competent viral vectors derived from adenovirus serotypes 4, 5, and 7 coding for Env or Gag induced both cellular and humoral responses (Prevec et al. 1991; Natuk et al. 1993; Lubeck et al. 1997; Buge et al. 1999; Patterson et al. 2004; Malkevitch et al. 2004). Similarly, vaccination with replication defective vectors was found to induce cellular and antibody responses (Bruce et al. 1999; Yoshida et al. 2001; Shiver et al. 2002; Vinner et al. 2003; Fitzgerald et al. 2003; Casimiro et al. 2003; Letvin et al. 2004; Santra et al. 2005; Seaman et al. 2005). To compare replicating and non-replicating vectors, E3- and E1/E3-deleted rAd5 and rAd7 constructs carrying an HIV-1 clade B *env* gene were constructed and used to immunise chimpanzees (Peng et al. 2005). Animals were vaccinated sequentially with the serologically distinct rAd5 and rAd7 followed by boosting with envelope protein. After the rAd vector immunisations, total antibody titres against a heterologous clade B virus were about 10-fold higher in animals vaccinated with replicating vector but these differences disappeared after the second protein boost. In contrast, NAbs against a heterologous virus were significantly higher in the replication competent vector vaccine group but there was no difference between the groups in NAb titre against the homologous virus. T-cell proliferative and interferon-γ (IFN-γ) ELISpot responses were higher throughout the immunisation schedule in the replication competent vaccine group. This may reflect higher levels of antigen over a longer period of time as suggested above but may also be due to cross presentation of antigen from infected apoptotic cells (Bevan 1976).

4.3 Mucosal/Systemic Responses and Prime Boost Strategies

HIV-1 is transmitted across mucosal surfaces in the genital tract or rectal tissue and shortly after infection the mucosal tissue of the gut becomes the major site of virus replication leading to the loss of up to 80% of the memory CD4 T-cell population (Mehandru et al. 2004; Li et al. 2005). Thus an optimal HIV-1 vaccine should provide an effective immune response in these tissues. Vaccination with rAd vectors at a mucosal site has been widely adopted to induce mucosal responses (Natuk et al. 1993; Lubeck et al. 1997; Patterson et al. 2004; Malkevitch et al. 2004); this may be particularly potent with replicating vectors as adenovirus infects and replicates in epithelial cells. An early study using chimpanzees vaccinated orally with replication competent rAd4, 5 or 7 vectors expressing either Env or Gag and followed by an intranasal boost with Env and/or Gag subunit vaccines induced low titres of neutralising antibodies in secretions (Natuk et al. 1993). However, concerns have been expressed with intranasal vaccination as virus was detected in the olfactory bulb of the CNS in mice vaccinated intranasally (Lemiale et al. 2003). To facilitate effective mucosal immunisation by the oral route E1-deleted rAd41 vectors have been constructed (Lemiale et al. 2007). Ad41 has a natural tropism for the gut and does not cause disease outside the gastrointestinal tract (Christensen 1989). The tropism of these viruses for the gastrointestinal tract is probably due to their increased resistance to acidic pH (Favier et al. 2004) and their unusual capsid structure including the presence of both long and short fibres (Yeh et al. 1994; Pieniazek et al. 1990). The long fibres mediate binding to CAR but the receptor for the short fibre is unknown (Roelvink et al. 1998; Schoggins et al. 2003). In addition there is no RGD motif in the penton base which can bind cellular integrins (Albinsson and Kidd 1999).

Most studies have used one or more priming vaccinations with one vector followed by one or more boosting vaccinations with a second vector. Vaccinations at mucosal surfaces have usually primed with a rAd vector followed by intramuscular boosting with Env protein (Lubeck et al. 1997; Patterson et al. 2004; Malkevitch et al. 2004; Gomez-Roman et al. 2005). Regimes using DNA vector have primed intramuscularly with DNA followed by intramuscular boosting with rAd vector (Shiver et al. 2002; Vinner et al. 2003; Mascola et al. 2005; Letvin et al. 2004). Although mucosal responses have not been analysed in all studies, they have been reported when vaccination has been through a mucosal surface.

In an attempt to improve the immune response, rhesus macaques have been vaccinated intramuscularly with Gag antigen with or without a TLR agonist, including TLR8, TLR7/8, and TLR9, followed by boosting with a rAd5-gag vector (Wille-Reece et al. 2006). After priming, all TLR agonists increased the number of IFN-γ and interleukin-2 (IL-2) positive cells and was further enhanced after vaccination with the rAd vector. Overall, the most marked improvement in the CD8 response was seen with the TLR7/8 agonist. Interestingly, HIV-specific CD8 cells were detected after priming with antigen plus the TLR7/8 agonist but not the other TLR ligands, suggesting that this ligand promoted cross-presentation.

4.4 Virus Challenge Studies

Challenge virus has been administered intravenously or via mucosal routes, either intravaginally or rectally. Traditionally vaccines have aimed to generate NAbs to protect against infection, while CD8 responses have been thought to be mainly involved in clearing virus after infection had become established. In a challenge study, chimpanzees were vaccinated intranasally with a replicating rAd vector containing an HIV-1 *env* gene and boosted by intramuscular injection of Env protein prior to intravenously challenge with a low dose of a heterologous HIV-1 isolate (Lubeck et al. 1997). All of four challenged animals developed low levels of HIV-specific CD8 T cells and three of the four had NAbs against the homologous virus whilst two had NAbs against the heterologous challenge virus. All animals were resistant to low dose challenge suggesting that CD8 T cells played a role in protection.

Challenge studies in macaques have been performed either after mucosal priming with rAd and intramuscular boosting with protein or following intramuscular DNA priming and intramuscular boosting with rAd. Envelope gene and Env protein have been used in mucosal vaccination regimes with or without *gag* gene in the rAd vector. Intramuscular DNA prime and rAd boost have used *gag* gene with and without other genes including *env, pol, nef,* and *tat*. Macaques vaccinated with rAd via the mucosal route, boosted with Env protein and challenged intravaginally with SIV, generally showed lower levels of SIV replication than non-immunised animals (Buge et al. 1997). However, the results were difficult to interpret with certainty because two out of six animals in both the control and vaccinated groups did not become infected. In a rhesus macaque study that used intravenous challenge with a SHIV, all non-vaccinated animals became infected (Shiver et al. 2002). Vaccinated animals were given DNA intramuscularly followed by intramuscular boosting with E1-deleted rAd5 containing an SIV *gag* gene. Vaccination-induced SIV-specific CD8 cells were identified by tetramer staining and although infection was not prevented, the level of virus in the blood in acutely infected animals was a log lower than in controls. As they progressed to the chronic stage of infection, virus loads were 100–1,000 fold lower than in unvaccinated animals. CD4 T-cell numbers were also about 10-fold higher than in controls at the chronic stage of infection. Approximately one year after challenge five out of six control animals developed AIDS-related illnesses whereas the rAd-vaccinated animals were all healthy at this time. In parallel experiments animals were primed with DNA and boosted with a modified vaccinia Ankara vector carrying the SIV *gag* gene. These animals showed slightly higher CD4 T-cell numbers than unvaccinated controls and lower levels of virus but this vaccination strategy was less effective than immunisation with the rAd vector. An SIV rectal challenge model suggested that vaccination with replication competent rAd-env followed by Env protein boosting was insufficient to afford protection (Patterson et al. 2004). However, addition of rAd-gag or rAd-nef to the vaccination regime resulted in lower virus loads and extended survival. In another DNA prime/rAd boost study, although rAd-env alone could not provide protection, addition of *env* gene components to a DNA/rAd *gag/pol/nef* vaccine protocol enhanced protection of rhesus macaques, challenged intravenously with a SHIV (Letvin et al.

2004). Addition of *env* improved maintenance of CD4 T-cells, resulted in better control of virus load and was not associated with NAbs but rather with an Env-specific cellular response. A possible contribution of NAbs was not ruled out by the authors who suggested that experimental numbers may not have been sufficient to detect significant differences.

5 Clinical HIV-1 Vaccine Trials

An early Phase I trial of an adenovirus-based vaccine vector used an E1-, E4-, part E3-deleted rAd5 construct (Catanzaro et al. 2006). HIV-1 seronegative volunteers were given a single intramuscular vaccination of a mixture of four vectors containing clade B *gag/pol*, clade A *env*, clade B *env* and clade C *env*. No adverse events were noted and 93% and 60% of vaccinees showed HIV-specific CD4 and CD8 T cell responses respectively. HIV-specific antibodies were detected by Western blotting in 93% of vaccinated volunteers but no NAbs were induced. An HIV-specific response was mounted by volunteers that had pre-existing NAbs to adenovirus but responses were about three-fold lower than in adenovirus seronegative individuals.

5.1 Merck Step HIV-1 Vaccine Trial

Development of rAd vectors as HIV-1 vaccines received a serious setback in the autumn of 2007 with the premature termination of the Merck HIV-1 Vaccine Step Trial because of lack of efficacy and the possibility that vaccination may have increased the risks of infection in some individuals. The trial involved volunteers from North and South America whose lifestyle gave them a higher risk of HIV-1 infection and included prostitutes and men who have sex with men. Three immunisations of a 1:1:1 ratio of 3 first generation rAd5 vectors carrying *gag, pol*, and *nef* genes were given. The consensus view was that vaccination was unlikely to prevent HIV-1 infection but, based on studies in non-human primates, it was hoped that virus load may be reduced and disease progression slowed or halted. Initially the trial only included individuals that were seronegative for Ad5 but later Ad5 seropositive volunteers were also included. A total of 3,000 volunteers were recruited between December 2004 and March 2007, one third of whom were women. By October 2007, 82 men and one woman had become infected. From the infected males, 49 belonged to the vaccinated group and 33 to the placebo group. These were further divided into individuals with high (>200) or low (<200) titres of Ad5 antibodies. In the group with Ad5 antibody titres <200, 28 cases of infection were in the vaccinated group and 24 infections were in the placebo group. For individuals with an Ad5 antibody titre >200, 21 infections were in vaccinated individuals whereas there were only nine infections in the placebo group. The placebo was saline rather than an empty rAd vector. Of note, 65% and 40% of men in the low and high Ad5 antibody groups respectively, were circumcised. There was no difference in virus load between the vaccinated and the unvaccinated group, indicating that vaccination had not induced an immune response able to control virus replication. Preliminary data from the study may be found at: http://www.hvtn.org/science/1107.html. Although the numbers are low there was concern that vaccination with rAd5 could increase the susceptibility to HIV-1 infection, possibly through the activation of memory Ad-specific CD4 T cells. However, preliminary data from analysis of blood samples from vaccinated individuals do not show increased expression of the HIV-1 co-receptor chemokine (C-C motif) receptor 5 (CCR5) on CD4 cells although crucially it was not possible to obtain cells from more relevant mucosal surfaces. These results are difficult to interpret in terms of activation of Ad-specific memory CD4 T cells, since different serotypes of Ad have cross-reactive CD4 and CD8 epitopes (Olive et al. 2002; Leen et al. 2008) and one might reasonably expect that, individuals who were seronegative for Ad5 would have encountered other Ad serotypes. The trial used first generation rAd5 vectors and the "leakiness" in Ad gene expression may have resulted in production and presentation to the immune system of *de novo* synthesised adenovirus proteins. In a human *in vitro* system a slightly higher level of Ad cytotoxicity was observed with target cells transduced with an empty first generation rAd vector than untransduced controls, suggesting that there was expression of some adenovirus genes (Butterfield et al. 1998). To determine whether memory T cells are responding to incoming proteins that constitute the vector or to newly synthesised adenovirus proteins, human monocyte-derived DC have been transduced with first generation vectors deleted in E1 or so-called "gutless" vectors that lack all adenovirus coding genes. Transduced DC were co-cultured with autologous lymphocytes and TNFα and IFN-γ production by Ad-specific CD4 and CD8 cells measured. Both first generation and the gutless vectors induced similar levels of CD4 and CD8 T-cell activation suggesting that the anti-vector responses are primarily directed against incoming vector protein entering the class II and cross presentation pathways (Roth et al. 2002).

Justification for the trial was based in part by encouraging results obtained in rhesus macaque challenge studies in which vaccinated animals were challenged with SHIVs. However, the infection with SHIVs does not closely mimic infection with HIV-1. In addition to being more readily neutralised, these chimeric viruses initially infect naïve CD4 cells through chemokine (C-X-C motif) receptor 4 (CXCR4) whereas HIV-1 initially infects and causes depletion of CD4 memory cells infecting through CCR5 (Nishimura et al. 2004). It is clear that although initial animal studies with rAd vaccines looked promising, major advances are still required before an effective rAd vaccine is developed.

References

Albinsson B, Kidd AH (1999) Adenovirus type 41 lacks an RGD alpha(v)-integrin binding motif on the penton base and undergoes delayed uptake in A549 cells. Virus Res 64:125–136

Banchereau J, Steinman RM (1998) Dendritic cells and the control of immunity. Nature 392:245–252

Barchet W, Price JD, Cella M, Colonna M, MacMillan SK, Cobb JP, Thompson PA, Murphy KM, Atkinson JP, Kemper C (2006) Complement-induced regulatory T cells suppress T-cell responses but allow for dendritic-cell maturation. Blood 107:1497–1504

Barouch DH, McKay PF, Sumida SM, Santra S, Jackson SS, Gorgone DA, Lifton MA, Chakrabarti BK, Xu L, Nabel GJ, Letvin NL (2003) Plasmid chemokines and colony-stimulating factors enhance the immunogenicity of DNA priming-viral vector boosting human immunodeficiency virus type 1 vaccines. J Virol 77:8729–8735

Barratt-Boyes SM, Soloff AC, Gao W, Nwanegbo E, Liu X, Rajakumar PA, Brown KN, Robbins PD, Murphey-Corb M, Day RD, Gambotto A (2006) Broad cellular immunity with robust memory responses to simian immunodeficiency virus following serial vaccination with adenovirus 5- and 35-based vectors. J Gen Virol 87:139–149

Bergelson JM, Cunningham JA, Droguett G, Kurt-Jones EA, Krithivas A, Hong JS, Horwitz MS, Crowell RL, Finberg RW (1997) Isolation of a common receptor for Coxsackie B viruses and adenoviruses 2 and 5. Science 275:1320–1323

Bevan MJ (1976) Cross-priming for a secondary cytotoxic response to minor H antigens with H-2 congenic cells which do not cross-react in the cytotoxic assay. J Exp Med 143:1283–1288

Borrow P, Lewicki H, Hahn BH, Shaw GM, Oldstone MB (1994) Virus-specific CD8+ cytotoxic T-lymphocyte activity associated with control of viremia in primary human immunodeficiency virus type 1 infection. J Virol 68:6103–6110

Borrow P, Lewicki H, Wei X, Horwitz MS, Peffer N, Meyers H, Nelson JA, Gairin JE, Hahn BH, Oldstone MB, Shaw GM (1997) Antiviral pressure exerted by HIV-1-specific cytotoxic T lymphocytes (CTLs) during primary infection demonstrated by rapid selection of CTL escape virus. Nat Med 3:205–211

Bruce CB, Akrigg A, Sharpe SA, Hanke T, Wilkinson GW, Cranage MP (1999) Replication-deficient recombinant adenoviruses expressing the human immunodeficiency virus Env antigen can induce both humoral and CTL immune responses in mice. J Gen Virol 80:2621–2628

Buge SL, Richardson E, Alipanah S, Markham P, Cheng S, Kalyan N, Miller CJ, Lubeck M, Udem S, Eldridge J, Robert-Guroff M (1997) An adenovirus-simian immunodeficiency virus env vaccine elicits humoral, cellular, and mucosal immune responses in rhesus macaques and decreases viral burden following vaginal challenge. J Virol 71:8531–8541

Buge SL, Murty L, Arora K, Kalyanaraman VS, Markham PD, Richardson ES, Aldrich K, Patterson LJ, Miller CJ, Cheng SM, Robert-Guroff M (1999) Factors associated with slow disease progression in macaques immunized with an adenovirus-simian immunodeficiency virus (SIV) envelope priming-gp120 boosting regimen and challenged vaginally with SIVmac251. J Virol 73:7430–7440

Burgert HG, Ruzsics Z, Obermeier S, Hilgendorf A, Windheim M, Elsing A (2002) Subversion of host defense mechanisms by adenoviruses. Curr Top Microbiol Immunol 269:273–318

Butterfield LH, Jilani SM, Chakraborty NG, Bui LA, Ribas A, Dissette VB, Lau R, Gamradt SC, Glaspy JA, McBride WH, Mukherji B, Economou JS (1998) Generation of melanoma-specific cytotoxic T lymphocytes by dendritic cells transduced with a MART-1 adenovirus. J Immunol 161:5607–5613

Casimiro DR, Chen L, Fu TM, Evans RK, Caulfield MJ, Davies ME, Tang A, Chen M, Huang L, Harris V, Freed DC, Wilson KA, Dubey S, Zhu DM, Nawrocki D, Mach H, Troutman R, Isopi L, Williams D, Hurni W, Xu Z, Smith JG, Wang S, Liu X, Guan L, Long R, Trigona W, Heidecker GJ, Perry HC, Persaud N, Toner TJ, Su Q, Liang X, Youil R, Chastain M, Bett AJ, Volkin DB, Emini EA, Shiver JW (2003) Comparative immunogenicity in rhesus monkeys of DNA plasmid, recombinant vaccinia virus, and replication-defective adenovirus vectors expressing a human immunodeficiency virus type 1 gag gene. J Virol 77:6305–6313

Catanzaro AT, Koup RA, Roederer M, Bailer RT, Enama ME, Moodie Z, Gu L, Martin JE, Novik L, Chakrabarti BK, Butman BT, Gall JG, King CR, Andrews CA, Sheets R, Gomez PL, Mascola JR, Nabel GJ, Graham BS (2006) Phase 1 safety and immunogenicity evaluation of a multiclade HIV-1 candidate vaccine delivered by a replication-defective recombinant adenovirus vector. J Infect Dis 194:1638–1649

Cheng C, Gall JG, Kong WP, Sheets RL, Gomez PL, King CR, Nabel GJ (2007) Mechanism of ad5 vaccine immunity and toxicity: fiber shaft targeting of dendritic cells. PLoS.Pathog 3:e25
Christensen ML (1989) Human viral gastroenteritis. Clin Microbiol Rev 2:51–89
Dhodapkar MV, Steinman RM, Krasovsky J, Munz C, Bhardwaj N (2001) Antigen-specific inhibition of effector T cell function in humans after injection of immature dendritic cells. J Exp Med 193:233–238
DiPaolo N, Ni S, Gaggar A, Strauss R, Tuve S, Li ZY, Stone D, Shayakhmetov D, Kiviat N, Toure P, Sow S, Horvat B, Lieber A (2006) Evaluation of adenovirus vectors containing serotype 35 fibers for vaccination. Mol Ther 13:756–765
Dorig RE, Marcil A, Chopra A, Richardson CD (1993) The human CD46 molecule is a receptor for measles virus (Edmonston strain). Cell 75:295–305
Edwards AD, Diebold SS, Slack EM, Tomizawa H, Hemmi H, Kaisho T, Akira S, Reise Sousa C (2003) Toll-like receptor expression in murine DC subsets: lack of TLR7 expression by CD8 alpha + DC correlates with unresponsiveness to imidazoquinolines. Eur J Immunol 33:827–833
Fallaux FJ, Bout A, van dV I, van den Wollenberg DJ, Hehir KM, Keegan J, Auger C, Cramer SJ, van Ormondt H, van der Eb AJ, Valerio D, Hoeben RC (1998) New helper cells and matched early region 1-deleted adenovirus vectors prevent generation of replication-competent adenoviruses. Hum Gene Ther 9:1909–1917
Farina SF, Gao GP, Xiang ZQ, Rux JJ, Burnett RM, Alvira MR, Marsh J, Ertl HC, Wilson JM (2001) Replication-defective vector based on a chimpanzee adenovirus. J Virol 75:11603–11613
Favier AL, Burmeister WP, Chroboczek J (2004) Unique physicochemical properties of human enteric Ad41 responsible for its survival and replication in the gastrointestinal tract. Virology 322:93–104
Fisher KD, Stallwood Y, Green NK, Ulbrich K, Mautner V, Seymour LW (2001) Polymer-coated adenovirus permits efficient retargeting and evades neutralising antibodies. Gene Ther 8:341–348
Fitzgerald JC, Gao GP, Reyes-Sandoval A, Pavlakis GN, Xiang ZQ, Wlazlo AP, Giles-Davis W, Wilson JM, Ertl HC (2003) A simian replication-defective adenoviral recombinant vaccine to HIV-1 gag. J Immunol 170:1416–1422
Gaggar A, Shayakhmetov DM, Lieber A (2003) CD46 is a cellular receptor for group B adenoviruses. Nat Med 9:1408–1412
Gomez-Roman VR, Patterson LJ, Venzon D, Liewehr D, Aldrich K, Florese R, Robert-Guroff M (2005) Vaccine-elicited antibodies mediate antibody-dependent cellular cytotoxicity correlated with significantly reduced acute viremia in rhesus macaques challenged with SIVmac251. J Immunol 174:2185–2189
Gorziglia MI, Lapcevich C, Roy S, Kang Q, Kadan M, Wu V, Pechan P, Kaleko M (1999) Generation of an adenovirus vector lacking E1, e2a, E3, and all of E4 except open reading frame 3. J Virol 73:6048–6055
He TC, Zhou S, da Costa LT, Yu J, Kinzler KW, Vogelstein B (1998) A simplified system for generating recombinant adenoviruses. Proc Natl Acad Sci USA 95:2509–2514
Jarrossay D, Napolitani G, Colonna M, Sallusto F, Lanzavecchia A (2001) Specialization and complementarity in microbial molecule recognition by human myeloid and plasmacytoid dendritic cells. Eur J Immunol 31:3388–3393
Juillard V, Villefroy P, Godfrin D, Pavirani A, Venet A, Guillet JG (1995) Long-term humoral and cellular immunity induced by a single immunization with replication-defective adenovirus recombinant vector. Eur J Immunol 25:3467–3473
Kadowaki N, Ho S, Antonenko S, Malefyt RW, Kastelein RA, Bazan F, Liu YJ (2001) Subsets of human dendritic cell precursors express different toll-like receptors and respond to different microbial antigens. J Exp Med 194:863–869
Koup RA, Safrit JT, Cao Y, Andrews CA, McLeod G, Borkowsky W, Farthing C, Ho DD (1994) Temporal association of cellular immune responses with the initial control of viremia in primary human immunodeficiency virus type 1 syndrome. J Virol 68:4650–4655

Krug A, Towarowski A, Britsch S, Rothenfusser S, Hornung V, Bals R, Giese T, Engelmann H, Endres S, Krieg AM, Hartmann G (2001) Toll-like receptor expression reveals CpG DNA as a unique microbial stimulus for plasmacytoid dendritic cells which synergizes with CD40 ligand to induce high amounts of IL-12. Eur J Immunol 31:3026–3037

Kuwata T, Igarashi T, Ido E, Jin M, Mizuno A, Chen J, Hayami M (1995) Construction of human immunodeficiency virus 1/simian immunodeficiency virus strain mac chimeric viruses having vpr and/or nef of different parental origins and their in vitro and in vivo replication. J Gen Virol 76:2181–2191

Leen AM, Christin A, Khalil M, Weiss H, Gee AP, Brenner MK, Heslop HE, Rooney CM, Bollard CM (2008) Identification of hexon-specific CD4 and CD8 T-cell epitopes for vaccine and immunotherapy. J Virol 82:546–554

Lemiale F, Kong WP, Akyurek LM, Ling X, Huang Y, Chakrabarti BK, Eckhaus M, Nabel GJ (2003) Enhanced mucosal immunoglobulin A response of intranasal adenoviral vector human immunodeficiency virus vaccine and localization in the central nervous system. J Virol 77:10078–10087

Lemiale F, Haddada H, Nabel GJ, Brough DE, King CR, Gall JG (2007) Novel adenovirus vaccine vectors based on the enteric-tropic serotype 41. Vaccine 25:2074–2084

Leopold PL, Kreitzer G, Miyazawa N, Rempel S, Pfister KK, Rodriguez-Boulan E, Crystal RG (2000) Dynein- and microtubule-mediated translocation of adenovirus serotype 5 occurs after endosomal lysis. Hum Gene Ther 11:151–165

Letvin NL, Huang Y, Chakrabarti BK, Xu L, Seaman MS, Beaudry K, Korioth-Schmitz B, Yu F, Rohne D, Martin KL, Miura A, Kong WP, Yang ZY, Gelman RS, Golubeva OG, Montefiori DC, Mascola JR, Nabel GJ (2004) Heterologous envelope immunogens contribute to AIDS vaccine protection in rhesus monkeys. J Virol 78:7490–7497

Li Q, Duan L, Estes JD, Ma ZM, Rourke T, Wang Y, Reilly C, Carlis J, Miller CJ, Haase AT (2005) Peak SIV replication in resting memory CD4+ T cells depletes gut lamina propria CD4 + T cells. Nature 434:1148–1152

Liniger M, Zuniga A, Naim HY (2007) Use of viral vectors for the development of vaccines. Expert Rev Vaccines 6:255–266

Lubeck MD, Natuk R, Myagkikh M, Kalyan N, Aldrich K, Sinangil F, Alipanah S, Murthy SC, Chanda PK, Nigida SM, Jr., Markham PD, Zolla-Pazner S, Steimer K, Wade M, Reitz MS, Jr., Arthur LO, Mizutani S, Davis A, Hung PP, Gallo RC, Eichberg J, Robert-Guroff M (1997) Long-term protection of chimpanzees against high-dose HIV-1 challenge induced by immunization. Nat Med 3:651–658

Malkevitch N, Rohne D, Pinczewski J, Aldrich K, Kalyanaraman VS, Letvin NL, Robert-Guroff M (2004) Evaluation of combination DNA/replication-competent Ad-SIV recombinant immunization regimens in rhesus macaques. AIDS Res Hum Retroviruses 20:235–244

Mascola JR, Sambor A, Beaudry K, Santra S, Welcher B, Louder MK, Vancott TC, Huang Y, Chakrabarti BK, Kong WP, Yang ZY, Xu L, Montefiori DC, Nabel GJ, Letvin NL (2005) Neutralizing antibodies elicited by immunization of monkeys with DNA plasmids and recombinant adenoviral vectors expressing human immunodeficiency virus type 1 proteins. J Virol 79:771–779

Matano T, Shibata R, Siemon C, Connors M, Lane HC, Martin MA (1998) Administration of an anti-CD8 monoclonal antibody interferes with the clearance of chimeric simian/human immunodeficiency virus during primary infections of rhesus macaques. J Virol 72:164–169

McChesney MB, Oldstone MB (1989) Virus-induced immunosuppression: infections with measles virus and human immunodeficiency virus. Adv Immunol 45:335–380

Mehandru S, Poles MA, Tenner-Racz K, Horowitz A, Hurley A, Hogan C, Boden D, Racz P, Markowitz M (2004) Primary HIV-1 infection is associated with preferential depletion of CD4 + T lymphocytes from effector sites in the gastrointestinal tract. J Exp Med 200:761–770

Mitani K, Graham FL, Caskey CT, Kochanek S (1995) Rescue, propagation, and partial purification of a helper virus-dependent adenovirus vector. Proc Natl Acad Sci USA 92:3854–3858

Miyazawa N, Crystal RG, Leopold PL (2001) Adenovirus serotype 7 retention in a late endosomal compartment prior to cytosol escape is modulated by fiber protein. J Virol 75:1387–1400

Molinier-Frenkel V, Prevost-Blondel A, Hong SS, Lengagne R, Boudaly S, Magnusson MK, Boulanger P, Guillet JG (2003) The maturation of murine dendritic cells induced by human adenovirus is mediated by the fiber knob domain. J Biol Chem 278:37175–37182
Morelli AE, Larregina AT, Ganster RW, Zahorchak AF, Plowey JM, Takayama T, Logar AJ, Robbins PD, Falo LD, Thomson AW (2000) Recombinant adenovirus induces maturation of dendritic cells via an NF-kappaB-dependent pathway. J Virol 74:9617–9628
Nanda A, Lynch DM, Goudsmit J, Lemckert AA, Ewald BA, Sumida SM, Truitt DM, Abbink P, Kishko MG, Gorgone DA, Lifton MA, Shen L, Carville A, Mansfield KG, Havenga MJ, Barouch DH (2005) Immunogenicity of recombinant fiber-chimeric adenovirus serotype 35 vector-based vaccines in mice and rhesus monkeys. J Virol 79:14161–14168
Natuk RJ, Lubeck MD, Chanda PK, Chengalvala M, Wade MS, Murthy SC, Wilhelm J, Vernon SK, Dheer SK, Mizutani S (1993) Immunogenicity of recombinant human adenovirus-human immunodeficiency virus vaccines in chimpanzees. AIDS Res Hum Retroviruses 9:395–404
Nishimura Y, Igarashi T, Donau OK, Buckler-White A, Buckler C, Lafont BA, Goeken RM, Goldstein S, Hirsch VM, Martin MA (2004) Highly pathogenic SHIVs and SIVs target different CD4 + T cell subsets in rhesus monkeys, explaining their divergent clinical courses. Proc Natl Acad Sci USA 101:12324–12329
O'Riordan CR, Lachapelle A, Delgado C, Parkes V, Wadsworth SC, Smith AE, Francis GE (1999) PEGylation of adenovirus with retention of infectivity and protection from neutralizing antibody in vitro and in vivo. Hum Gene Ther 10:1349–1358
Okada N, Tsukada Y, Nakagawa S, Mizuguchi H, Mori K, Saito T, Fujita T, Yamamoto A, Hayakawa T, Mayumi T (2001) Efficient gene delivery into dendritic cells by fiber-mutant adenovirus vectors. Biochem Biophys Res Commun 282:173–179
Olive M, Eisenlohr L, Flomenberg N, Hsu S, Flomenberg P (2002) The adenovirus capsid protein hexon contains a highly conserved human CD4+ T-cell epitope. Hum Gene Ther 13:1167–1178
Ophorst OJ, Kostense S, Goudsmit J, De Swart RL, Verhaagh S, Zakhartchouk A, Van Meijer M, Sprangers M, Van Amerongen G, Yuksel S, Osterhaus AD, Havenga MJ (2004) An adenoviral type 5 vector carrying a type 35 fiber as a vaccine vehicle: DC targeting, cross neutralization, and immunogenicity. Vaccine 22:3035–3044
Parks RJ, Chen L, Anton M, Sankar U, Rudnicki MA, Graham FL (1996) A helper-dependent adenovirus vector system: removal of helper virus by Cre-mediated excision of the viral packaging signal. Proc Natl Acad Sci USA 93:13565–13570
Patterson LJ, Malkevitch N, Venzon D, Pinczewski J, Gomez-Roman VR, Wang L, Kalyanaraman VS, Markham PD, Robey FA, Robert-Guroff M (2004) Protection against mucosal simian immunodeficiency virus SIV(mac251) challenge by using replicating adenovirus-SIV multigene vaccine priming and subunit boosting. J Virol 78:2212–2221
Peng B, Wang LR, Gomez-Roman VR, Davis-Warren A, Montefiori DC, Kalyanaraman VS, Venzon D, Zhao J, Kan E, Rowell TJ, Murthy KK, Srivastava I, Barnett SW, Robert-Guroff M (2005) Replicating rather than nonreplicating adenovirus-human immunodeficiency virus recombinant vaccines are better at eliciting potent cellular immunity and priming high-titer antibodies. J Virol 79:10200–10209
Phillips RE, Rowland-Jones S, Nixon DF, Gotch FM, Edwards JP, Ogunlesi AO, Elvin JG, Rothbard JA, Bangham CR, Rizza CR (1991) Human immunodeficiency virus genetic variation that can escape cytotoxic T cell recognition. Nature 354:453–459
Philpott NJ, Nociari M, Elkon KB, Falck-Pedersen E (2004) Adenovirus-induced maturation of dendritic cells through a PI3 kinase-mediated TNF-alpha induction pathway. Proc Natl Acad Sci USA 101:6200–6205
Pieniazek NJ, Slemenda SB, Pieniazek D, Velarde J, Jr., Luftig RB (1990) Human enteric adenovirus type 41 (Tak) contains a second fiber protein gene. Nucleic Acids Res 18:1901
Prevec L, Christie BS, Laurie KE, Bailey MM, Graham FL, Rosenthal KL (1991) Immune response to HIV-1 gag antigens induced by recombinant adenovirus vectors in mice and rhesus macaque monkeys. J Acquir Immune Defic Syndr 4:568–576
Ranieri E, Herr W, Gambotto A, Olson W, Rowe D, Robbins PD, Kierstead LS, Watkins SC, Gesualdo L, Storkus WJ (1999) Dendritic cells transduced with an adenovirus vector encod-

ing Epstein-Barr virus latent membrane protein 2B: a new modality for vaccination. J Virol 73:10416–10425

Rea D, Schagen FH, Hoeben RC, Mehtali M, Havenga MJ, Toes RE, Melief CJ, Offringa R (1999) Adenoviruses activate human dendritic cells without polarization toward a T-helper type 1-inducing subset. J Virol 73:10245–10253

Reyes-Sandoval A, Fitzgerald JC, Grant R, Roy S, Xiang ZQ, Li Y, Gao GP, Wilson JM, Ertl HC (2004) Human immunodeficiency virus type 1-specific immune responses in primates upon sequential immunization with adenoviral vaccine carriers of human and simian serotypes. J Virol 78:7392–7399

Roberts DM, Nanda A, Havenga MJ, Abbink P, Lynch DM, Ewald BA, Liu J, Thorner AR, Swanson PE, Gorgone DA, Lifton MA, Lemckert AA, Holterman L, Chen B, Dilraj A, Carville A, Mansfield KG, Goudsmit J, Barouch DH (2006) Hexon-chimaeric adenovirus serotype 5 vectors circumvent pre-existing anti-vector immunity. Nature 441:239–243

Roelvink PW, Lizonova A, Lee JG, Li Y, Bergelson JM, Finberg RW, Brough DE, Kovesdi I, Wickham TJ (1998) The coxsackievirus-adenovirus receptor protein can function as a cellular attachment protein for adenovirus serotypes from subgroups A, C, D, E, and F. J Virol 72:7909–7915

Roth MD, Cheng Q, Harui A, Basak SK, Mitani K, Low TA, Kiertscher SM (2002) Helper-dependent adenoviral vectors efficiently express transgenes in human dendritic cells but still stimulate antiviral immune responses. J Immunol 169:4651–4656

Rozis G, de Silva S, Benlahrech A, Papagatsias T, Harris J, Gotch F, Dickson G, Patterson S (2005) Langerhans cells are more efficiently transduced than dermal dendritic cells by adenovirus vectors expressing either group C or group B fibre protein: implications for mucosal vaccines. Eur J Immunol 35:2617–2626

Santoro F, Kennedy PE, Locatelli G, Malnati MS, Berger EA, Lusso P (1999) CD46 is a cellular receptor for human herpesvirus 6. Cell 99:817–827

Santra S, Seaman MS, Xu L, Barouch DH, Lord CI, Lifton MA, Gorgone DA, Beaudry KR, Svehla K, Welcher B, Chakrabarti BK, Huang Y, Yang ZY, Mascola JR, Nabel GJ, Letvin NL (2005) Replication-defective adenovirus serotype 5 vectors elicit durable cellular and humoral immune responses in nonhuman primates. J Virol 79:6516–6522

Schmitz JE, Kuroda MJ, Santra S, Sasseville VG, Simon MA, Lifton MA, Racz P, Tenner-Racz K, Dalesandro M, Scallon BJ, Ghrayeb J, Forman MA, Montefiori DC, Rieber EP, Letvin NL, Reimann KA (1999) Control of viremia in simian immunodeficiency virus infection by CD8+ lymphocytes. Science 283:857–860

Schoggins JW, Gall JG, Falck-Pedersen E (2003) Subgroup B and F fiber chimeras eliminate normal adenovirus type 5 vector transduction in vitro and in vivo. J Virol 77:1039–1048

Schumacher L, Ribas A, Dissette VB, McBride WH, Mukherji B, Economou JS, Butterfield LH (2004) Human dendritic cell maturation by adenovirus transduction enhances tumor antigen-specific T-cell responses. J Immunother 1997 27:191–200

Seaman MS, Xu L, Beaudry K, Martin KL, Beddall MH, Miura A, Sambor A, Chakrabarti BK, Huang Y, Bailer R, Koup RA, Mascola JR, Nabel GJ, Letvin NL (2005) Multiclade human immunodeficiency virus type 1 envelope immunogens elicit broad cellular and humoral immunity in rhesus monkeys. J Virol 79:2956–2963

Shayakhmetov DM, Li ZY, Ternovoi V, Gaggar A, Gharwan H, Lieber A (2003) The interaction between the fiber knob domain and the cellular attachment receptor determines the intracellular trafficking route of adenoviruses. J Virol 77:3712–3723

Shiver JW, Emini EA (2004) Recent advances in the development of HIV-1 vaccines using replication-incompetent adenovirus vectors. Annu Rev Med 55:355–372

Shiver JW, Fu TM, Chen L, Casimiro DR, Davies ME, Evans RK, Zhang ZQ, Simon AJ, Trigona WL, Dubey SA, Huang L, Harris VA, Long RS, Liang X, Handt L, Schleif WA, Zhu L, Freed DC, Persaud NV, Guan L, Punt KS, Tang A, Chen M, Wilson KA, Collins KB, Heidecker GJ, Fernandez VR, Perry HC, Joyce JG, Grimm KM, Cook JC, Keller PM, Kresock DS, Mach H, Troutman RD, Isopi LA, Williams DM, Xu Z, Bohannon KE, Volkin DB, Montefiori DC, Miura A, Krivulka GR, Lifton MA, Kuroda MJ, Schmitz JE, Letvin NL, Caulfield MJ, Bett

AJ, Youil R, Kaslow DC, Emini EA (2002) Replication-incompetent adenoviral vaccine vector elicits effective anti-immunodeficiency-virus immunity. Nature 415:331–335

Smith A, Santoro F, Di Lullo G, Dagna L, Verani A, Lusso P (2003) Selective suppression of IL-12 production by human herpesvirus 6. Blood 102:2877–2884

Smith CA, Woodruff LS, Rooney C, Kitchingman GR (1998) Extensive cross-reactivity of adenovirus-specific cytotoxic T cells. Hum Gene Ther 9:1419–1427

Smith SG, Patel PM, Selby PJ, Jackson AM (2001) The response of human dendritic cells to recombinant adenovirus, recombinant Mycobacterium bovis Bacillus Calmette Guerin and biolistic methods of antigen delivery: different induction of contact-dependant and soluble signals. Immunol Lett 76:79–88

Sumida SM, Truitt DM, Kishko MG, Arthur JC, Jackson SS, Gorgone DA, Lifton MA, Koudstaal W, Pau MG, Kostense S, Havenga MJ, Goudsmit J, Letvin NL, Barouch DH (2004) Neutralizing antibodies and CD8 + T lymphocytes both contribute to immunity to adenovirus serotype 5 vaccine vectors. J Virol 78:2666–2673

Sumida SM, Truitt DM, Lemckert AA, Vogels R, Custers JH, Addo MM, Lockman S, Peter T, Peyerl FW, Kishko MG, Jackson SS, Gorgone DA, Lifton MA, Essex M, Walker BD, Goudsmit J, Havenga MJ, Barouch DH (2005) Neutralizing antibodies to adenovirus serotype 5 vaccine vectors are directed primarily against the adenovirus hexon protein. J Immunol 174:7179–7185

Tatsis N, Fitzgerald JC, Reyes-Sandoval A, Harris-McCoy KC, Hensley SE, Zhou D, Lin SW, Bian A, Xiang ZQ, Iparraguirre A, Lopez-Camacho C, Wherry EJ, Ertl HC (2007) Adenoviral vectors persist in vivo and maintain activated CD8 + T cells: implications for their use as vaccines. Blood 110:1916–1923

Vinner L, Wee EG, Patel S, Corbet S, Gao GP, Nielsen C, Wilson JM, Ertl HC, Hanke T, Fomsgaard A (2003) Immunogenicity in Mamu-A*01 rhesus macaques of a CCR5-tropic human immunodeficiency virus type 1 envelope from the primary isolate (Bx08) after synthetic DNA prime and recombinant adenovirus 5 boost. J Gen Virol 84:203–213

Vogels R, Zuijdgeest D, van Rijnsoever R, Hartkoorn E, Damen I, de Bethune MP, Kostense S, Penders G, Helmus N, Koudstaal W, Cecchini M, Wetterwald A, Sprangers M, Lemckert A, Ophorst O, Koel B, van Meerendonk M, Quax P, Panitti L, Grimbergen J, Bout A, Goudsmit J, Havenga M (2003) Replication-deficient human adenovirus type 35 vectors for gene transfer and vaccination: efficient human cell infection and bypass of preexisting adenovirus immunity. J Virol 77:8263–8271

Weiss RA, Clapham PR, Weber JN, Dalgleish AG, Lasky LA, Berman PW (1986) Variable and conserved neutralization antigens of human immunodeficiency virus. Nature 324:572–575

Wickham TJ, Mathias P, Cheresh DA, Nemerow GR (1993) Integrins alpha v beta 3 and alpha v beta 5 promote adenovirus internalization but not virus attachment. Cell 73:309–319

Wille-Reece U, Flynn BJ, Lore K, Koup RA, Miles AP, Saul A, Kedl RM, Mattapallil JJ, Weiss WR, Roederer M, Seder RA (2006) Toll-like receptor agonists influence the magnitude and quality of memory T cell responses after prime-boost immunization in nonhuman primates. J Exp Med 203:1249–1258

Worgall S, Busch A, Rivara M, Bonnyay D, Leopold PL, Merritt R, Hackett NR, Rovelink PW, Bruder JT, Wickham TJ, Kovesdi I, Crystal RG (2004) Modification to the capsid of the adenovirus vector that enhances dendritic cell infection and transgene-specific cellular immune responses. J Virol 78:2572–2580

Yang Y, Ertl HC, Wilson JM (1994) MHC class I-restricted cytotoxic T lymphocytes to viral antigens destroy hepatocytes in mice infected with E1-deleted recombinant adenoviruses. Immunity 1:433–442

Yang Y, Li Q, Ertl HC, Wilson JM (1995) Cellular and humoral immune responses to viral antigens create barriers to lung-directed gene therapy with recombinant adenoviruses. J Virol 69:2004–2015

Yang ZY, Wyatt LS, Kong WP, Moodie Z, Moss B, Nabel GJ (2003) Overcoming immunity to a viral vaccine by DNA priming before vector boosting. J Virol 77:799–803

Yeh HY, Pieniazek N, Pieniazek D, Gelderblom H, Luftig RB (1994) Human adenovirus type 41 contains two fibers. Virus Res 33:179–198

Yoshida T, Okuda K, Xin KQ, Tadokoro K, Fukushima J, Toda S, Hagiwara E, Hamajima K, Koshino T, Saito T (2001) Activation of HIV-1-specific immune responses to an HIV-1 vaccine constructed from a replication-defective adenovirus vector using various combinations of immunization protocols. Clin Exp Immunol 124:445–452
Youil R, Toner TJ, Su Q, Chen M, Tang A, Bett AJ, Casimiro D (2002) Hexon gene switch strategy for the generation of chimeric recombinant adenovirus. Hum Gene Ther 13:311–320
Zhong L, Granelli-Piperno A, Choi Y, Steinman RM (1999) Recombinant adenovirus is an efficient and non-perturbing genetic vector for human dendritic cells. Eur J Immunol 29:964–972

IFN-alpha in the Generation of Dendritic Cells for Cancer Immunotherapy

Stefano Maria Santini, Caterina Lapenta, Laura Santodonato, Giuseppina D'Agostino, Filippo Belardelli, and Maria Ferrantini

Contents

Abstract Dendritic cells (DCs) play a crucial role in linking innate and adaptive immunity, by virtue of their unique ability to take up and process antigens in the peripheral blood and tissues and, upon migration to draining lymph nodes, to present antigen to resting lymphocytes. Notably, these DC functions are modulated by cytokines and chemokines controlling the activation and maturation of these cells, thus shaping the response towards either immunity or tolerance.

An ensemble of recent studies have emphasized an important role of type I IFNs in the DC differentiation/activation, suggesting the existence of a natural alliance between these cytokines and DCs in linking innate and adaptive immunity. Herein, we will review how type I IFNs can promote the *ex vivo* differentiation of human DCs and orient DC functions towards the priming and expansion of protective antitumor

S.M. Santini (✉)
Section of Experimental Immunotherapy, Department of Cell Biology and Neurosciences, Istituto Superiore di Sanità, Viale Regina Elena, 299, 00161 Rome, Italy
stefano.santini@iss.it

G. Lombardi, Y. Riffo-Vasquez (eds.), *Dendritic Cells,* Handbook of Experimental Pharmacology 188,

immune responses. We will also discuss how the knowledge on type I IFN-DC interactions could be exploited for the design of more selective and effective strategies of cancer immunotherapy.

1 Introduction

Immunotherapy of cancer is aimed at eliciting immune responses against tumor cell associated antigens, in order to recognize and eradicate neoplastic cells or to control tumor growth. Such therapeutic approach would have the potential to eradicate neoplastic cells, especially in patients with minimal residual disease after tumor bulk resection, eventually resulting in prolongation of patients' survival and in a substantial improvement of patients' quality of life. Recently, an increasing interest has been focused on immunotherapeutic approaches utilizing dendritic cells (DCs), as cellular adjuvants, to effectively sensitize lymphocytes towards tumor antigens. DCs represent the key cells linking innate and adaptive immune responses, acting at the interface between the environment and the immune system by virtue of their role of professional antigen presenting cells.

A series of recent papers has revealed that type I IFNs, namely IFN-α and IFN-β, are capable of promoting the conversion of blood monocytes into highly active DCs. IFN-α and IFN-β are currently the most used cytokines in clinics, especially in the treatment of cancer and certain infectious diseases. Early studies had reported multiple effects of IFN-α/β on the immune system, including the enhancement of macrophage functions and of natural killer (NK) cell activity (Belardelli 1995; Belardelli and Gresser 1996; Belardelli and Ferrantini 2002). Besides its well known role in innate immunity (Belardelli 1995), type I IFNs are considered to play a role in the shaping of adaptive immunity, as previously demonstrated in mouse tumor models (Belardelli and Gresser 1996), and more recently by a series of papers highlighting the role of type I IFNs, and in particular of IFN-α, in the modulation of T cell functions, including the polarization of T-helper cells toward the TH-1 type of immune response. and the generation/activation of cytotoxic T lymphocytes (CTL) (Belardelli and Ferrantini 2002; Ferrantini et al. 2007). Over the last years, it has become apparent that many of the effects of type I IFNs on adaptive immunity are mediated by effects of these cytokines on macrophages and DCs. In particular, type I IFNs have been shown as potent inducers of DC differentiation from monocytes (IFN-DCs).

In this review article, we provide an overview of the existing knowledge on the ability of type I IFNs to induce the differentiation of human DCs *ex vivo* and to modulate DC functions towards the generation of an antitumor adaptive immunity. We will also summarize and discuss the main results obtained in clinical trials based on the treatment of cancer patients with therapeutic vaccines comprising autologous type I IFN-induced-DCs as cellular adjuvants.

2 Biology of Dendritic Cells and Their Role in Linking Innate and Adaptive Immunity

DCs are considered as the best professional antigen presenting cells (APCs), capable of efficiently priming naïve T cells toward microbial and tumor antigens (Steinman and Banchereau 2007). DCs act as an interface between the environment and the immune system, representing an important link between innate and adaptive immune response and determining the quality of the immune response to incoming pathogens. DCs represent 0.5–1.5% of circulating human mononuclear cells. Based on the relative expression of specific surface markers, different subsets of DC precursors can be distinguished in human blood (Liu 2001): a major CD1a+/CD11c+ and CD1a−/CD11c+population, expressing the CD13, CD33 and GM-CSF-receptor (referred as myeloid DCs), and a CD1a−/CD11c− population expressing high levels of CD123 (IL-3Rα), known as plasmacytoid DCs (pDCs), which represent the major source of type I IFN upon virus challenge (Siegal et al. 1999; Cella et al. 1999). The major pool of myeloid DC precursors is represented by monocytes, which give origin to interstitial DCs or tissue-resident DCs and Langherhans cells (LCs) (Caux et al. 1996).

Circulating immature DCs migrate to peripheral non-lymphoid tissues by the extravasation process to continuously replenish the pool of tissue-resident myeloid DCs. Immature DCs are endowed with an efficient capability to capture and internalize a wide spectrum of antigens, bacteria, viruses, apoptotic bodies and necrotic cells by different mechanisms such as conventional phagocytosis, macropinocytosis and receptor-mediated endocytosis via C-type lectin receptors, such as mannose receptor, DEC-205, DC-SIGN (CD209), FCγ receptors type I (CD64) and type II (CD32).

Exposure of immature DCs to inflammatory cytokines, bacterial and virus-derived molecules, such as LPS, double strand RNA, poly I:C and DNA promotes their maturation that is characterized by phenotypic and functional changes (Bell et al. 1999; Sallusto et al. 2000).

Following maturation, DCs loose the capacity to phagocytose and migrate to the T cell areas of lymphoid tissues (Heath and Carbone 2001) as a direct consequence of the switch of their chemokine receptor set. In fact, mature DCs loose their sensitivity to inflammatory chemokines (i.e., CCL3, CCL4 and CCL5) and become responsive to CCL20 and CCL21 chemokines. Moreover, mature DCs upregulate the membrane expression of accessory molecules, such as CD80, CD86 and CD40, MHC class I and II antigens and exhibit a strong capability to prime an immune response. Of note, DCs are capable to exploit peculiar MHC class I-restricted antigen presentation pathways. Besides the classical presentation of endogenous peptides derived from intracellular proteins and pathogens, DCs are capable of presenting MHC class I-restricted epitopes derived from exogenous antigens by unconventional antigen processing pathways, ensuring the efficient "cross priming" of cytotoxic $CD8^+$ T cells (Heath and Carbone 2001; Albert et al. 1998). Of interest, the adaptive immune response is biased during the process of antigen presentation by DCs and is affected by the cytokine milieu (Steinman and Hemmi 2006). Inflammatory cytokines generally promote DC activation, favoring a TH-1 type of immune response through the production of IL-12 and of both IL-23 and IL-27, the newly discovered members of IL-12 cytokine family (Hunter 2005). Pathogens can directly interact with DCs through an array of receptors known as Toll-like receptors (TLRs) inducing the production of IL-12 and IL-23 (Napolitani et al. 2005). In contrast, exposure of immature DCs to IL-10 results in impairment of the up-regulation of co-stimulatory molecules and CD83 as well as in the inhibition of the development of a fully mature DC phenotype. These effects of IL-10 can promote the induction of anergic T cells, characterized by reduced IL-2 and IFN-γ production and low CD25 expression (Steinbrink et al. 1997, 1999). The availability of defined cell culture conditions for generating relatively large numbers of DCs from cell precursors has allowed an impressive advance in our comprehension of DC biology. DCs can be obtained from CD34+ stem cells and expanded and differentiated in vitro upon exposure to cytokine cocktails, including GM-CSF, IL-4 and TNF-α (Caux et al. 1992; Luft et al. 1998a). Although blood monocytes can differentiate into macrophages endowed with scavenging activity, they represent a pool of DC precursors. The fate of monocytes mostly depends on the cytokine environment. In fact, large numbers of immature DCs can be obtained by cultivating monocytes in the presence of GM-CSF and IL-4 for 5–7 days (Sallusto and Lanzavecchia 1994). GM-CSF is required to ensure monocyte survival, whereas IL-4 exerts an inhibitory activity on macrophage differentiation, promoting the generation of immature DCs (Romani et al. 1994). Maturation/activation of DCs is reached through a further culture step with maturation stimuli, such as Toll-like receptor (TLR) ligands (such as LPS, poly-I:C, etc.), pro-inflammatory cytokines (such as TNF-α), CD40L or the so-called "gold standard" (IL-1β, TNF-α, IL-6 and prostaglandin E2), also known as monocyte-conditioned medium (MCM) mimic or cytokine cocktail (Jonuleit et al. 1997a).

Even though the IL-4/GM-CSF culture method has allowed to perform many important studies on DC biology, this pathway of DC differentiation may not reflect the physiological process by which monocytes differentiate into DCs in vivo, as high levels of IL-4 are unlikely to be present in the course of a natural immune response to infections. Since type I IFNs are rapidly produced in response to viruses and other stimuli, these cytokines could represent early danger signals ensuring an efficient link between innate and adaptive immunity, thus acting as physiological factors involved in DC differentiation. In the following sections, we will review the recently obtained information on the effects of IFN-α and IFN-β on the differentiation and activation of human DCs.

3 Type I IFNs and Ex Vivo Generation of Dendritic Cells

It has been clearly demonstrated that in monocytes and B cells both IFN-α and IFN-β can up-regulate in a few hours the surface expression of molecules commonly recognized as markers of antigen-presenting cell activation, such as CD86 and MHC class I and MHC class II molecules, and can induce a new set of chemokines and chemokine receptors (Pogue et al. 2004).

Paquette and colleagues (1998) provided the first evidence that IFN-α, in combination with GM-CSF, is capable to drive the full differentiation of human blood monocytes into DCs. Soon after, this group demonstrated that monocytes exposed to IFN-α together with GM-CSF acquired the features of fully functional partially mature DCs (IFN-DCs) after not more than 3 days of culture (Santini et al. 2000). Since then, a number of studies have investigated the effects of IFN-α and of IFN-β on the differentiation of human DCs. In spite of some contrasting results probably due to the experimental setting, the timing and culture conditions, several groups have independently demonstrated that type I IFNs efficiently promote the differentiation of peripheral blood monocytes into DCs.

In the following sections, we will review the existing evidence on the effects of type I IFNs on the differentiation and activation of human DCs, discussing possible explanations for the conflicting results obtained in different studies. We will then illustrate the features exhibited by DCs differentiated from monocytes in a single-step culture with GM-CSF and IFN-α (IFN-DCs), according to the method developed by our group (Santini et al. 2000). In this context, we will also describe the effects of some variations of culture conditions as well as of the treatment with maturation stimuli on the phenotypic and functional features of IFN-DCs.

3.1 Effects of Type I IFNs on the Differentiation and Activation of Human Dendritic Cells

IFN-α and IFN-β have been demonstrated to differently modulate the activation/maturation of DCs, depending on the experimental model and culture conditions (Luft et al. 1998b, 2002; Bartholomè et al. 1999; McRae et al. 2000a, b; Radvanyi et al. 1999; Santini et al. 2000; Huang et al. 2001; Hussien et al. 2001; Ito et al. 2001; Padovan et al. 2002; Wiesemann et al. 2002). Terminal differentiation of immature DCs obtained from $CD34^+$ progenitors has been shown to be accelerated by both IFN-α and IFN-β (Luft et al. 1998b), while low levels of endogenous IFN was demonstrated to be released in culture supernatants of spontaneously maturing DCs (Luft et al. 1998b). Likewise, Ito and colleagues (2001) have showed that IFN-α can markedly enhance the maturation of $CD11c^+$ DCs. However, some contrasting results have emerged from studies published by different research groups. In fact, although the majority of studies on the effects of type I IFNs on DCs have emphasized a promoting effect on differentiation/activation (Paquette et al. 1998; Santini et al. 2000; Parlato et al. 2001; Mazouz et al. 2005; Renneson et al. 2005; Santodonato et al. 2003; Gabriele et al. 2004), some authors have shown inhibitory activities on DC functions, including a decreased IL-12 production (Detournay et al. 2005; Carbonneil et al. 2003, 2004; Della Bella et al. 2004; Luft et al. 1998b). McRae and coworkers (2000a) reported an inhibitory effect of both IFN-α and IFN-β on the yield of monocyte-derived DCs as compared to DCs generated in the presence of only IL-4 and GM-CSF, a decreased IL-12 production and an impaired capability to stimulate and support naïve T cell proliferation and IFN-γ production as well. Similarly, Bartholomè and colleagues (1999) have reported that the addition of IFN-β to monocyte cultures differentiated in the presence of GM-CSF and IL-4 for 6–7 days negatively affected both the spontaneous and CD40L-triggered production of IL-12 p40 and p70, resulting in decreased IFN-γ production in Mixed Lymphocyte reaction (MLR) cultures. To this regard, it is worth mentioning that different and contrasting observations have been reported on IL-12 production by DCs differentiated in the presence of type I IFNs, depending on the experimental model used. IFN-α-induced DCs have been shown to release low amounts of IL-12 and to induce T helper cells producing both TH-1 and TH-2 cytokines (Della Bella et al. 2004). Interestingly, IFN-α was shown to enhance the IL-12 p70 expression upon stimulation of freshly isolated monocytes with LPS and *Staphylococcus aureus Cowan* I strain (SAC), even though the IL-12 p40 release was inhibited (Hermann et al. 1998). In keeping with these findings, the amount of IL-12-producing IFN-α-induced DCs has been found comparable to conventional IL-4-DCs or even higher after SAC stimulation (Carbonneil et al. 2003). Of note, although DCs differentiated with GM-CSF and IL-4 and then exposed to IFN-α as a maturation stimulus exhibited a lower basal level of IL-12 production as compared to conventional mature DCs, a significant boost of IL-12 secretion has been shown upon their interaction with T cells during antigen presentation (Padovan et al. 2002). McRae's group (2000a) has shown that the IL-12 secretion dependent upon CD40 triggering was down regulated by IFN-β in monocyte-derived DCs, while the LPS-induced IL-12 secretion was not affected. Exposure to IFN-β during DC differentiation, has been also shown to inhibit CD40L-induced IL-12 p40 production by another group (Hussien et al. 2001), even though the production of the bioactive IL-12 p70 was not tested.

On the whole, IFN-β has been described to have opposite effects on DCs, depending on their differentiation stage, selectively enhancing functional activity at late stage of DC maturation, but exerting an opposite effect on DC functions when given at early stages of DC differentiation (Wiesemann et al. 2002). However, it should be kept in mind that the scenario is far more complex than expected. The timing of DC exposure to IFN-β determines, whether it exerts negative or positive effects on the generation of TH-1 cells from naïve CD4+ T lymphocytes (Nagai et al. 2003). In fact, exposure to IFN-β during DC maturation enhances the capacity to generate TH-1 cells producing IFN-γ, while its addition at the time of the interaction of naïve lymphocytes with DCs exerts an opposite effect by promoting the generation of IL-10-producing cells and inhibiting TH-1 polarization. This phenomenon has been found to involve the participation of the IL-12 family cytokines (IL-12, IL-23 and IL-27) as well as of IL-18 and other cytokines/chemokines (Nagai et al. 2003). In this regard, it is worth noting that the kinetics and the regulation of IL-12 production are finely regulated during DC activation. Thus, in the latest stages of maturation, the capability of secreting IL-12 by DCs is eventually lost (Kalinski et al. 1999), so that, stimulated DCs produce IL-12 only transitorily and become refractory to further stimulation (Langenkamp et al. 2000). However, it should be pointed out that the contradictory dual role of IFN-β in the generation of active mature DCs might have a functional explanation. In fact, the negative regulation of IL-12 production by IFN-β observed in some studies (McRae et al. 2000a, b; Bartholomè et al. 1999; Hussien et al. 2001) could represent a beneficial regulatory mechanism preventing excessive immune activation and tissue damage.

The apparently contradictory results reported above on the effects of type I IFNs on the differentiation and functional activation of DCs might be explained by the use of different IFN subtypes, the timing of type I IFN addition, the differences in the culture conditions or the presence of unknown cofactors.

Most importantly, the interpretation of results from experiments where both IL-4 and type I IFNs were concomitantly utilized for DC differentiation/activation should be carefully evaluated because of the complex interactions between type I IFNs and other cytokines, synergy or reciprocal regulation or possible interference between the corresponding intracellular signaling pathways, which influence DC functions and cytokine production. For instance, type I IFN-mediated suppression of STAT-6 activity has been shown to inhibit IL-4 inducible gene expression in human monocytes (Dickensheets and Donnelly 1999). Similarly, treatment of monocytes with IL-4 may result in DCs exhibiting an impaired functional activity (Thurnher et al. 2001). Interestingly, an antagonism between IFN-α-induced cellular gene expression and IL-4 has been reported (Larner et al. 1993), possibly linked to negative regulation of STAT-1-dependent transcription (Ohmori and Hamilton 1998). Thus, the results obtained by using monocyte-derived DCs generated in the presence of GM-CSF, IL-4, and type I IFNs cannot directly be compared to those obtained with DCs differentiated with type I IFNs in the absence of IL-4 (Santini et al. 2000; Parlato et al. 2001; Santodonato et al. 2003; Lapenta et al. 2003). Moreover, possible modulations of cytokine receptors occurring during the differentiation/maturation process of DCs after exposure to different stimuli should be taken into consideration. Gauzzi and colleagues (2002) have reported a marked down regulation of the expression of type I IFN receptors shortly after LPS-induced maturation of DCs generated from human monocytes treated with IL-4 and GM-CSF. This effect was linked to a low responsiveness to type I IFNs.

On the other hand, a number of studies reported a synergy between type I IFNs and other factors in inducing DC terminal maturation. In fact, IFN-α has been shown to act synergistically with TNF-α to induce DC maturation (Radvanyi et al. 1999). IFN-α has also been found to synergize with double-stranded RNA in enhancing the production of TNF-α and IL-12 by DCs (Barnes et al. 2004). Likewise, Luft and colleagues (2002) have reported that IFN-α powerfully enhances CD40L-mediated DC activation by inducing an increase of the IL-12-p70/p40 ratio towards the bioactive p70 form as well as IL-12 secretion. Interestingly, it has been reported that immature DCs generated in the presence of IL-4 and then exposed to IFN-α produce high amounts of CXCL10 and CXCL9, exerting a chemotactic effect on CD8+ T effector cells and promoting MHC-class I-restricted responses (Padovan et al. 2002). Furthermore, it has been reported that when monocytes are exposed to IFN-β and IL-3 they differentiate into DCs endowed with potent helper T-cell stimulatory activity (Buelens et al. 2002). These cells closely resemble IFN-α-induced DCs and are similarly endowed with potent functional activities and are capable of expanding peptide specific CTL secreting high amounts of IFN-γ when pulsed with an HLA-A2-restricted Melan-A peptide (Mazouz et al. 2005).

Importantly, IFN-β/IL-3 DCs matured by TLR-3 or CD40 ligation have been found to efficiently prime Melan-A specific $CD8^+$ T cells similarly to GM-CSF/IL-4 DCs. Activated antigen-specific $CD8^+$ T cells were demonstrated to produce IFN-γ and to exert potent cytotoxic activity against peptide-pulsed target cells (Renneson et al. 2005).

Moreover, the release of IL-6 by DCs generated by IL-3 and IFN-β has been shown to contrast the suppressive effect of regulatory T cells on IFN-γ production (Detournay et al. 2005).

3.2 Differentiation of Highly Active Dendritic Cells from Human Peripheral Blood by a Single-Step 3-Day Culture with IFN-α

As mentioned in the previous Sect. 3, our group has shown that human peripheral blood monocytes differentiate into highly active, partially mature DCs in three days of culture with IFN-α and GM-CSF (Santini et al. 2000; Parlato et al. 2001) (Fig. 1). We demonstrated that, these IFN-DCs undergo an early loss of adhesion

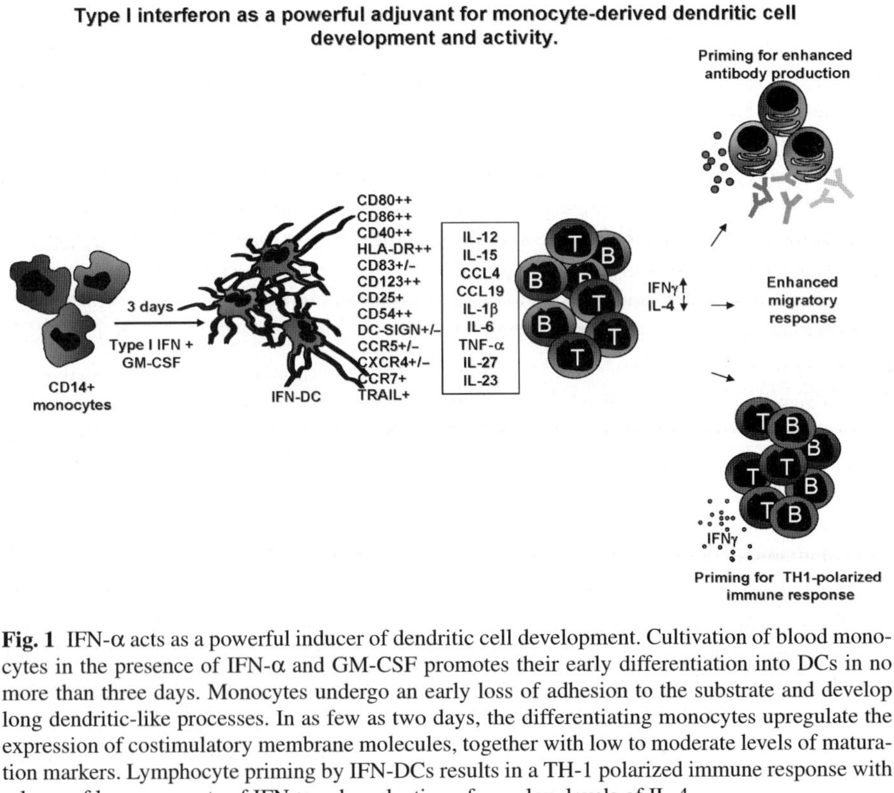

Fig. 1 IFN-α acts as a powerful inducer of dendritic cell development. Cultivation of blood monocytes in the presence of IFN-α and GM-CSF promotes their early differentiation into DCs in no more than three days. Monocytes undergo an early loss of adhesion to the substrate and develop long dendritic-like processes. In as few as two days, the differentiating monocytes upregulate the expression of costimulatory membrane molecules, together with low to moderate levels of maturation markers. Lymphocyte priming by IFN-DCs results in a TH-1 polarized immune response with release of large amounts of IFN-γ and production of very low levels of IL-4

to the substrate and attitude to form large cell clusters, developing long dendritic-like processes in a couple of days. The expression of membrane molecules such as CD80, CD86 and CD40, the intercellular adhesion molecule, ICAM-1 (CD54) and HLA-DR is rapidly enhanced, while low levels of CD14 are retained all through the differentiation process together with significant levels of CD123, typical of plasmacytoid DCs. Even though the majority of DCs generated in the presence of IFN-α displayed features of immature DCs, markers of activated/mature DCs, such as CD83 and CD25, could be unexpectedly detected in a variable percentage (12–40%) of fully differentiated IFN-DCs, concomitantly with high levels of costimulatory molecule expression.

Consistently with their partially activated phenotype and in agreement with the attribution of IL-15 production to CD83-expressing DCs (Jonuleit et al. 1997b), IFN-DCs produce significant amounts of IL-15 in the culture supernatant (Santini et al. 2000; Parlato et al. 2001). Interestingly, IFN-DCs were found to markedly express the molecule TRAIL (TNF-related apoptosis-inducing ligand) and to specifically kill TRAIL-sensitive tumor cell lines (Santini et al. 2000; Korthals et al. 2007; Papewalis et al. 2008a). To this regard, very recent studies have shown that monocyte-derived IFN-α-induced DCs combine features of NK cells and mature DCs, as demonstrated by anti-CD56 antibody staining (Papewalis et al. 2008a) and microarray gene expression profiling that revealed a higher expression of genes coding for DC maturation markers and molecules linked to DC migration to the lymph nodes, like DC-LAMP, CCR7 and CD49d, as well as for markers of NK cells, including granzymes and TRAIL (Korthals et al. 2007). Of note, in the study by Papewalis and colleagues (2008a) the TRAIL-dependent cytolytic activity of IFN-α-DCs was attributed to the $CD56^+$ fraction.

IFN-DCs also exhibit an enhanced chemotactic response and migration activity. They expressed very high levels of CCR5 and exhibit an enhanced response to its ligands CCL5, CCL3 and CCL4, while a remarkable fraction of IFN-DCs expresses CCR7, shows a migratory response to CCL19 and expresses significant levels of CCL19 themselves, together with CCL18 and CXCL10 (Parlato et al. 2001).

IFN-DCs are able to stimulate the proliferative response of allogeneic T cells and the production of high levels of IFN-γ in mixed lymphocyte reactions even at very low stimulator/responder ratios (Santini et al. 2000). A typical feature of professional APCs is their ability of successfully priming naïve T cells and of inducing an effective immune response. In vitro priming of autologous T cells with antigen pulsed IFN-DCs has been shown to induce a strong lymphocyte proliferation and a Th1 polarized response, as revealed by production of high levels of IFN-γ and the virtual absence of IL-4 in the culture upon restimulation (Santini et al. 2000; Parlato et al. 2001; Lapenta et al. 2003; Tosi et al. 2004). It is not clear which are the factors involved in the stronger capacity of IFN-DCs to bias the T helper response toward the TH1 type. Perhaps, several mediators might be implicated, including cytokines belonging to the IL-12 cytokine family, such as IL-23 and IL-27 (Lapenta et al. 2006), as well as IL-18 and unknown mediators. Moreover, we can speculate that IFN-DCs are inclined to TH1 polarization by virtue of their capacity to produce IFN-γ by themselves, as recently shown by Papewalis and colleagues (2008a) by intracytoplasmatic cytokine staining. To this regard, Mohty and colleagues (2003) demonstrated that the TH-1 response can be independent from IL-12p70 and IL-18 production and substantially inhibited by IFN-γ neutralization.

By using the chimeric model of SCID mice reconstituted with the human-peripheral blood lymphocytes (Hu-PBL-SCID), we found that IFN-DC-based vaccination against HIV-1 resulted in a superior human humoral response toward the whole spectrum of viral proteins, with antibodies belonging mainly to the IgG1 isotype, as compared to the response elicited by conventional immature monocyte-derived DCs (Santini et al. 2000; Parlato et al. 2001). When DCs were pulsed with inactivated HIV-1 and injected into hu-PBL-SCID mice, the frequency of virus-specific $CD8^+$ T cells was markedly higher in animals immunized with IFN-DCs than in mice immunized with CD40L-matured IL-4-DCs (Lapenta et al. 2003). Of note, when the hu-PBL-SCID mice immunized with antigen-pulsed IFN-DCs were infected with HIV-1, inhibition of virus infection was observed as compared with control animals (Lapenta et al. 2003).

More recently we reported that, in spite of similar antigen uptake and endosomal processing capabilities of IFN-DCs and conventional immature IL-4-DCs, cross-priming with IFN-DCs resulted in the induction of higher numbers of IFN-γ-producing cells as compared to IL-4-DCs, as evidenced by enzyme-linked immunospot assays (Lapenta et al. 2006). Although both DC types efficiently cross-presented soluble HCV NS3 protein to a specific $CD8^+$ T cell clone, IFN-DCs proved more efficient in cross-presenting low amounts of viral antigens (Lapenta et al. 2006). Of interest, in experiments with purified $CD8^+$ T cells, IFN-DCs have been found superior with respect to CD40L-matured IL-4-DCs in inducing in vitro cross-priming of HIV-specific $CD8^+$ T cells, suggesting that IFN-DCs are directly licensed for an efficient $CD8^+$ T cell priming (Lapenta et al. 2006).

3.3 *Effects of Variation of Culture Conditions on the Phenotype and Functional Features of IFN-DCs*

Over the years, we have attempted to optimize the protocol for the generation of IFN-DCs to be used as cellular adjuvants of therapeutic vaccines upon loading with the relevant antigens. In this section, we report the results of a comparison of different culture conditions for the generation of IFN-DCs from human monocytes. IFN-DCs were initially generated by culturing monocytes in RPMI1640 medium supplemented with FCS (Santini et al. 2000; Parlato et al. 2001). Then, phenotype and functions of IFN-DCs generated in parallel by culturing monocytes in RPMI supplemented with fetal calf serum (FCS) or human serum AB or in serum-free AIM-V medium containing GM-CSF and IFN were compared. We found that cell density affects cell recovery when IFN-DCs are generated with AIM-V medium. Infact, the seeding of monocytes at 0.4×10^6 c/ml resulted in a lower DC recovery (13%) with respect to that obtained (72%) seeding monocytes at 2×10^6 c ml^{-1} (Fig. 2, panel **(a)**). As for phenotype, IFN-DCs generated by using different media,

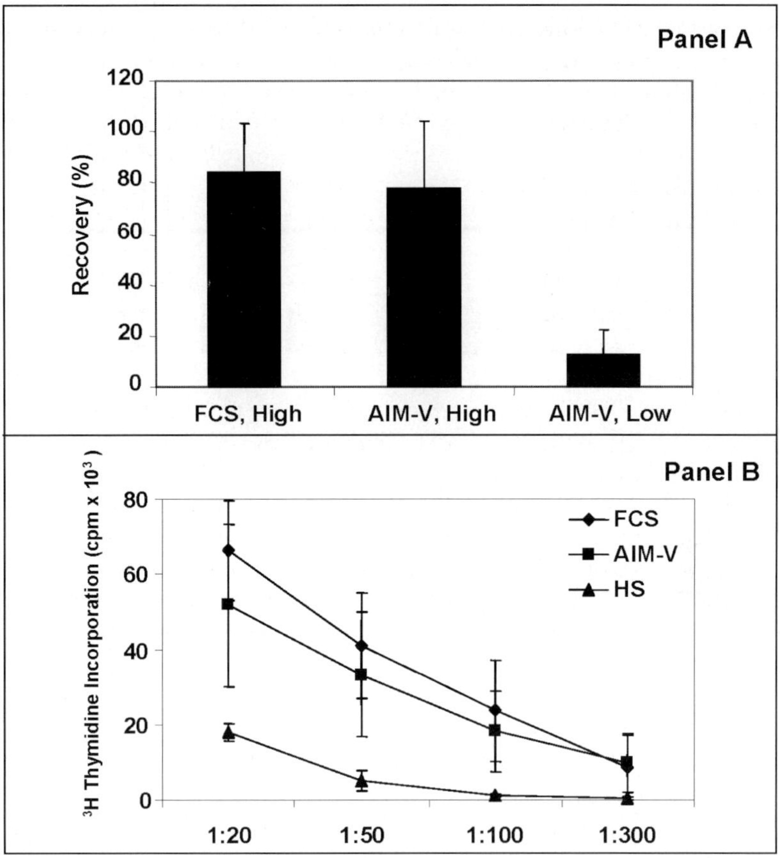

Fig. 2 Comparison of recovery and allostimulatory capacity of IFN-DCs differentiated in different culture conditions. **(a)** Recovery of IFN-DCs generated by culturing monocytes at the density of $2 \times 10^6\,c\,ml^{-1}$ in RPMI1640 medium supplemented with FCS compared to the recovery of IFN-DCs generated by culturing monocytes at the density of $2 \times 10^6\,c\,ml^{-1}$ or $0.4 \times 10^6\,c\,ml^{-1}$ in serum-free AIM-V medium. **(b)** Allostimulatory capacity of IFN-DCs generated by using RPMI1640 supplemented with FCS (*filled diamond*), human serum AB (HS) (*filled triangle*) or by using AIM-V medium (*filled square*)

showed similar expression of the CD14, CD83, CD40, CD86, HLA-DR, CD1a and CD80 markers (not shown). However, IFN-DCs differentiated in FCS-containing RPMI medium or in serum-free AIM-V medium exhibited a higher capability of stimulating MLR reactivity in allogeneic T lymphocytes with respect to IFN-DCs generated in RPMI medium containing human serum (Fig. 2b).

We also comparatively evaluated different clinical grade human type I IFNs, namely leukocyte IFN-α (Alfaferone, Wassermann), IFN-β (Serobif, Serono), IFN-α2b (IntronA, ScheringPlough), in terms of their ability to induce the differentiation of IFN-DCs from purified $CD14^+$ monocytes. The analysis of the IFN-DC phenotype (not shown) and functional activity, evaluated as the ability of stimulating a

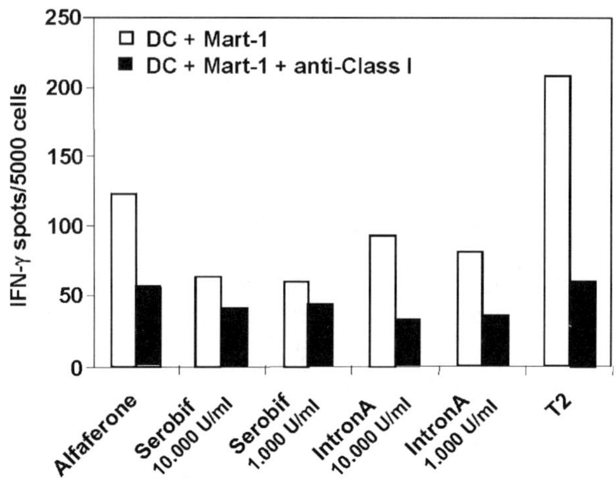

Fig. 3 Comparison of different clinical grade type I IFNs for their ability to induce DC differentiation. Purified $CD14^+$ monocytes were cultured for 3 days with AIM-V in the presence of GM-CSF and different clinical grade type I IFNs (Alfaferone, Wassermann; Serobif, Serono; IntronA, ScheringPlough). The figure shows the numbers of cells of the A42 MART-1_{27-35}-specific $CD8^+$ T-cell clone secreting IFN-γ, as assessed in ELISPOT assays, upon stimulation, in the absence (*white bars*) or in the presence (*black bars*) of anti-HLA class I antibodies, with the IFN-DCs generated in 3 days of culture with the different type I IFNs, and pulsed with the HLA-2.1-restricted Mart-1_{27-35} peptide

$CD8^+$ T cell clone specific for the HLA2.1-restricted Mart-1_{27-35} epitope (Rivoltini et al. 1995), after pulsing with the cognate peptide, indicated that Alfaferone and IntronA at the dose of 10.000 IU/ml are equally effective and superior to IFN-β in inducing the differentiation of highly functional DCs (Fig. 3).

3.4 Evaluation of Different Clinical Grade DC Maturation Factors/Cocktails for Their Effects on IFN-DCs

In order to evaluate the effects of inducing a full maturation of IFN-DCs, the following agents and cocktails, all known to be DC maturation stimuli, were initially used: CD40L, Bacillus Calmette-Guérin (BCG), Ribomunyl (RBL) $\pm$ IFN-γ (Boccaccio et al. 2002) and FMKp $\pm$ IFN-γ. The choice of these agents was based on their availability as clinical grade products and on the use of two of them, namely BCG and RBL, as adjuvants for human treatment. In addition, RBL, an immunostimulatory drug composed of membrane fractions of *Klebsiella pneumoniae* and purified ribosomes from four respiratory pathogens (Dussourd d'Hinterland et al. 1980), was shown to induce a significant enhancement of allostimulatory abilities and cytokine production by DCs differentiated in the presence of GM-CSF and IL-13 (Boccaccio et al. 2002), the "so-called" Dendritophages, a DC type sharing a number of phenotypic and functional features with IFN-DCs (unpublished observations). The addition of IFN-γ to Ribomunyl was found to trigger in only 6 h of treatment an irreversible further maturation of Dendritophages and, interestingly, to modulate their cytokine secretion, resulting in higher levels of bioactive interleukin-12 concomitant with lower levels of interleukin-10 (Boccaccio et al. 2002). Effects similar to those exerted by RBL on Dendritophages were observed using FMKp, a membrane fraction from the gram-negative bacteria *Klebsiella pneumoniae* (for details, visit http://www.cipf.com), either as single agent or in combination with IFN-γ (unpublished observations). Based on these effects, the association of Ribomunyl or FMKp with IFN-γ might represent a preferable cocktail for the *ex vivo* maturation of monocyte-derived DCs highly efficient in promoting a potent type 1 immune response.

Concerning the functional activity of matured vs non-matured IFN-DCs, the main results can be summarized as follows. Stimulation of a MART-$1_{27–35}$-specific $CD8^+$ clone (Rivoltini et al. 1995) with peptide-pulsed IFN-DCs indicated that IFN-DCs exposed for 6 h to the various maturation stimuli were stronger stimulators, except for BCG-matured IFN-DCs, than non-matured IFN-DCs, as assessed by ELISPOT assays (not shown). The stimulatory ability of matured IFN-DCs further increased after 20 h of treatment with the maturation agents, with the CD40L-matured-IFN-DCs showing the best activity (Fig. 4, panel **(a)**). The addition of IFN-γ to RBL or FMKp had no consequence on the ability of either agent to induce functional maturation of IFN-DCs (Fig. 4, panel **(a)**). Concerning the profile of cytokine secretion, the levels of IL-12 and IL-10 in the culture supernatant were assessed by ELISA assays before as well as 20 h after addition of the maturation inducers. In the absence of IFN-γ, low to undetectable amounts of IL-12 were secreted by IFN-DCs in response to the different maturation agents, whereas high amounts of IL-10 were produced following treatment of IFN-DCs with RBL or FMKp (Fig. 4, panel **b**). Interestingly, among the maturation inducers tested as single agents, CD40L induced the production of the highest levels of IL-12 and of the lowest levels of IL-10 in IFN-DCs (Fig. 4, panel **b**). In the presence of IFN-γ, the balance between IL-12 and IL-10 secreted by IFN-DCs was reversed, because of a strong increase in the levels of IL-12 and a parallel reduction of those of IL-10 (Fig. 4, panel **b**). The addition of IFN-γ to RBL or FMKp further augmented the secretion of IL-15 (Fig. 4, panel **b**). Overall, the combination FMKp + IFN-γ proved superior to the RBL + IFN-γ in inducing the production of IL-12p70 in IFN-DCs. In a parallel set of experiments, the PGE2 + IL6 + IL-1β + TNF-α maturation cocktail (Jonuleit et al. 1997a) was also tested. In particular, the DCs were characterized, as described below, after a 6 h treatment with medium or different maturation stimuli (CD40L, CD40L + IFN-γ, FMKp + IFN-γ and PGE2 + IL6 + IL-1β + TNF-α). Both the non-matured and the matured DCs were frozen and further characterized at 2 and 20 h after thawing, in terms of viability and expression of DC maturation markers, by flow cytometry, and of allostimulatory activity in MLR assays. The treatment with CD40L + IFN-γ or FMKp + IFN-γ resulted in a dramatic decrease of the percentage of viable IFN-DCs (ranging from 5 to 10%) with respect to IFN-DCs either non-matured (38–44%) or matured with CD40L alone (15–19%) or PGE2 + IL-6 + IL-1β + TNF-α cocktail (28%). Indeed, the addition of IFN-γ resulted in an increase

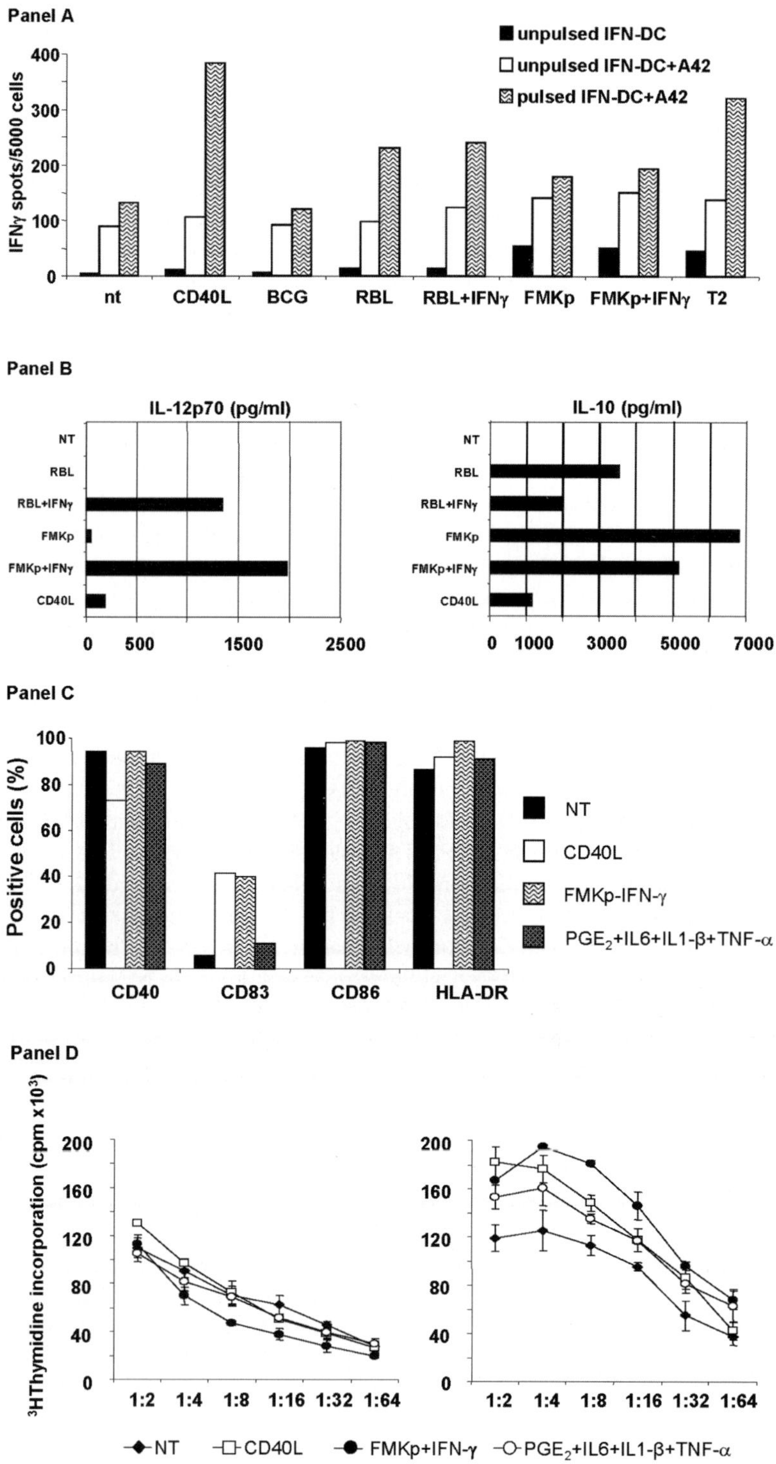
Panel A
unpulsed IFN-DC
unpulsed IFN-DC+A42
pulsed IFN-DC+A42
IFNγ spots/5000 cells
0
100
200
300
400
nt
CD40L
BCG
RBL
RBL+IFNγ
FMKp
FMKp+IFNγ
T2
Panel B
IL-12p70 (pg/ml)
IL-10 (pg/ml)
NT
RBL
RBL+IFNγ
FMKp
FMKp+IFNγ
CD40L
0
500
1500
2500
0
1000
3000
5000
7000
Panel C
Positive cells (%)
0
20
40
60
80
100
CD40
CD83
CD86
HLA-DR
NT
CD40L
FMKp-IFN-γ
PGE2+IL6+IL1-β+TNF-α
Panel D
3HThymidine incorporation (cpm x10³)
0
40
80
120
160
200
1:2
1:4
1:8
1:16
1:32
1:64
NT
CD40L
FMKp+IFN-γ
PGE2+IL6+IL1-β+TNF-α

of Annexin V-positive DCs, as assessed by FACS analysis (not shown). As for the immunophenotype, not-matured and matured IFN-DCs showed similar expression of costimulatory molecules (CD40, CD86 and HLA-DR) whereas, the expression of CD83 was higher in IFN-DCs matured with CD40L or FMKp + IFN-γ (Fig. 4, panel **c**). The allostimulatory activity of matured IFN-DCs was higher as compared to that exhibited by non-matured IFN-DCs 20 h after thawing, whereas it was similar two hours after thawing (Fig. 4 d). A similar allostimulatory activity was exerted by IFN-DCs matured with CD40L or PGE2 + IL-6 + IL-1β + TNF-α cocktail (Fig. 4, panel **d**). Interestingly, the FMKp + IFN-γ-matured IFN-DCs induced the strongest proliferation of allogeneic T lymphocytes, in spite of the dramatically reduced viability, suggesting their high functional efficiency.

Overall, these results indicate that CD40L may represent the stimulus to be preferably used for inducing the full maturation of IFN-DCs, taking into consideration its effects on different IFN-DC functional features such as viability, balance of IL-12 vs. IL-10 secretion, and efficiency in the stimulation of the MART-1_{27-35}-specific T cell clone and of allogeneic primary T lymphocytes.

Further studies are warranted in order to assess the need and advantage of inducing the full maturation of IFN-DCs to potentiate their ability to prime and expand a potentially protective and long-lasting immune response.

4 Type I IFN-Induced DCs as Candidate Cellular Adjuvants of Therapeutic Vaccines

Over the last years, a remarkable interest has been focused on the attempts to use DCs in the development of therapeutic vaccines against cancer (Gilboa 2007). The DC-based immunotherapy approach most commonly used so far is based on the *ex vivo* generation of DCs, their loading with tumor antigens and re-injection into the patient for stimulating cell-mediated immunity, taking advantage of the ability of DCs to migrate to the T-cell areas of lymphoid organs. Cytokines have represented invaluable tools for the ex vivo differentiation and activation of DCs from their precursors, and thus for the development of DC-based vaccines (Ferrantini et al. 2008). More than ten years have elapsed since the first "proof of concept" clinical

Fig. 4 Comparison of different clinical grade DC maturation factors/cocktails for their effects on IFN-DCs. **(a)** The figure shows the numbers of cells of the A42 MART-1_{27-35}-specific $CD8^+$ T-cell clone secreting IFN-γ, as assessed in ELISPOT assays, upon stimulation with unpulsed- or MART-1_{27-35}-pulsed- IFN-DCs exposed for 6 hours to the various maturation stimuli (CD40L, BCG, RBL, RBL + IFN-γ, FMKp and FMKp + IFN-γ). **(b)** ELISA assays assessing the levels of IL-12 and IL-10 secreted before as well as 20 h after addition of the maturation inducers. **(c)** and **(d)** Both the non-matured and the matured DCs were frozen and further characterized at 2 and 20 h after thawing. **(c)** Flow cytometry assay performed on non matured or matured IFN-DCs 20 h after thawing. **(d)** MLR assays performed 2 and 20 h after thawing on non matured (filled *diamond*) or matured IFN-DCs (*open square* CD40L; *filled circle*, FMKp + IFN-γ; *open circle*, PGE2 + IL-6 + IL1-β + TNF-α)

trials using DC-based therapeutic cancer vaccines (Gilboa 2007). Nevertheless, in spite of all the knowledge acquired through these and subsequent studies, there is no *consensus* yet on the methods to be used for the generation of fully competent DCs for the development of vaccines capable of inducing both immune and clinical responses in cancer patients. As for the cytokines or cytokine combinations to be preferred for the *ex vivo* differentiation and activation of DCs, we still need to improve our knowledge particularly concerning those DC-targeting cytokines with a long record of clinical use, such as IFN-α and GM-CSF.

In recent years a growing body of evidence has indicated that IFN-α can exert important effects on the differentiation and function of DCs and that such effects may play major roles in the induction of IFN-induced antitumor immunity and autoimmunity. Important insights to this regard have been provided by the studies carried out by Banchereau's group, reviewed by Banchereau and Pascual (2006). The presence of increased levels of IFN-α in the serum of Systemic Lupus Erythematosus (SLE) patients as well as the appearance of some autoimmunity symptoms after long-term IFN treatment are well known observations (Durelli et al. 1999; Preziati et al. 1995; Ronnblom et al. 1991). Banchereau and colleagues reported that a 24–72 h exposure to serum from SLE patients induces blood monocytes to differentiate into highly potent DCs, and that this differentiation is dependent on the action of IFN-α (Blanco et al. 2001). DCs in the blood of the SLE patients, strongly resembling IFN-DCs, can play a major role in breaking peripheral tolerance (Steinman 2003) and autoimmunity, through inappropriate antigen presentation leading to a pathologic immune response to self antigens in these patients (Blanco et al. 2001). Of interest, these studies also led to the suggestion of a possible role of IFN-DC interactions in the pathogenesis of autoimmune diseases (Banchereau and Pascual 2006). Consistent with the hypothesis of a possible role of IFN-DCs in the pathogenesis of autoimmune responses are the results of a recent study describing a striking correlation between clinical response to IFN-α and autoimmune manifestations in melanoma patients treated with the high dose IFN-α regimen (Gogas et al. 2006).

A possible association between the effects of in vivo administration of IFN-α on monocyte/dendritic cell precursors and the activation of tumor-specific $CD8^+$ T cells is suggested by the results of a pilot phase I-II trial that we recently carried out to determine the effects of IFN-α, administered as an adjuvant of Melan-A/MART-1:26–35(27L) and gp100:209–217(210M) peptides, on immune responses in stage IV melanoma patients (Di Pucchio et al. 2006). In 5 out of the 7 evaluable patients, a consistent enhancement of $CD8^+$ T cells recognizing modified and native MART-1 and gp100 peptides and MART-1^+ gp100^+ melanoma cells was observed. Moreover, vaccination induced a raise in $CD8^+$ T-cell binding to HLA tetramers containing the relevant peptides and an increased frequency of $CD45RA^+$ $CCR7^-$ (terminally differentiated effectors) and $CD45RA^-CCR7^-$ (effector memory) cells. Interestingly, in all patients the treatment augmented significantly the percentage of $CD14^+$ monocytes, and particularly of the $CD14^+$ $CD16^+$ cell fraction. Notably, post-vaccination monocytes from 2 out of the 3 patients showing stable disease or long disease-free survival showed an enhanced APC function and capability to secrete CXCL10 when tested in MLR assays, associated to a boost of antigen and melanoma-specific $CD8^+$ T cells.

Altogether, these findings support the rationale of using IFN-α-induced DCs as cellular adjuvants of therapeutic cancer vaccines.

The ensemble of results illustrated in the previous sections indicating that highly active DCs could be generated from human precursors by exposure to type I IFNs, has prompted the clinical testing of these practical powerful cellular adjuvants in DC-based therapeutic vaccines for the treatment of cancer patients.

The first clinical trial using type I IFN-induced DC-based vaccine was performed by Banchereau and colleagues (2005), who reported on the vaccination of stage IV melanoma patients with DCs differentiated from $CD34^+$ progenitors in the presence of IFN-α and loaded with peptides derived from four melanoma tissue differentiation antigens (MART-1, tyrosinase, MAGE-3, and gp100) and influenza matrix peptide (Flu-MP). Although none of the analyzed patients showed the expansion of melanoma-peptide-specific circulating effector memory T cells capable of secreting IFN-γ in direct ex vivo ELISPOT assays, tumor Ag-specific recall memory CD8 + T cells able to secrete IFN-γ and to proliferate could be detected in the majority of patients. The overall results of this trial suggested that DCs generated from $CD34^+$ precursors by IFN-α, although safe, elicit only limited immune responses. Moreover, no objective clinical responses were observed. Subsequently, Trakatelli and colleagues (2006) vaccinated a group of stage III/IV melanoma patients with IFN-DCs obtained with IFN-β and IL-3, activated by poly I: C, and pulsed with the tumor-specific antigen NA17.A2. Tetramer labeling indicated that three out of eight patients mounted a $CD8^+$ T cell response against the melanoma peptide and isotopic imaging demonstrated that IFN-DCs migrate to the draining lymph nodes.

A very recent clinical trial was carried out in five patients with metastasized medullary thyroid carcinoma, who were immunized with IFN-α-DCs pulsed with the tumor-specific antigenic peptide calcitonin (Papewalis et al. 2008a). Interestingly, after a long term follow-up all patients are alive. These patients showed an increase of tumor-specific T cells secreting IFN-γ and a strong $CD8^+$ T lymphocyte infiltration upon DTH skin test, suggesting that IFN-DCs induce Ag-specific $CD8^+$ T cells. In two patients who responded to therapy a large increase of antigen-specific IFN-γ-secreting $CD4^+$ cells as well as an increase of granzyme B positive $CD8^+$ cells in the peripheral blood was found. In parallel, a decrease of $CD4^+/CD25^+/FoxP3^+$ regulatory T cells was observed (Papewalis et al. 2008b).

5 Final Remarks

On the whole, the results on IFN-α-DC interactions support the concept that IFN-α represents a powerful natural adjuvant for the connection between innate and adaptive immunity by acting on DC differentiation/activation. This knowledge supports the use of this cytokine for the in vitro generation of IFN-DCs from cancer patient's monocytes. Then, following the DC-based immunotherapy approach most commonly used so far, these IFN-DCs would be loaded with the relevant tumor-associated antigen(s) (TAA) and reinfused into the patient (Fig. 5).

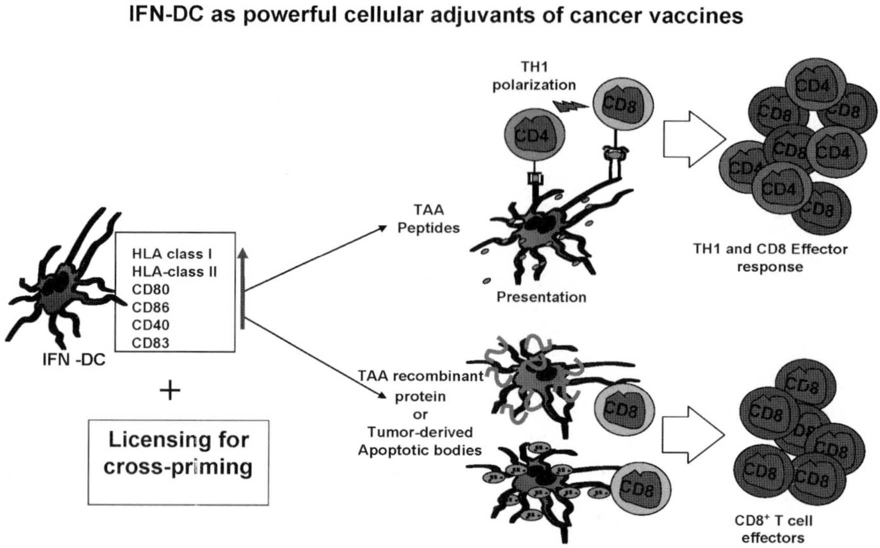

Fig. 5 IFN-DC as powerful cellular adjuvants of cancer vaccines. IFN-DCs efficiently cross-present exogenous soluble proteins and even very low amounts peptide to the specific $CD8^+$ T cells. Of interest, in experiments with purified $CD8^+$ T cells, IFN-DCs have been found superior with respect to CD40L-matured IL-4-DCs in inducing in vitro cross-priming of $CD8^+$ T cells, suggesting that IFN-DCs are directly licensed for an efficient $CD8^+$ T cell priming and suitable for efficient stimulation of an antitumor immune response

Based on certain peculiar functional features exhibited by IFN-DCs and on the emerging concept of immunogenic cell death induced by defined chemotherapeutic agents as well as by radiotherapy and photodynamic therapy (Melero et al. 2006; Tesniere et al. 2008), an alternative use of IFN-DCs for immunotherapy of cancer can be envisaged. In mouse models, the injection of DCs into tumor lesions following treatments inducing immunogenic cell death has been shown to result in an augmented therapeutic effectiveness (for references, see (Melero et al. 2006). In spite of their partially mature phenotype, IFN-DCs appear to be particularly effective in taking up apoptotic bodies (our unpublished results) and in inducing the cross-priming of $CD8^+$ T cells against defined antigens. Thus, thank to this peculiar attitude of IFN-DCs, the intratumoral injection of IFN-DCs in patients pre-treated with chemotherapy, radiotherapy, or photodynamic therapy, may represent a potentially advantageous strategy for achieving the cross-priming against immunogenic TAA and for the induction of a tumor-specific and potentially effective TH-1 immune response.

Acknowledgements We are grateful to Mrs. Alessandra Mariani for excellent secretarial assistance. Work in the authors' laboratory was supported in part by grants provided by the European Union (6th Framework Programme, LSHB-CT-2003-503583) and AIRC.

References

Albert ML, Sauter B, Bhardwaj N (1998) Dendritic cells acquire antigen from apoptotic cells and induce class I-restricted CTLs. Nature 392:86–89

Banchereau J, Pascual V (2006) Type I IFN in systemic lupus erythematosus and other autoimmune diseases. Immunity 25:383–392

Banchereau J, Ueno H, Dhodapkar M, Connolly J, Finholt JP, Klechevsky E, Blanck JP, Johnston DA, Palucka AK, Fay J (2005) Immune and clinical outcomes in patients with stage IV melanoma vaccinated with peptide-pulsed dendritic cells derived from $CD34^+$ progenitors and activated with type I interferon. J Immunother 28:505–516

Barnes E, Salio M, Cerundolo V, Medlin J, Murphy S, Dusheiko G, Klenerman P (2004) Impact of alpha interferon and ribavirin on the function of maturing dendritic cells. Antimicrob Agents Chemother 48:3382–3389

Bartholomé EJ, Willems F, Crusiaux A, Thielemans K, Schandene L, Goldman M (1999) IFN-beta interferes with the differentiation of dendritic cells from peripheral blood mononuclear cells: selective inhibition of CD40-dependent interleukin-12 secretion. J Interf Cytok Res 19:471–478

Belardelli F (1995) Role of interferons and other cytokines in the regulation of the immune response. APMIS 103:161–179

Belardelli F, Ferrantini M (2002) Cytokines as a link between innate and adaptive antitumor immunity. Trends Immunol 23:201–208

Belardelli F, Gresser I (1996) The neglected role of type I interferon in the T-cell response: implications for its clinical use. Immunol Today 17:369–372

Bell D, Young JW, Banchereau J (1999) Dendritic cells. Adv Immunol 72:255–324

Blanco P, Palucka AK, Gill M, Pascual V, Banchereau J (2001) Induction of dendritic cell differentiation by IFN-alpha in systemic lupus erythematosus. Science 294:1540–1543

Boccaccio C, Jacod S, Kaiser A, Boyer A, Abastado JP, Nardin A (2002) Identification of a clinical-grade maturation factor for dendritic cells. J Immunother 25:88–96

Buelens C, Bartholome EJ, Amraoui Z, Boutriaux M, Salmon I, Thielemans K, Willems F, Goldman M (2002) Interleukin-3 and interferon beta cooperate to induce differentiation of monocytes into dendritic cells with potent helper T-cell stimulatory properties. Blood 99:993–998

Carbonneil C, Aouba A, Burgard M, Cardinaud S, Rouzioux C, Langlade-Demoyen P, Weiss L (2003) Dendritic cells generated in the presence of granulocyte-macrophage colony-stimulating factor and IFN-alpha are potent inducers of HIV-specific CD8 T cells. AIDS 17:1731–1740

Carbonneil C, Saidi H, Donkova-Petrini V, Weiss L (2004) Dendritic cells generated in the presence of interferon-alpha stimulate allogeneic CD4+ T-cell proliferation: modulation by autocrine IL-10, enhanced T-cell apoptosis and T regulatory type 1 cells. Int Immunol 16:1037–1052

Caux C, Dezutter-Dambuyant C, Schmitt D, Banchereau J (1992) GM-CSF and TNF-alpha cooperate in the generation of dendritic Langerhans cells. Nature 360:258–261

Caux C, Vanbervliet B, Massacrier C, Dezutter-Dambuyant C, de Saint-Vis B, Jacquet C, Yoneda K, Imamura S, Schmitt D, Banchereau J (1996) CD34+ hematopoietic progenitors from human cord blood differentiate along two independent dendritic cell pathways in response to GM-CSF + TNF alpha. J Exp Med 184:695–706

Cella M, Jarrossay D, Facchetti F, Alebardi O, Nakajima H, Lanzavecchia A, Colonna M (1999) Plasmacytoid monocytes migrate to inflamed lymph nodes and produce large amounts of type I interferon. Nat Med 5:919–923

Della Bella S, Nicola S, Riva A, Biasin M, Clerici M, Villa ML (2004) Functional repertoire of dendritic cells generated in granulocyte macrophage-colony stimulating factor and interferon-alpha. J Leukoc Biol 75:106–116

Detournay O, Mazouz N, Goldman M, Toungouz M (2005) IL-6 produced by type I IFN DC controls IFN-gamma production by regulating the suppressive effect of CD4 + CD25+ regulatory T cells. Hum Immunol 66:460–468

Dickensheets HL, Donnelly RP (1999) Inhibition of IL-4-inducible gene expression in human monocytes by type I and type II interferons. Leukoc Biol 65:307–312

Di Pucchio T, Pilla L, Capone I, Ferrantini M, Montefiore E, Urbani F, Patuzzo R, Pennacchioli E, Santinami M, Cova A, Sovena G, Arienti F, Lombardo C, Lombardi A, Caporaso P, D'Atri S, Marchetti P, Bonmassar E, Parmiani G, Belardelli F, Rivoltini L (2006) Immunization of stage IV melanoma patients with Melan-A/MART-1 and gp100 peptides plus IFN-α results in the activation of specific CD8$^+$ T cells and monocyte/dendritic cell precursors. Cancer Res 66:4943–4951

Durelli L, Ferrero B, Oggero A, Verdun E, Bongioanni MR, Gentile E, Isoardo GL, Ricci A, Rota E, Bergamasco B, Durazzo M, Saracco G, Biava MA, Brossa PC, Giorda L, Pagni R, Aimo G (1999) Autoimmune events during interferon beta-1b treatment for multiple sclerosis. J Neurol Sci 162:74–83

Dussourd d'Hinterland L, Normier G, Durand J (1980) Ribosomal vaccines: preparation of subcellular fractions. Arzneimittelforschung 30:126–132

Ferrantini M, Capone I, Belardelli F (2007) Interferon-alpha and cancer: mechanisms of action and new perspectives of clinical use. Biochimie 89:884–893

Ferrantini M, Capone I, Belardelli F (2008) Dendritic cells and cytokines in immune rejection of cancer. Cytokine Growth Factor Rev 19:93–107

Gabriele L, Borghi P, Rozera C, Sestili P, Andreotti M, Guarini A, Montefusco E, Foà R, Belardelli F (2004) IFN-alpha promotes the rapid differentiation of monocytes from patients with chronic myeloid leukemia into activated dendritic cells tuned to undergo full maturation after LPS treatment. Blood 103:980–987

Gauzzi MC, Canini I, Eid P, Belardelli F, Gessani S (2002) Loss of type I IFN receptors and impaired IFN responsiveness during terminal maturation of monocyte-derived human dendritic cells. J Immunol 169:3038–3045

Gilboa E (2007) DC-based cancer vaccines. J Clin Invest 117:1195–1203

Gogas H, Ioannovich J, Dafni U, Stavropoulou-Giokas C, Frangia K, Tsoutsos D, Panagiotou P, Polyzos A, Papadopoulos O, Stratigos A, Markopoulos C, Bafaloukos D, Pectasides D, Fountzilas G, Kirkwood JM (2006) Prognostic significance of autoimmunity during treatment of melanoma with interferon. N Engl J Med 354:709–718

Heath WR, Carbone FR (2001) Cross-presentation, dendritic cells, tolerance and immunity. Annu Rev Immunol 19:47–64

Hermann P, Rubio M, Nakajima T, Delespesse G, Sarfati M (1998) IFN-alpha priming of human monocytes differentially regulates gram-positive and gram-negative bacteria-induced IL-10 release and selectively enhances IL-12p70, CD80, and MHC class I expression. J Immunol 161:2011–2018

Huang YM, Kouwenhoven M, Jin YP, Press R, Huang WX, Link H (2001) Dendritic cells derived from patients with multiple sclerosis show high CD1a and low CD86 expression. Mult Scler 7:95–99

Hunter CA (2005) New IL-12-family members: IL-23 and IL-27, cytokines with divergent functions. Nat Rev Immunol 5:521–531

Hussien Y, Sanna A, Soderstrom M, Link H, Huang YM (2001) Glatiramer acetate and IFN-beta act on dendritic cells in multiple sclerosis. J Neuroimmunol 121:102–110

Ito T, Amakawa R, Inaba M, Ikehara S, Inaba K, Fukuhara S (2001) Differential regulation of human blood dendritic cell subsets by IFNs. J Immunol 166:2961–2969

Jonuleit H, Kühn U, Müller G, Steinbrink K, Paragnik L, Schmitt E, Knop J, Enk AH (1997a) Proinflammatory cytokines and prostaglandins induce maturation of potent immunostimulatory dendritic cells under fetal calf serum-free conditions. Eur J Immunol 27:3135–3142

Jonuleit H, Wiedemann K, Müller G, Degwert J, Hoppe U, Knop J, Enk AH (1997b) Induction of IL-15 messenger RNA and protein in human blood-derived dendritic cells: a role for IL-15 in attraction of T cells. J Immunol 158:2610–2615

Kalinski P, Schuitemaker JHN, Hilkens CMU, Wierenga EA, Kapsenberg ML (1999) Final maturation of dendritic cells is associated with impaired responsiveness to IFN-gamma and to bacterial IL-12 inducers: decreased ability of mature dendritic cells to produce IL-12 during the interaction with Th cells. J Immunol 162:3231–3236

Korthals M, Safaian N, Kronenwett R, Maihöfer D, Schott M, Papewalis C, Diaz Blanco E, Winter M, Czibere A, Haas R, Kobbe G, Fenk R (2007) Monocyte derived dendritic cells generated by IFN-alpha acquire mature dendritic and natural killer cell properties as shown by gene expression analysis. J Transl Med 5:46

Langenkamp A, Messi M, Lanzavecchia A, Sallusto F (2000) Kinetics of dendritic cell activation: impact on priming of TH1, TH2 and nonpolarized T cells. Nat Immunol 1:311–316

Lapenta C, Santini SM, Logozzi M, Spada M, Andreotti M, Di Pucchio T, Parlato S, Belardelli F (2003) Potent immune response against HIV-1 and protection from virus challenge in hu-PBL-SCID mice immunized with inactivated virus-pulsed dendritic cells generated in the presence of IFN-alpha. J Exp Med 198:361–367

Lapenta C, Santini SM, Spada M, Donati S, Urbani F, Accapezzato D, Franceschini D, Andreotti M, Barnaba V, Belardelli F (2006) IFN-alpha-conditioned dendritic cells are highly efficient in inducing cross-priming CD8(+) T cells against exogenous viral antigens. Eur J Immunol 36:2046–2060

Larner AC, Petricoin EF, Nakagawa Y, Finbloom DS (1993) IL-4 attenuates the transcriptional activation of both IFN-alpha and IFN-gamma-induced cellular gene expression in monocytes and monocytic cell lines. J Immunol 150:1944–1950

Liu YJ (2001) Dendritic cell subsets and lineages, and their functions in innate and adaptive immunity. Cell 106:259–262

Luft T, Pang KC, Thomas E, Bradley CJ, Savoia H, Trapani J, Cebon J (1998a) A serum-free culture model for studying the differentiation of human dendritic cells from adult CD34+ progenitor cells. Exp Hematol 26:489–500

Luft T, Pang KC, Thomas E, Hertzog P, Hart DN, Trapani J, Cebon J (1998b) Type I IFNs enhance the terminal differentiation of dendritic cells. J Immunol 161:1947–1953

Luft T, Luetjens P, Hochrein H, Toy T, Masterman KA, Rizkalla M, Maliszewski C, Shortman K, Cebon J, Maraskovsky E (2002) IFN-alpha enhances CD40 ligand-mediated activation of immature monocyte-derived dendritic cells. Int Immunol 14:367–380

Mazouz N, Detournay O, Buelens C, Renneson J, Trakatelli M, Lambermont M, Goldman M, Toungouz M (2005) Immunostimulatory properties of human dendritic cells generated using IFN-beta associated either with IL-3 or GM-CSF. Cancer Immunol Immunother 54:1010–1017

McRae BL, Beilfuss BA, van Seventer GA (2000a) IFN-beta differentially regulates CD40-induced cytokine secretion by human dendritic cells. J Immunol 164:23–28

McRae BL, Nagai T, Semnani RT, van Seventer JM, van Seventer GA (2000b) Interferon-alpha and -beta inhibit the in vitro differentiation of immunocompetent human dendritic cells from CD14(+) precursors. Blood 96:210–217

Melero I, Arina A, Murillo O, Dubrot J, Alfaro C, Pérez-Gracia JL, Bendandi M, Hervás-Stubbs S (2006) Immunogenic cell death and cross-priming are reaching the clinical immunotherapy arena. Clin Cancer Res 12:2385–2389

Mohty M, Vialle-Castellano A, Nunes JA, Isnardon D, Olive D, Gaugler B (2003) IFN-alpha skews monocyte differentiation into Toll-like receptor 7-expressing dendritic cells with potent functional activities. J Imm 171:3385–3393

Nagai T, Devergne O, Mueller TF, Perkins DL, van Seventer JM, van Seventer GA (2003) Timing of IFN-beta exposure during human dendritic cell maturation and naive Th cell stimulation has contrasting effects on Th1 subset generation: a role for IFN-beta-mediated regulation of IL-12 family cytokines and IL-18 in naive Th cell differentiation. J Immunol 171:5233–5243

Napolitani G, Rinaldi A, Bertoni F, Sallusto F and Lanzavecchia A (2005) Selected Toll-like receptor agonist combinations synergistically trigger a T helper type 1-polarizing program in dendritic cells. Nat Immunol 6:769–776

Ohmori Y, Hamilton TA (1998) STAT6 is required for the anti-inflammatory activity of interleukin-4 in mouse peritoneal macrophages. J Biol Chem 273:29202–29209

Padovan E, Spagnoli GC, Ferrantini M, Heberer M (2002) IFN-alpha2a induces IP-10/CXCL10 and MIG/CXCL9 production in monocyte-derived dendritic cells and enhances their capacity to attract and stimulate CD8+ effector T cells. J Leuk Biol 71:669–676

Papewalis C, Jacobs B, Wuttke M, Ullrich E, Baehring T, Fenk R, Willenberg HS, Schinner S, Cohnen M, Seissler J, Zacharowski K, Scherbaum WA, Schott M (2008a) IFN-alpha skews monocytes into CD56+-expressing dendritic cells with potent functional activities in vitro and in vivo. J Immunol 180:1462–1470

Papewalis C, Wuttke M, Jacobs B, Domberg J, Willenberg H, Baehring T, Cupisti K, Raffel A, Chao L, Fenk R, Seissler J, Scherbaum WA, Schott M (2008b) Dendritic cell vaccination induces tumor epitope-specific Th1 immune response in medullary thyroid carcinoma. Horm Metab Res 40:108–116

Paquette RL, Hsu NC, Kiertscher SM, Park AN, Tran L, Roth MD, Glaspy JA (1998) Interferon-alpha and granulocyte-macrophage colony-stimulating factor differentiate peripheral blood monocytes into potent antigen-presenting cells. J Leukoc Biol 64:358–367

Parlato S, Santini SM, Lapenta C, Di Pucchio T, Logozzi M, Spada M, Giammarioli AM, Malorni W, Fais S, Belardelli F (2001) Expression of CCR-7, MIP-3beta, and Th-1 chemokines in type I IFN-induced monocyte-derived dendritic cells: importance for the rapid acquisition of potent migratory and functional activities. Blood 98:3022–3029

Pogue SL, Preston BT, Stalder J, Bebbington CR, Cardarelli PM (2004) The receptor for type I IFNs is highly expressed on peripheral blood B cells and monocytes and mediates a distinct profile of differentiation and activation of these cells. J Interferon Cytokine Res 24:131–139

Preziati D, La Rosa L, Covini G, Marcelli R, Rescalli S, Persani L, Del Ninno E, Meroni PL, Colombo M, Beck-Peccoz P (1995) Autoimmunity and thyroid function in patients with chronic active hepatitis treated with recombinant interferon alpha-2a. Eur J Endocrinol 132:587–593

Radvanyi LG, Banerjee A, Weir M, Messner H (1999) Low levels of interferon-alpha induce CD86 (B7.2) expression and accelerates dendritic cell maturation from human peripheral blood mononuclear cells. Scand J Immunol 50:499–509

Renneson J, Salio M, Mazouz N, Goldman M, Marchant A, Cerundolo V (2005) Mature dendritic cells differentiated in the presence of interferon-beta and interleukin-3 prime functional antigen-specific CD8 T cells. Clin Exp Immunol 139:468–475

Rivoltini L, Barracchini KC, Viggiano V, Kawakami Y, Smith A, Mixon A, Restifo NP, Topalian SL, Simonis TB, Rosenberg SA, Francesco MM (1995) Quantitative correlation between HLA class I allele expression and recognition of melanoma cells by antigen-specific cytotoxic T lymphocytes. Cancer Res 55:3149–3157

Romani N, Gruner S, Brang D, Kampgen E, Lenz A, Trockenbacher B, Konwalinka G, Fritsch PO, Steinman RM, Schuler G (1994) Proliferating dendritic cell progenitors in human blood. J Exp Med 180:83–93

Ronnblom LE, Alm GV, Oberg K (1991) Autoimmune phenomena in patients with malignant carcinoid tumors during interferon-alpha treatment. Acta Oncol 30:537–540

Sallusto F, Lanzavecchia A (1994) Efficient presentation of soluble antigen by cultured human dendritic cells is maintained by granulocyte/macrophage colony-stimulating factor plus interleukin 4 and downregulated by tumor necrosis factor alpha. J Exp Med 179:1109–1118

Sallusto F, Mackay CR, Lanzavecchia A (2000) The role of chemokine receptors in primary, effector, and memory immune responses. Annu Rev Immunol 18:593–620

Santini SM, Lapenta C, Logozzi M, Parlato S, Spada M, Di Pucchio T, Belardelli F (2000) Type I interferon as a powerful adjuvant for monocyte-derived dendritic cell development and activity in vitro and in Hu-PBL-SCID mice. J Exp Med 191:1777–1788

Santodonato L, D'Agostino G, Nisini R, Mariotti S, Monque DM, Spada M, Lattanzi L, Perrone MP, Andreotti M, Belardelli F, Ferrantini M (2003) Monocyte-derived dendritic cells generated after a short-term culture with IFN-alpha and granulocyte-macrophage colony-stimulating factor stimulate a potent Epstein-Barr virus-specific CD8+ T cell response. J Immunol 170:5195–5202

Siegal FP, Kadowaki N, Shodell M, Fitzgerald-Bocarsly PA, Shah K, Ho S, Antonenko S, Liu YJ (1999) The nature of the principal type 1 interferon-producing cells in human blood. Science 284:1835–1837

Steinbrink K, Wolfl M, Jonuleit H, Knop J, Enk AH (1997) Induction of tolerance by IL-10-treated dendritic cells. J Immunol 159:4772–4780

Steinbrink K, Jonuleit H, Muller G, Schuler G, Knop J, Enk AH (1999) Interleukin-10-treated human dendritic cells induce a melanoma-antigen-specific anergy in CD8(+) T cells resulting in a failure to lyse tumor cells. Blood 93:1634–1642

Steinman RM (2003) The control of immunity and tolerance by dendritic cell. Pathol Biol 51:59–60

Steinman RM, Banchereau J (2007) Taking dendritic cells into medicine. Nature 449:419–426

Steinman RM, Hemmi H (2006) Dendritic cells: translating innate to adaptive immunity. Curr Top Microbiol Immunol 311:17–58

Tesniere A, Panaretakis T, Kepp O, Apetoh L, Ghiringhelli F, Zitvogel L, Kroemer G (2008) Molecular characteristics of immunogenic cancer cell death. Cell Death Differ 15:3–12

Thurnher M, Zelle-Rieser C, Ramoner R, Bartsch G, Holtl L (2001) The disabled dendritic cell. Faseb J 15:1054–1061

Tosi D, Valenti R, Cova A, Sovena G, Huber V, Pilla L, Arienti F, Belardelli F, Parmiani G, Rivoltini L (2004) Role of cross-talk between IFN-alpha-induced monocyte-derived dendritic cells and NK cells in priming CD8+ T cell responses against human tumor antigens. J Immunol 172:5363–5370

Trakatelli M, Toungouz M, Blocklet D, Dodoo Y, Gordower L, Laporte M, Vereecken P, Sales F, Mortier L, Mazouz N, Lambermont M, Goldman S, Coulie P, Goldman M, Velu T (2006) A new dendritic cell vaccine generated with interleukin-3 and interferon-beta induces CD8+ T cell responses against NA17-A2 tumor peptide in melanoma patients. Cancer Immunol Immunother 55:469–474

Wiesemann E, Sonmez D, Heidenreich F, Windhagen A (2002) Interferon-beta increases the stimulatory capacity of monocyte-derived dendritic cells to induce IL-13, IL-5 and IL-10 in autologous T-cells. J Neuroimmunol 123:160–169

Dendritic Cell-Based Immunotherapy in Myeloid Leukaemia: Translating Fundamental Mechanisms into Clinical Applications

A.A. van de Loosdrecht, W. van den Ancker, I. Houtenbos, G.J. Ossenkoppele, and T. M. Westers

Contents

Abstract Immunotherapy for leukaemia patients, aiming at the generation of anti-leukaemic T cell responses, could provide a new therapeutic approach to eliminate minimal residual disease (MRD) cells in acute myeloid leukaemia (AML).

A.A. van de Loosdrecht (✉)
Department of Haematology, VU-Institute of Cancer and Immunology, VU University Medical Center, De Boelelaan 1117, 1081 HV, Amsterdam, The Netherlands
A.vandeloosdrecht@vumc.nl

G. Lombardi, Y. Riffo-Vasquez (eds.), *Dendritic Cells,* Handbook of Experimental Pharmacology 188,

Leukaemic blasts harbour several ways to escape the immune system including deficient MHC class II expression, low levels of co-stimulatory molecules and suppressive cytokines. Therapeutic vaccination with dendritic cells (DC) is now recognized as an important investigational therapy. Due to their unique antigen presenting capacity, immunosuppressive features of the leukaemic blasts can be circumvented. DC can be successfully cultured from leukaemic blasts in 60–70% of patients and show functional potential in vivo. Alternatively, monocyte derived DC obtained at time of complete remission loaded with leukaemia-specific antigens can be used as vaccine. Several sources of leukaemia-associated antigen and different methods of loading antigen onto DC have been used in an attempt to optimize antitumour responses including apoptotic cells, necrotic cell lysates and tumour-associated peptides. Currently, the AML-derived cell line MUTZ-3, an immortalized equivalent of $CD34^+$ DC precursor cells, is under investigation for vaccination purposes. For effective DC vaccination the intrinsic tolerant state of the patient must be overcome. Therefore, the development of efficient and safe adjuvants in antigen specific immunotherapeutic programs should be encouraged.

1 Introduction

Although intensive chemotherapy-based approaches induce complete remission (CR) in 80% of patients with acute myeloid leukaemia (AML), a lot of patients ultimately relapse due to persistence of minimal residual disease (MRD) cells, resulting in survival percentages of 30–40% (Lowenberg et al. 1999). Immunotherapy for leukaemia patients, aiming at the generation of anti-leukaemic T cell responses could provide a new therapeutic approach to eliminate MRD cells in leukaemia (van de Loosdrecht 2007; van de Loosdrecht and Beelen 2006). Considerable data point out the critical role played by T cell immunity in the control of leukaemia. Most well-known is the re-induction of CR after donor lymphocyte infusion (DLI) for patients with relapsed leukaemia, after allogeneic stem cell transplantation (Kolb et al. 1995; Mackinnon et al. 1995). T cells present in DLI are held responsible for this graft-versus-leukaemia effect. Already in the early seventies it was shown that a combination of chemotherapy and immunotherapy, consisting of vaccination with irradiated autologous AML blasts, resulted in an increased survival of patients as compared to treatment with chemotherapy alone (Powles et al. 1973). More recent data emphasize a possible role for immunotherapy in the eradication of MRD cells by exploring vaccination strategies (Fujii et al. 1999; Houtenbos et al. 2006a, c; Li et al. 2006; Litzow et al. 2006; Ossenkoppele et al. 2003; Roddie et al. 2006).

Dendritic cells (DC) are known for their unique antigen (Ag) presenting capacity and their ability to activate naïve T cells thereby orchestrating the primary immune response (Banchereau and Steinman 1998; Hart 1997). DC reside in peripheral tissues in an immature state, where they capture and process Ags for presentation in the context of Major Histocompatibility Complex (MHC) molecules (Banchereau et al. 2000). Upon the encounter with microbial agents, inflammatory stimuli or T cell derived stimuli, a complex process of morphological, phenotypical and functional changes is induced, commonly referred to as DC maturation (Caux et al. 1997; Cella et al. 1996). Attracted by lymphoid chemokines, mature DC migrate towards T cell areas in the lymph nodes (LN) where they activate naïve T cells; this makes DC ideal candidates for cellular immunotherapy (Randolph 2001). With the development of recombinant cytokines and advances in cell culture techniques, optimal culture conditions could be established for the in vitro generation of DC. The in vitro culture of $CD34^+$ progenitor cells and $CD14^+$ monocytes, in presence of GM-CSF and interleukin-4 (IL-4), results in differentiation into immature DC in 5–7 days (Caux et al. 1997; Romani et al. 1994; Sallusto and Lanzavecchia 1994). Activation of various signal transduction pathways caused by, for example, the cytokines tumour necrosis factor α (TNF-α), CD40 ligand (CD40L) or interferon-γ (IFN-γ), the microbial products lipopolysaccharide (LPS), CpG oligonucleotides and polyriboinosinic polyribocyticylic acid (poly-(I:C)) and inflammatory agents such as IL-1β and prostaglandin E2 (PGE2), leads to the induction of DC maturation. Cultured DC can be fused with target cells and pulsed or transformed with target Ags. Although considerable progress has been made in identifying relevant tumour Ags, for the majority of human cancers it remains unclear which Ags represent the most important tumour rejection Ags (Renkvist et al. 2001). Leukaemic blasts express tumour Ags, capable of eliciting high avidity T cell responses. Unfortunately, these Ags are not uniformly expressed by each leukaemia subtype. The unique property of leukaemic blasts to be able to differentiate into DC, provides therefore a distinctive opportunity to generate Ag presenting cells (APC) which harbour the full range of potential, including unidentified tumour Ags. Leukaemia-derived DC have shown the capacity to induce leukaemia-specific T cell responses in vitro as well as in vivo, thus offering a potential new immunotherapeutic modality for patients with AML and Chronic Myeloid Leukaemia (CML) with MRD (Engels et al. 1999; Harrison et al. 2001; Houtenbos et al. 2003b; Westers et al. 2003).

2 Immunogenicity of Leukaemic Blasts

2.1 The Immunological Synapse

When T cells and APC encounter, a defined sequence of cellular and molecular interactions follows. Contact between APC and T cells can be either adhesive and static or dynamic and migratory. Migratory contacts are driven by the active amoeboid T cell crawling across the APC surface, for example, during the initial scanning phase of T cells. After this initial scanning, Ag recognition by the T cell receptor (TCR) and development of TCR-derived signals such as calcium influx takes place and the T cell stops crawling (Friedl and Storim 2004). Interaction of T cells with APC results in the formation of a contact zone called the immunological synapse (IS). Assembly of the IS occurs in several stages. MHC molecules interacting with TCR are first seen to accumulate in a ring surrounding a central cluster of the interacting adhesion molecules LFA-1 and ICAM-1; together with other adhesion molecules such as DC-SIGN, interacting with ICAM-2 and ICAM-3, the immature synapse is formed. This synapse later inverts in a way that a central zone of TCR termed the central-supramolecular activating complex (c-SMAC) is surrounded by a peripheral ring of adhesion molecules (Dustin et al. 2004; Geijtenbeek et al. 2000a, b). Subsequently, the T cell polarizes towards the APC to optimize signalling between the cells. The function of this highly organized structure remains controversial. Initially the synapse was thought to represent a structure necessary for initiating signals (Lee et al. 2002). Clustering of TCR in the central region might also function to balance signalling. This was shown by T cells lacking LFA-2 adaptor protein thus being unable to form a stable mature IS. These T cells were unable to down regulate TCR and were hypersensitive to presented Ags (Lee et al. 2003; Monks et al. 1998). Several other functions have been ascribed to the immunological synapse, such as directing secretion of cytokines, enhanced signalling and the balancing of enhancing and terminating signals to maintain agonist-triggered signals in T cells (Jacobelli et al. 2004).

Although adhesion molecules are clearly expressed in AML, expression of most of these molecules is low and heterogeneous, as seen for ICAM-1. Therefore, AML blasts are likely to be limited in their ability to develop stable contacts with T cells. Though, not one single adhesion molecule is responsible for stable encounters with T cells, rather the combination of these molecules plays a crucial role in the recognition of leukaemic cells by T cells (Brouwer et al. 2000b) Moreover, a mature IS is only formed on recognition of peptides presented by the MHC and constitutes "signal one" in DC-T cell interaction.

2.2 Leukaemia-Specific Antigens in Acute Myeloid Leukaemia

In AML, leukaemia associated Ags (LAA) can be qualified either as tumour-rejection or as tumour-regression Ags based on their ability to elicit high-avidity T cell responses and to recruit a large number of T cells with a diversity in TCR (Galea-Lauri 2002). The fusion proteins BCR-ABL, PML/RARα and ETO/AML1 resulting from the chromosomal translocations t(9;22), t(15;17) and t(8;21) respectively, provide potential targets for immunotherapy. Additionally, normal proteins overexpressed in leukaemic progenitors such as WT1 (Wilms' tumour-gene product), PRAME (preferentially expressed Ag of melanoma), RHAMM (receptor for hyaluronic acid mediated motility), PR1 (a proteinase 3 derived peptide), hTERT (human telomerase reverse transcription Ag) and Survivin, can be efficiently processed and presented by MHC-class I molecules (Gao et al. 2000; Molldrem et al. 1996). WT1-specific antibodies are identified in 15–25% of AML patients (Gaiger et al. 2000, 2001) Furthermore, cytotoxic responses elicited by WT1 and PR1 have been observed (Scheibenbogen et al. 2002). MUC1, an epithelial mucin, over expressed in many epithelial malignancies has also been shown to be over expressed on AML blasts and to be capable of inducing Cytotoxic T Lymphocyte (CTL) responses (Brossart et al. 2001). These characteristics make AML blasts potential inducers of T cell immunity.

2.3 MHC Class I and MHC Class II Antigen Presentation

A successful antitumour T cell response requires two effector arms of the immune system. $CD4^{+}$ T helper (Th) cells generate T cell help upon activation by MHC class II-Ag complexes and $CD8^{+}$ CTL provide the specific kill of tumour cells upon recognition of MHC class I-Ag complexes. In the past decade, failure of the MHC class I Ag presentation was demonstrated to contribute to tumour immune escape phenomena in a number of malignancies. In addition, data are accumulating that point to the necessity of effective MHC class II Ag presentation to establish effective antitumour immune responses. The absence of T cell help can lead to abortive CTL induction and subsequent tolerance. Moreover, T cell help is required for the maintenance of CTL responses, which is essential in diseases such as cancer (Zajac et al. 1998). However, essential insight is lacking about the mechanisms by which malignant cells might circumvent immune surveillance through obstruction of MHC class II Ag presentation. B cells seem to be important Ag presenting cells in the process of T cell mediated antitumor immunity. Presentation of tumour Ags by B cells induces tolerance and ineffective antitumour immunity by shifting T helper cells towards a Th2-type response instead of the required Th1 response. (Ackerman and Cresswell 2004; Chaturvedi et al. 2000; Kloetzel 2004; Watts 2004).

2.4 Class II-Associated Invariant Chain Peptide (CLIP) in Acute Myeloid Leukaemia

MHC class II molecules bind exogenous Ags generated in the endosomal/lysosomal pathway of the cell. After synthesis, the MHC class II molecule is directed into this pathway by associating to the Invariant Chain (Ii) (Lotteau et al. 1990; Neefjes et al. 1990). During transport to the Ag-loading compartments, the Ii is proteolytically cleaved, leaving only a small fragment, termed CLIP, in the class II peptide binding groove (Roche and Cresswell 1990; Romagnoli and Germain 1994). Release of CLIP or other non-stable binding peptides is catalysed by the specialised chaperone HLA-DM (DM), a MHC-like molecule (Armstrong et al. 1997; Sloan et al. 1995; Ullrich et al. 1997). Consequently, DM acts as a peptide editor, favouring presentation of stable binding Ags. HLA-DO (DO) regulates the action of DM. DO reduces MHC class II-mediated presentation of antigenic peptides in general and modulates the antigenic peptide repertoire by facilitating presentation of certain Ags, while suppressing others. DO therefore both limits and skews the class II-presented antigenic peptide repertoire in B cells (Chalouni et al. 2003; Chen et al. 2002; Denzin et al. 1997; Glazier et al. 2002; Kropshofer et al. 1998; Roucard et al. 2001; Van Ham et al. 1997, 2000; van Lith M. et al. 2001). Thus, the balance between DO and DM is a key factor in controlling Ag presentation in B cells, which may explain why DO and DM expression is very consistent and seemingly tightly regulated. Aberrant over expression of DO compared to DM could lead to a generalized reduction in class II-mediated Ag presentation. In addition, a DO/DM imbalance may skew the peptide repertoire such that presentation of tumour-specific antigenic peptides is prevented. This could lead to the aberrant or deficient T helper cell responses in malignancy.

AML blasts consistently show a high expression of MHC class I molecules, whereas MHC class II molecules are variably expressed. A high amount of CLIP expressed on AML blasts might serve as a tumour escape mechanism; in a recent study in AML patients, CLIP expression was shown to be variable. In AML patients, most relapses occur within 2 years. Significant lower relative CLIP amount was observed in patients with prolonged remission compared to patients who relapsed before 2 years. A cut-off level of 35% of CLIP positive cells resulted in strongly deviating Kaplan Meier curves ($p = 0.01$) that clearly demonstrates the survival advantage for $DR^+/CLIP^-$ patients. A multivariate analysis of cytogenetic risk group combined with relative CLIP amount revealed that cytogenetic risk profile becomes a non-significant variable. Patients with a favourable risk profile had significant lower relative CLIP amount compared to patients with an adverse profile. It is hypothesized that in the favourable cytogenetic risk group, tumour-specific Ags e.g. fusion proteins might be more immunogenic through efficient Ag processing in the absence of CLIP. Within the standard cytogenetic risk group, patients with $>35\%$ of $CLIP^+$ leukaemic blasts showed a significant shorter disease free survival (DFS) as compared to patients with $<35\%$ $CLIP^+$, similar as observed for the whole group (Chamuleau et al. 2004). Finally, evidence is provided that CLIP expression on MRD cells supports the hypothesis that CLIP positive MRD cells might escape immune surveillance (Chamuleau et al. 2006).

Preliminary data show that upon leukaemic DC differentiation, the relative amount of CLIP was down-regulated whereas in other samples no changes in relative CLIP expression were observed; in two samples obtained from patients at relapse, the relative amount of CLIP was increased upon leukaemic DC differentiation. [Data not published]. These data indicate that leukamic DC differentiation modulates immunogenicity; this subject is under investigation.

2.5 Costimulatory Signals

The second signal that is crucial to sustain T cell activation is the interaction of costimulatory molecules and their ligands. In this respect, CD28 is the most important costimulatory molecule expressed on naïve T cells that interacts with CD80 and CD86 on APC. Data showing recruitment of CD28 to the immunological synapse suggest that CD28 regulates events that occur soon after T cell-APC interaction (Bromley et al. 2001). CD28 engagement leads to the initiation and maintenance of the calcium signal within the first 60 s of that signal and contributes to the formation of stable TCR-MHC couples (Andres et al. 2004). Therefore it seems that CD28 has a function in the early immature synapse before the formation of the c-SMAC. In contrast to CD28, its inhibitory counterpart CTLA-4, is recruited into the synapse during the late stages of T cell stimulation. The extent to which this recruitment takes place depends on the high level of T cell activation, emphasizing its function as a negative feedback system (Egen and Allison 2002). Furthermore, the expression of costimulatory molecules, such as CD80, CD86 and CD40, on AML blasts has been described. Attempts to increase the expression of costimulatory molecules on AML blasts have been made, for example by transfecting AML blasts with genes encoding for CD80 (Hirano et al. 1997; Hirst et al. 1997)

2.6 Cytokine Secretion

An important function of the IS might be the direction of signalling towards a Th1 or Th2 type response through colocalization of cytokine receptors and cytokine secretion, often referred as T cell-polarizing "signal three". The observation that the IFN-γ receptor colocalizes with the TCR in the c-SMAC suggests, that the function of such copolarisation might include the concentration of cytokine receptors at the actual sites where cytokines are produced. For naïve T cells, the IS could provide a platform for cytokine presentation of activating and polarizing factors such as IL-2, IFN-γ or IL-12 derived from APC. In these studies it was observed that IL-4 prevented colocalization of IFN-γ and TCR and thereby prevented a Th1 response (Maldonado et al. 2004).

AML blasts are able to produce IFN-γ (Panoskaltsis et al. 2003). Though, it has been shown that cytokines act locally rather than at a distance (Poo et al. 1988). The inability to form a functional IS in AML might hamper efficient T cell responses. Another mechanism by which tumours could potentially escape elimination by the immune system is by secretion of cytokines that suppress cells involved in immune surveillance (Buggins et al. 2001; Orleans-Lindsay et al. 2001). The production of factors such as vascular endothelial growth factor (VEGF), IL-6, GM-CSF, IL-10 and TGFβ are associated with inhibited DC function and maturation (de Bont et al., 2002; Menetrier-Caux et al. 1998). It was shown that the U937 leukaemic cell line generates tumour supernatant which inhibits Ag presentation and subsequent T cell secretion of IFN-γ and IL-2 (Buggins et al. 1999).

3 Development of Dendritic Cell-Based Vaccines in Leukaemia

3.1 Culture of Leukaemic DC

Culture of leukaemic blasts in presence of various combinations of cytokines, including GM-CSF, TNF-α and IL-4 results in the differentiation towards leukaemic DC-like APC (Brouwer et al. 2000a; Charbonnier et al. 1999; Choudhury et al. 1997; Cignetti et al. 1999; Harrison et al. 2001; Houtenbos et al. 2003b; Oehler et al. 2000; Panoskaltsis et al. 2002; Robinson et al. 1998; Westers et al. 2003;

Woiciechowsky et al. 2001). Maturation of cytokine-cultured AML-DC, can be achieved by incubation with a mixture of inflammatory cytokines TNF-α, IL-1β, IL-6 and PGE2 or by the addition of CD40L (Cignetti et al. 2004; Westers et al. 2005a). Apart from monocytes and $CD34^+$ haematopoietic progenitors also CML cells as well as AML blasts are able to respond to calcium-mobilizing agents such as calcium ionophores (CI), thereby bypassing receptor mediated signalling (Czerniecki et al. 1997; Engels et al. 1999; Koski et al. 1999; Waclavicek et al. 2001; Westers et al. 2003). The acquisition of dendritic features upon CI incubation occurs far more rapidly though their viability was less as compared to cytokine cultured AML-DC (Westers et al. 2003). In a direct comparative study it was shown that the serum-free culture of AML-DC is feasible by the cytokine-based culture method as well as the CI-based culture method, and that these DC are comparable to serum-enriched cultured AML-DC with regard to morphological, phenotypical and functional features (Houtenbos et al. 2003b). Thus, AML-DC are suitable for the development of clinical vaccination programs that comply with good clinical practice demands.

In order to elicit an adequate T cell response in vivo, AML-DC have to be able to migrate from the injection site towards the lymph nodes. In migration assays, mature AML-DC and also CML-DC, exhibited potent migratory capacity towards the lymph node-associated chemokines SDF-1 (CXCL12) and MIP-3β (CCL19), implying their ability to migrate towards the lymph nodes (Westers et al. 2005b). Upon arrival in the lymph nodes AML-DC should be capable of stimulating T cells. AML-DC proved to be potent inducers of T cell stimulation in alloreactivity tests (Choudhury et al. 1999; Panoskaltsis et al. 2002; Robinson et al. 1998; Westers et al. 2003). AML-DC were shown to evoke a Th1 response; Th1 cells are capable of stimulating $CD8^+$ cytotoxic T cells, important for antitumour immunity (Cignetti et al. 2004; Westers et al. 2003). Most importantly, T cells primed with autologous AML-DC demonstrated cytolytic capacity towards autologous AML blasts as assessed by cytotoxicity assays (Choudhury et al. 1999; Harrison et al. 2001; Westers et al. 2003). To avoid the risk of infusing residual leukaemic cells potentially causing relapse of the disease, AML-DC vaccines should be irradiated before injection. ^{3}[H] thymidine incorporation assays indicate that irradiated blasts as well as AML-DC are unable to proliferate, while AML-DC retain their capacity to induce T cell proliferation. AML-DC maintain migratory capacity upon irradiation (Westers et al. 2005b). All together, these data confirm safety and the functional potential of AML-DC that are instrumental in vaccination regimens to stimulate autologous cytotoxic T cell responses.

3.2 Prediction of Feasibility to Culture Leukaemic DC

Reflecting the heterogeneity of the disease, selection of the most optimal DC culture method for each individual AML patient at diagnosis is of great importance. Surprisingly, in a large cohort of patients it was found that DC differentiation capacity is independent from the French-American-British (FAB) classification subtype. In particular, no significant differences were found between the monocytic subtypes, M4 and M5, and other subtypes (Houtenbos et al. 2006e). It is possible to predict AML-DC culture outcome by the expression of defined surface markers on AML blasts (Houtenbos et al. 2004; Mohty et al. 2002; Re et al. 2002). It was described that $CD14^{+}$ blasts represent the population that can be induced in vitro into DC whereas, the $CD14^{-}$ population could not (Mohty et al. 2002). In addition, high TNFα-RI expression on AML blasts is predictive for the DC differentiation capacity of blasts when cultured in presence of cytokines (Houtenbos et al. 2004). Interestingly, induction of DC differentiation in $CD14^{-}$ blasts is possible if these blasts express TNFα-RI (Houtenbos et al. 2003a). Alternative culture methods, for example the CI-based method, can be used to induce DC differentiation in CD14- and TNFα-RI- AML samples. The presence of CD86 on AML blasts has also been associated with the ability to differentiate into AML-DC (Re et al. 2002). Besides the expression of these surface markers, the presence of a Flt-3 internal tandem duplication (ITD), that causes a block in myeloid differentiation (Zheng et al. 2002), is strongly associated with a diminished DC differentiation capacity in both cytokine and CI DC culture methods (Houtenbos et al. 2006d).

Using these selection parameters the most optimal protocol for the generation of AML-DC can be identified for each individual patient. Although the fact remains that in only 60–70% of the cases AML blasts can be cultured into leukaemic DC. Therefore monocyte derived DC cultured at the time of complete remission, loaded with tumour specific peptides or patients' tumour material frozen at onset of the disease may serve as an alternative.

3.3 DC Loading Strategies in Acute Myeloid Leukaemia

3.3.1 Peptides as Tumour Associated Antigens

Several protocols have been described to deliver Ags to monocyte derived DC (MoDC), mostly in solid malignancies. In these solid tumours, known tumour associated Ags (TAA) are already used in clinical trials (Dunn et al. 2004).

The restricted number of TAA known in AML is a major disadvantage for the use as peptides. Other limitations in peptide vaccination are: the low affinity of peptides that bind to the MHC class I molecules; the short time peptides reside on the surface of DC; the diversity of the HLA profiles and the bypassing of T helper cells via MHC class- II molecules (Amoscato et al. 1998; Rosenberg et al. 1998). Moreover, there is a risk that, targeting a single Ag may result in immunologic pressure against expression of the parent protein, resulting in selection of Ag-loss variants. Therefore, other approaches utilizing whole tumours as source of Ag, containing known and unknown Ags, have been developed. This allows HLA molecules to select epitopes from a tumour Ag's entire sequence. Possibilities for Ag loading onto DC containing whole cell Ags are apoptotic cells, lysates, RNA/DNA or eluted peptides as discussed below.

3.3.2 Eluted Peptides

AML peptides can be eluted from the cell surface with citrate phosphate (CP) or trifluoroacetic acid (TFA). These peptides represent a pool of naturally processed peptides. It was shown in AML that TFA-eluted peptides loaded onto MoDC were able to generate significant anti-leukaemia $CD4^+$ and cytotoxic $CD8^+$ T cell responses. (Delluc et al. 2006) In a murine model using DC pulsed with acid-eluted tumour peptides, a superior immune response could be shown as compared to DC pulsed with tumour cell lysates. (Delluc et al. 2005).

3.3.3 Apoptotic Cells

Physiologic cell death occurs primarily through a form of cell suicide termed apoptosis. The decision of a cell to undergo apoptosis can be influenced by a wide variety of extracellular and intracellular signals. Extracellular pro-apoptotic signals include hormones, growth factors, nitric oxide or cytokines. Intracellular apoptotis is initiated in response to stress, the binding of glucocorticoids to nuclear receptors, heat, radiation, nutrient deprivation, viral infection and hypoxia. Hereby, subtle alterations in the plasma membrane take place such as translocation of soluble molecules phosphatidylserine and calreticulin to the plasma membrane or the adsorption of soluble proteins from outside the cell such as C1q and thrombospondin These changes are associated with an enhanced uptake of the dying cell by DC (Obeid et al. 2007). For vaccination purposes, the induction of apoptosis of AML blasts should be immunogenic. In colon carcinoma for instance, the upregulation of calreticulin by radiation with UV light or by treatment with antracyclins is associated with immunogenic apoptosis (Blachere et al. 2005; Obeid et al. 2007). In myeloma, the proteosome inhibitor Bortezomib® can enhance DC-mediated induction of immunity via exposure of heat shock protein (HSP) 90 (Spisek et al. 2007). The best approach to induce apoptosis is not clarified yet.

Phagocytosis of apoptotic cells is believed to be less efficient as compared to microbial cells, due to the fact that microbial cells also supply danger signals. Danger signals induce Ag uptake, DC maturation and activation of inflammatory responses. Examples of these danger signals are ligands for Toll Like Receptors (TLR) that will be discussed in 4.1 (Blander and Medzhitov 2006). Leukaemic blasts transfected with double-stranded (ds) RNA, TLR3 ligand, poly(I:C), mimicking viral infection showed an enhanced expression of MHC and co-stimulatory molecules and production of IFNs. This resulted in an enhanced uptake by the DC, an increased Th1 polarizing capacity and higher production of proinflammatory cytokines (Smits et al. 2007). Another strategy to enhance phagocytosis is to coat the cells with IgG antibodies that targets apoptotic cells via Fcγ receptors into DC. Hereby cross-presentation of various exogenous Ags into MHC class I molecules is encouraged. In a B cell lymphoma model this resulted in a better tumour protection. (Amigorena 2002; Franki et al. 2007)

3.3.4 Lysate or Necrotic Tumour Cells

Necrosis is defined as a brisk plasma membrane rupture. It has long been hypothesized that apoptotic cell death is poorly immunogenic, or even tolerogenic, whereas necrotic cell death is immunogenic (Steinman et al. 2000). In contrast, necrosis is also associated with local immunosuppression in solid tumours (Vakkila and Lotze 2004). On the other hand, evidence is provided that necrotic, but not apoptotic tumour cells, provide signals for DC resulting in the upregulation of maturation-specific markers as well as optimal expression of co-stimulatory molecules (Sauter et al. 2000; Steinman et al. 2000). Cell lysates, generated by freeze/thaw cycles, cover the whole range of tumour Ags and therefore cover all known and unknown TAA. A disadvantage could be that whole cell lysates, as is also the case for apoptotic cells, harbour normal peptides and therefore could increase the risk of autoimmunity (Nestle et al. 2005; Roskrow et al. 1999).

In AML, cell lysates might contain a complex mixture of peptides including intracellular proteases with inhibitory activity and immunosuppressive cytokines, such as TGF-β, that could impair the induction of Th1 immune responses or favour transient IL-12 secretion insufficient to maintain T cell activation with loss of leukaemic cell lysis (Delluc et al. 2006; Galea-Lauri et al. 2004; Schui et al. 2002). Nevertheless, a direct comparison of DC loaded with freeze-thaw lysates, trifluoroacetic acid lysates, extracted membranes, affinity-purified MHC class I- and class II-presented peptides, acid-eluted peptides all from an EBV transduced B lymphoblastoid cell line showed that lysates were most potent in inducing an immune response as compared to eluted peptides (Herr et al. 2000).

3.3.5 Whole Cell RNA/DNA

Whole cell RNA or DNA molecules encode for all cellular peptides and therefore cover all known and unknown TAA. These peptides are produced intracellular and are processed onto MHC class I molecules and may be the optimal source of Ags for DC loading strategies in AML (Jarnjak-Jankovic et al. 2005). As described above, $CD4^+$ T cells are of crucial importance in inducing effective immune responses. Reverse cross-presentation is needed, whereby endogenously produced Ags are presented to MHC class-II molecules as well. (Dissanayake et al. 2005) It was shown that loading of MoDC with RNA and lysates from AML blasts is even supplementary; both intracellular and extracellular Ags are introduced thereby enhancing Ag loading onto both MHC class I and II molecules (Decker et al. 2006).

4 Modulation of DC and T Cell Interaction

In order to take full advantage of the potential of the AML-DC to induce a T cell response in vitro and in vivo through the formation of an IS, additional strategies can be explored that increase the AML-DC yield and its functional effects.

4.1 Adjuvants

In many of the current DC vaccination protocols Bacillus Calmette Guérin (BCG) and keyhole limpet haemocyanin (KLH) are added to vaccines in order to enhance immune responses. Innovative molecular techniques are now instrumental to replace bacterial adjuvants by more sophisticated ways to increase the immunogenicity of cancer cells. Genetically modified AML blasts that express immunomodulatory cytokines used to enhance antigenicity, such as IL-12 or GM-CSF proved to be potent vaccines that are able to cure leukaemia in mice (Bramson et al. 1996; Dranoff et al. 1993; Levitsky et al. 1996; Saudemont et al. 2002; Vereecque et al. 2000). Analogous to this approach, the transduction of DC with genes encoding for GM-CSF and IL-12 could also provide a way to enhance T cell stimulation as shown by the induction of strong T cell responses in a murine melanoma model (Okada et al. 2005). Transient production of IL-12, caused by exhaustion of cytokine production by DC, limits the T cell activation capacity (Langenkamp et al. 2000). This finding implies that prolonged interaction of DC and T cells could increase the immune response. A strategy to extend the contact time between DC and T cells would be the targeting of CD40 on DC. Targeting CD40 not only enhances DC maturation state but also increases the expression of anti-apoptotic molecules (Miga et al. 2001). DC transfected with a drug-inducible CD40 receptor induced prolonged T cell activation and enhanced antitumour responses (Hanks et al. 2005). Also in vivo targeting of CD40 leads to sustained antitumour responses. Thus, increased potentiation of an AML-DC vaccine could be achieved by simultaneously targeting CD40 (Stumbles et al. 2004; Van Mierlo et al. 2002).

Similar to CD40 targeting, it was found that persistent co-administration of TLR ligands enhances DC-based vaccines through prolongation of DC lifespan (Hou and Van Parijs 2004). TLR are a family of pattern-recognition receptors that detects conserved pathogen-associated molecular patterns, a product unique for micro-organisms. TLR can act as adjuvant receptors. They are able to skew specific immune responses towards the Th1 or the Th2 types according to the antigenic stimulation involved. In DC, TLR stimulation can enhance migration into lymph nodes, Ag presentation, cytokine secretion and subsequent activation of adaptive immunity (Schnare et al. 2001). Human myeloid DC express TLR1, 2, 3, 4, 5, 6 and 8; plasmacytoid DC express TLR7 and TLR9 (Seya et al. 2006).

Double-stranded RNA has been shown to act as a viral danger signal to DC recognised through TLR3. TLR3 signalling is important in eliciting cross priming of exogenous Ag (Seya et al. 2006).

TLR4 agonist LPS is frequently used for maturation of DC in vitro. Since LPS itself is not clinically applicable, an analog has to be used. Components of the frequently applied adjuvant BCG also act as TLR2/4 agonists leading to cross-priming of Ag (Seya et al. 2006). Dosage of these kind of agonists is important, because high concentrations can be immunosuppressive as has been shown in systemic infection in which the MHC class II and MHC class I cross-presentation is impaired (Wilson et al. 2006).

Clinical experiences with CpG oligodeoxynucleotides, that target TLR9, are accumulating. Synthetic CpG oligonucleotides mimic immunostimulatoty bacterial DNA. CpG motifs are thought to be responsible for initiating a potent immune response: activate DC, lead to up regulation of co-stimulatory molecules and stimulate secretion of pro-inflammatory cytokines. Potent anti-leukaemia effects were observed when CpG was administered as a single agent in mice (Weigel et al. 2006). CpG are currently in clinical trials for the treatment of lymphoma and lung carcinoma as well as adjuvant therapy for vaccines. CpG can overcome tumour-inhibition of DC-activation in vivo at the tumour site when administered intratumoural (Furumoto et al. 2004). CpG administration activates endogenous DC; whether CpG has any effect on already mature DC in DC-based immunotherapy is questionable. In mice, CpG was administered after maturation of DC; the numbers of leukaemia-reactive CTL modestly increased in vivo, albeit not significant as compared to without additional CpG (Weigel et al. 2006). Important in this respect is that human myeloid DC do not express TLR9 (Seya et al. 2006).

The natural ligand of TLR7 and TLR8 is single stranded RNA. This may represent a better adjuvant than CpG as TLR7 and TLR8 are more broadly expressed. It has been shown that R848 (TLR7/8 agonist) and imiquimod (TLR7 agonist) increase IFNα production in plasmacytoid DC and even induce perforin and Granzyme B expression in myeloid DC. The latter indicates the possibility of direct cytotoxic immune responses and tumour destruction by myeloid DC (Stary et al. 2006).

4.2 Co-stimulatory Pathways

For effective DC vaccination, the vaccine must overcome the intrinsic tolerant state of the patient. It has been shown that especially MRD cells upregulate certain co-stimulatory pathways that could protect them from the patients' immune response. For example, B7-H1, a ligand for programmed death receptor 1 (PD1), was upregulated in MRD cells generated in an acute myeloid leukaemia mouse model (Saudemont and Quesnel 2004). Blocking this pathway increased CTL-mediated killing and enhanced the production of IFN-γ by effector T cells. Enhanced IFN-γ and decreased IL-10 production have also been reported after PD1 blockade in myeloid DC (Brown et al. 2003; Curiel et al. 2003). These findings suggest that modulation of co-stimulatory pathways might improve leukaemic DC vaccine efficacy.

T cells co-cultured with AML blasts in presence of the CD28 antibody showed increased proliferative capacity. In addition, co-stimulation could be further enhanced synergistically by the addition of IL-12 (Orleans-Lindsay et al. 2003). Since AML-DC display a heterogeneous expression of CD80 and CD86; direct targeting of CD28, thereby circumventing interaction via CD80 and CD86, could provide a way to increase T cell responses. Next to that, blocking of CTLA-4, the most important inhibitory co-stimulating pathway, results in rejection of immunogenic transplanted tumour cell lines in vivo, including colorectal carcinoma, renal carcinoma and lymphoma (Leach et al. 1996; Sotomayor et al. 1999). Weak immune responses elicited by tumours can be potentiated, once the inhibitory effect of CTLA-4 is diminished. However, susceptibility appears to be correlated with the inherent immunogenicity of the tumour. Therefore, a combined approach of increasing immunogenicity, combined with CTLA-4 blockade as could be the case in AML-DC vaccination protocols, seems preferable. CTLA-4 is not only expressed by T cells, AML blasts have been reported to express CTLA-4 as well (Pistillo et al. 2003). Anti-CTLA-4 immunotoxins were able to induce apoptosis of AML blasts suggesting a possible role for CTLA-4 as a target molecule for immunotherapeutic strategies. It can also be hypothesized that CTLA-4^+ AML blasts might interact with CD80 and CD86 on APC with potential transduction of an immune inhibitory signal, thus proposing another possible advantage of CTLA-4 blockade.

4–1BB, a member of the TNFα receptor family, represents an important co-stimulatory pathway necessary for the development of CTL (Hellstrom and Hellstrom 2003). Triggering of this pathway increases expansion of Ag specific T cells and could prevent activation induced cell death of $CD8^+$T cells. 4–1BB ligation prevents and even restores T cell anergy in vivo (Wilcox et al. 2004). Also the combined approach of DC-based vaccines potentiated with co-administration of the 4–1BB antibody proved to improve antitumour responses (Ito et al. 2004). In vitro studies show that the combination of T cell priming by AML-DC with 4–1BB targeting results in increased proliferation of $CD8^+$T cells capable of producing IFN-γ, without IL-4 production (Houtenbos et al. 2007). Thus addition of 4–1BB targeting to AML-DC vaccination protocols might augment anti-leukaemic T cell responses. However, to obtain optimal responses upon 4–1BB targeting it might be necessary to simultaneously block the B7-H1 pathway since it was shown that expression of B7-H1 confers resistance to 4–1BB costimulation, while blocking this pathway rescues antitumour responses (Hirano et al. 2005).

5 Clinical Application of Leukaemic and Non-Leukaemic DC-Based Vaccines

5.1 Clinical Studies on Leukaemic DC-Based Vaccination

DC-based immunotherapy has shown promising results in the treatment of cancer (Hsu et al. 1996; Nestle et al. 1998). Moreover, several clinical trials for cancer patients indicate that DC-vaccines are safe with minimal side effects. The first clinical studies on leukaemia-derived DC vaccination were performed in CML patients. In 1999, infusion of leukaemic DC in a single patient with chronic phase caused activation of CTL in vivo and resulted in a decreased BCR-ABL^+ cells in the peripheral blood and bone marrow (Fujii et al. 1999). In 2000, a small phase I study was performed in which autologous CML-derived DC were administered intradermally in three patients in late chronic phase CML. Despite the presumed functional deficiencies of CML-derived DC, an anti-leukaemia immune response was observed as demonstrated by a strong delayed type of hypersensitivity (DTH) response. In one patient immunological responses to autologous leukaemic cells were detected even two years post-vaccination (Ossenkoppele et al. 2003). In another phase I study six CML patients in late chronic phase or accelerated phase were injected with mature CML-derived DC; four of these patients were treated concurrently with Imatinib (Glivec). After vaccination T cells were more responsive to CML-DC in vitro indicating immune effectiveness of the vaccine though significant clinical responses were not observed (Litzow et al. 2006). These data underscore that DC-based immunotherapy might provide a tool to control or eradicate MRD in CML.

In order to establish whether DC vaccination was feasible and safe in AML, a phase I study (2002–2005) was undertaken in 15 AML patients in second CR. DC differentiation from the total leukaemic cell population, harvested at relapse prior to start of chemotherapy, was successfully induced in nine patients. However, the majority of these patients did not reach CR or relapsed shortly thereafter and vaccines were not administered. In one patient, only two vaccines were administered due to limited DC numbers. DTH responses were not observed (Houtenbos et al. 2006a).

Another study on DC vaccination was performed in a group of five AML patients, all vaccinated second or third line in a palliative setting. Autologous AML-derived DC were cultured from adherent monocytoid cells out of leukapheresis products. Three of these patients completed the treatment of four biweekly vaccinations and remained in stable condition for 5–13 months, two patients died from progressive disease. No adverse side effects and no signs of autoimmunity were observed. Immunological responses were analysed in vitro. The cytokine levels in patient's serum changed towards a Th1 type and increased T cell numbers were detected that specifically recognized a PRAME-derived peptide (Li et al. 2006).

Roddie et al. (2006) performed a phase I/II study on vaccination with AML-DC. Twenty-one patients were enrolled of which 14 de novo AML, six relapses and two Myelodysplastic Syndromes (MDS) in transformation. Leukaemia cells were harvested from blood or bone marrow prior to start of induction chemotherapy. Five patients, four de novo and one relapse, achieved both CR and had leukaemia cells that underwent DC differentiation; these patients were vaccinated. In general, vaccination was well tolerated although one patient developed extensive eczema and an increased anti-nuclear factor indicating induction of autoimmunity. DTH responses were either minimal or absent. In vitro analysis showed increased anti-leukaemia T cell responses in four patients. MRD was monitored by RT-PCR for WT1 gene expression. Two patients relapsed shortly after start of vaccination which was mirrored by a rise in the level of WT1 expression; the remaining patients had relatively constant WT1 expression levels following vaccination. Two patients remained in remission more than 12 months post-vaccination (Roddie et al. 2006).

All leukaemia-derived DC vaccines were stated to be prepared under Good Manufacturing Process conditions. Yet the majority of the trials include serum supplementation when culturing DC. In a large DC vaccination trial in melanoma 10% of the patients experienced reaction towards human serum albumin (Schuler 2006).

The number of patients in the leukaemia vaccination trials might be too small to be able to detect such phenomena.

In the clinical trials described above insufficient cell numbers in the initial leukaemia cell harvest, failure of leukaemia cells to undergo DC differentiation and failure to achieve CR, progressive disease or death before vaccination were the main problems in exploring vaccination regimens in myeloid leukaemia. From these data it is concluded that leukaemia-derived DC-based vaccination is only feasible in a subgroup of patients.

5.2 Tumour Specific T Cells are Induced upon Allogeneic DC Vaccination

An alternative approach to autologous DC vaccination is the use of allogeneic DC (alloDC). A major advantage of the use of alloDC is the feasibility of preparing large clinical-grade batches, thus providing a more standardized DC vaccine in terms of phenotype and maturation status. Furthermore, AML patients can be vaccinated immediately after (second) remission increasing patient accrual since relapses frequently occur before preparation and quality control of the autologous DC vaccine is achieved. Although seemingly counter-intuitive, from a theoretical point of view alloDC-based vaccines might even induce a stronger vaccine-specific immune response than autologous DC (Fabre 2001). Since an estimated 1–10% of the circulating T cell repertoire is directed against allo-Ags, alloDC may be expected to trigger a broad T cell response with two possible advantages: (1) activation of tumour-reactive T cells through fortuitous cross-reactivity and (2) allo-Ags on the DC may provide Th epitopes aiding in the optimal activation of CTL against the tumour-related vaccine payload. Although several clinical trials have been carried out to validate the use of alloDC-based tumour vaccination, results so far have been controversial. (Holtl et al. 2005; Hus et al. 2005; Neves et al. 2005; Tamir et al. 2007; Trefzer et al. 2000–2005) All studies showed the tolerability and safety of this approach, with some partial clinical responses, accompanied by evidence of tumour-specific T cell activation. On the whole, alloDC based vaccines appeared less effective than autologous DC used in previous trials. (Trefzer et al. 2000, 2005). Allo-MHC class II molecules may provide beneficial Th activity. It is likely that for a sufficient CTL response at least partial MHC class I matching is required. Of note, most favourable results in murine models were obtained with "semi-allogeneic" DC, i.e. alloDC that were partially MHC-matched (Hus et al. 2005). This was recently confirmed by a vaccination study in colorectal cancer patients, showing that tumour lysate-loaded DC with one haplotype miss-match induced stronger antitumour immune responses as compared to fully autologous DC (Tamir et al. 2007). These studies clearly demonstrate the feasibility of generating TAA-specific T cell responses in an allogeneic-background.

5.2.1 The MUTZ-3 Cell Line: A Source of Functional Allogeneic Leukaemic DC

It was shown recently that the $CD34^+$ human AML derived cell line MUTZ-3 behaves as the immortalized equivalent of $CD34^+$ DC precursor cells (Masterson et al. 2002). Upon stimulation with specific cytokine cocktails, MUTZ-3 progenitors acquire a phenotype consistent with either DC or langerhans cells (LC) with characteristic and mutually exclusive expression of DC-SIGN or Langerin and birbeck granules (Santegoets et al. 2006a). MUTZ-3-DC display the full range of functional MHC- and CD1d-mediated Ag processing and presentation pathways, and express CD83 upon maturation (induced by cocktails comprising IL-6, PGE2, TNFα, IL-1β, IFNα, or Poly:IC). MUTZ-3-DC migrated towards LN-derived chemokines CCL19 and CCL21 confirming their LN homing potential which was shown to be comparable to MoDC. This is in line with their CCR7 expression and suggestive of their in vivo ability to reach the paracortical T cell areas of LN. Functional (i.e. tumour cell-recognizing) CTL clones could be generated against multiple tumour-associated epitopes by stimulating $CD8\beta^+$ CTL precursors with peptide-loaded allogeneic HLA-A2-matched MUTZ-3-DC. Importantly, a consistent induction capacity, as determined by MHC tetramer (Tm) binding, was found in multiple donors and at an efficiency comparable to autologous peptide-loaded MoDC (Santegoets et al. 2006b). In vitro functions of MUTZ-3-DC suggest an ability to induce anti-AML T-cells in vivo, making the MUTZ-3 cell line an universal source of $HLA\text{-}A2^+/HLA\text{-}A3^+$ DC for AML-specific CTL priming in an allogeneic setting.

5.3 Standardization of Clinical Vaccination Protocols

In order to enable comparison of DC vaccination trials, standardization of clinical protocols and immune monitoring techniques is essential (Houtenbos et al. 2006b). Minimal quality criteria regarding DC vaccines are mainly focused on the necessity to vaccinate with mature DC, defined morphologically and immunophenotypically, as well as functionally (Figdor et al. 2004). In vitro and in vivo studies provided evidence that Ag-loaded immature DC silence T cells either by deleting them or by expanding regulatory T cells (Dhodapkar et al. 2001; Hawiger et al. 2001; Jonuleit et al. 2000). In a comparative study on the use of mature versus immature peptide-pulsed MoDC for the vaccination of advanced-stage melanoma patients it was evident that an immunological response could only be detected after vaccination with mature DC. The absence of a T cell response could partly be explained by the observation that immature MoDC are unable to efficiently migrate to the T cell areas of the lymph nodes (de Vries et al. 2003). However, considering relevant cytokine secretion, the maturation state of DC is still a matter of debate. Kinetic studies showed that shortly after activation, DC secrete higher amounts of cytokines and that prolonged maturation periods result in exhaustion of DC with considerable less cytokine production and impaired capacity to stimulate Th1 responses (Camporeale et al. 2003). Although leukaemic DC meet most proposed quality criteria, it is not yet known which level of maturation needs to be achieved to elicit an optimal immune response and whether leukaemic DC are capable of attaining a fully mature state in vivo upon vaccination (Figdor et al. 2004). Another unresolved question in DC vaccination therapy is the optimal route of administration. Intradermal or subcutaneous injections may lead to improved T cell responses as compared with intravenous (IV) administration (Butterfield et al. 2003; Fong et al. 2001) However, these routes of administration rely on the capacity of injected DC to migrate towards the lymph nodes. Intranodal administration circumvents this problem and allows delivery of a known amount of DC to the desired anatomic region, potentially leading to increased T cell immunity (Bedrosian et al. 2003). On the other hand, intranodal vaccination requires technical expertise and includes the risk of damaging the architecture of the lymph node. Additionally, route of administration could determine the location of the primary immune response, the distribution of memory cells, and the ability to control the outgrowth of tumours at different sites in the body (Mullins et al. 2003).

5.4 Minimal Residual Disease and Immunotherapy

Immunotherapy is thought to be most effective in a MRD situation. Detection of leukaemic MRD cells, as characterized by the presence of a leukaemia associated phenotype, is highly predictive for the occurrence of a relapse. A cut off percentage of 0.1% detectable MRD cells after the third course of chemotherapy identifies patients at risk for a fast-developing relapse. Patients with a MRD percentage less than 0.1% should be monitored each 3 months in order to anticipate a possible relapse (Feller et al. 2004). Thus, selection of patients that may benefit from additional immunotherapy might be based on MRD percentages. However, the need for reconstitution of lymphocyte populations and lymphoid tissue after chemotherapy and SCT treatment is likely to influence the effect of immunotherapy. For example, after SCT $CD8^+$ T cells reappear more rapid, i.e. within 6 months, as compared to $CD4^+$ T cells which show low levels even after 1 year. Different immune responses were observed after in vitro priming with AML-DC at different time points during remission. During early remission immune responses seem to be largely MHC-restricted whereas during a later time it was observed that the immune response shifted towards non-MHC restricted as detected in a cytotoxicity assay (Westers et al. 2005b). Thus, time of vaccination should take into account the pace of immune reconstitution in order to obtain efficient immune responses.

5.5 Immunomonitoring of Efficacy

From early clinical studies on DC vaccination it is clear that monitoring the immune response is complex but of great importance (Fong et al. 2001; Nestle et al. 2005). Most techniques represent indirect measurement of cytolytic activity of effector cells. Effector T cells can be isolated either from peripheral blood, lymph node biopsies or DTH reactions. Several clinical vaccination studies in cancer patients have reported T cell responses in peripheral blood but usually only in a minority of patients or after prolonged antigenic restimulation in vitro (Brossart et al. 2000; Coulie et al. 2001; Lau et al. 2001; Valmori et al. 2002). DTH-infiltrated T lymphocytes are able to show Ag specific responses after short term in vitro cultures without the need for Ag restimulation (de Vries et al. 2003). The tetramer technology enables the sensitive detection of Ag specific T cells. Also for leukaemia, LAA have been identified for which tetramers can be developed. However, for a large proportion of the leukaemias, the TAAs are unknown and T cell specificity needs to be determined in a more indirect way. CTL activity can be analysed using a classical ^{51}Cr release assay or by a more sophisticated flow cytometric assay, that uses a Syto-16/7-AAD staining able to detect early apoptosis and secondary necrosis in heterogeneous cell populations such as AML (Westers et al. 2005b). Other immune monitoring methods involve the detection of cytokines released by CTL, by ELISPOT or ELISA, to establish the type of T cell responses.

6 Concluding Remarks and Future Perspectives

The induction of a long-lasting immune response may provide a novel strategy for eradication of residual disease. AML blasts, though being potentially immunogenic, often fail to induce an effective immune response, because they harbour several ways to escape immune surveillance. Nevertheless, the presence of CTLs directed against leukaemic blasts emphasizes their suitability as immunological targets. Increased immunogenicity of AML blasts can be achieved by the induction of differentiation into leukaemic DC. Encouraging results have been obtained by the in vivo application of CML-derived DC and AML-derived DC. (Houtenbos et al. 2006a; Li et al. 2006; Ossenkoppele et al. 2003; Roddie et al. 2006; Westers et al. 2006, 2007).

Important lessons can be learnt from early DC-based vaccines targeting other types of malignancies, such as melanoma, colon carcinoma or prostate carcinoma. In a review on the first 1000 DC vaccinees data are summarized on the types of DC vaccines, route of administration, reported side effects and clinical efficacy (Ridgway 2003). From these data an important conclusion was that side effects were minimal indicating that DC vaccines can be administered safely. Concerning clinical responses, data seem rather disappointing with antitumour responses observed in approximately half of the trials (Nestle et al. 2005; Ridgway 2003). However, it should be taken into account that treated patients often were in end-stage disease. Additional strategies might be required to optimize efficacy of DC vaccines as was outlined above. The combined strength of increasing immunogenicity of AML blasts by differentiation into leukaemic DC and enhancement of T cell responses by immunomodulating agents could represent a new powerful treatment for AML patients. However clinical trials utilizing AML-DC are hampered by patient inclusion criteria. One of the main problems in current clinical trials is, application of vaccination in a late stage of the disease with a high tumour load and a disabled immune system (Houtenbos et al. 2006a). Meaningful clinical responses provoked by DC vaccines are most likely to occur during early stage of disease. Immunotherapy is thought to be most effective in a MRD situation, ideally after achieving first CR. From these data, it is anticipated that intensive fundamental and pre-clinical research of active specific immunotherapy with DC might lead to control progression or even might cure leukaemia.

References

Ackerman AL, Cresswell P (2004) Cellular mechanisms governing cross-presentation of exogenous antigens. Nat Immunol 5:678–684

Amigorena S (2002) Fc gamma receptors and cross-presentation in dendritic cells. J Exp Med 195:F1–F3

Amoscato AA, Prenovitz DA, Lotze MT (1998) Rapid extracellular degradation of synthetic class I peptides by human dendritic cells. J Immunol 161:4023–4032

Andres PG, Howland KC, Dresnek D, Edmondson S, Abbas AK, Krummel MF (2004) CD28 signals in the immature immunological synapse. J Immunol 172:5880–5886

Armstrong TD, Clements VK, Martin BK, Ting JP, Ostrand-Rosenberg S (1997) Major histocompatibility complex class II-transfected tumor cells present endogenous antigen and are potent inducers of tumor-specific immunity. Proc Natl Acad Sci USA 94:6886–6891

Banchereau J, Steinman RM (1998) Dendritic cells and the control of immunity. Nature 392: 245–252

Banchereau J, Briere F, Caux C, Davoust J, Lebecque S, Liu YJ, Pulendran B, Palucka K (2000) Immunobiology of dendritic cells. Annu Rev Immunol 18:767–811

Bedrosian I, Mick R, Xu S, Nisenbaum H, Faries M, Zhang P, Cohen PA, Koski G, Czerniecki BJ (2003) Intranodal administration of peptide-pulsed mature dendritic cell vaccines results in superior CD8+ T-cell function in melanoma patients. J Clin Oncol 21:3826–3835

Blachere NE, Darnell RB, Albert ML (2005) Apoptotic cells deliver processed antigen to dendritic cells for cross-presentation. PLoS Biol 3:1070–1086

Blander JM, Medzhitov R (2006) On regulation of phagosome maturation and antigen presentation. Nat Immunol 7:1029–1035

Bramson JL, Hitt M, Addison CL, Muller WJ, Gauldie J, Graham FL (1996) Direct intratumoral injection of an adenovirus expressing interleukin-12 induces regression and long-lasting immunity that is associated with highly localized expression of interleukin-12. Hum Gene Ther 7:1995–2002

Bromley SK, Iaboni A, Davis SJ, Whitty A, Green JM, Shaw AS, Weiss A, Dustin ML (2001) The immunological synapse and CD28-CD80 interactions. Nat Immunol 2:1159–1166

Brossart P, Wirths S, Stuhler G, Reichardt VL, Kanz L, Brugger W (2000) Induction of cytotoxic T-lymphocyte responses in vivo after vaccinations with peptide-pulsed dendritic cells. Blood 96:3102–3108

Brossart P, Schneider A, Dill P, Schammann T, Grunebach F, Wirths S, Kanz L, Buhring HJ, Brugger W (2001) The epithelial tumor antigen MUC1 is expressed in hematological malignancies and is recognized by MUC1-specific cytotoxic T-lymphocytes. Cancer Res 61:6846–6850

Brouwer RE, van der Hoorn MA, Kluin-Nelemans HC, van Zelderen-Bhola S, Willemze R, Falkenburg JH (2000a) The generation of dendritic-like cells with increased allostimulatory function from acute myeloid leukemia cells of various FAB subclasses. Hum Immunol 61:565–574

Brouwer RE, Zwinderman KH, Kluin-Nelemans HC, van Luxemburg-Heijs SA, Willemze R, Falkenburg JH (2000b) Expression and induction of costimulatory and adhesion molecules on acute myeloid leukemic cells: implications for adoptive immunotherapy. Exp Hematol 28: 161–168

Brown JA, Dorfman DM, Ma FR, Sullivan EL, Munoz O, Wood CR, Greenfield EA, Freeman GJ (2003) Blockade of programmed death-1 ligands on dendritic cells enhances T cell activation and cytokine production. J Immunol 170:1257–1266

Buggins AG, Lea N, Gaken J, Darling D, Farzaneh F, Mufti GJ, Hirst WJ (1999) Effect of costimulation and the microenvironment on antigen presentation by leukemic cells. Blood 94:3479–3490

Buggins AG, Milojkovic D, Arno MJ, Lea NC, Mufti GJ, Thomas NS, Hirst WJ (2001) Microenvironment produced by acute myeloid leukemia cells prevents T cell activation and proliferation by inhibition of NF-kappaB, c-Myc, and pRb pathways. J Immunol 167:6021–6030

Butterfield LH, Ribas A, Dissette VB, Amarnani SN, Vu HT, Oseguera D, Wang HJ, Elashoff RM, McBride WH, Mukherji B, Cochran AJ, Glaspy JA, Economou JS (2003) Determinant spreading associated with clinical response in dendritic cell-based immunotherapy for malignant melanoma. Clin Cancer Res 9:998–1008

Camporeale A, Boni A, Iezzi G, Degl'Innocenti E, Grioni M, Mondino A, Bellone M (2003) Critical impact of the kinetics of dendritic cells activation on the in vivo induction of tumor-specific T lymphocytes. Cancer Res 63:3688–3694

Caux C, Massacrier C, Vanbervliet B, Dubois B, de Saint-Vis B, zutter-Dambuyant C, Jacquet C, Schmitt D, Banchereau J (1997) CD34+ hematopoietic progenitors from human cord blood differentiate along two independent dendritic cell pathways in response to GM − CSF + TNF alpha. Adv Exp Med Biol 417:21–25

Cella M, Scheidegger D, Palmer-Lehmann K, Lane P, Lanzavecchia A, Alber G (1996) Ligation of CD40 on dendritic cells triggers production of high levels of interleukin-12 and enhances T cell stimulatory capacity: T-T help via APC activation. J Exp Med 184:747–752

Chalouni C, Banchereau J, Vogt AB, Pascual V, Davoust J (2003) Human germinal center B cells differ from naive and memory B cells by their aggregated MHC class II-rich compartments lacking HLA-DO. Int Immunol 15:457–466

Chamuleau FN, Kelder A, van de Loosdrecht AA, Ossenkoppele GJ (2006) High CLIP (Class II Associated Invariant Chain Peptide) Expression on Minimal Residual Disease Cells Is Associated with High Relapse Rate in AML Patients. 108: Abstract 2300

Chamuleau ME, Souwer Y, Van Ham SM, Zevenbergen A, Westers TM, Berkhof J, Meijer CJ, van de Loosdrecht AA, Ossenkoppele GJ (2004) Class II-associated invariant chain peptide expression on myeloid leukemic blasts predicts poor clinical outcome. Cancer Res 64:5546–5550

Charbonnier A, Gaugler B, Sainty D, Lafage-Pochitaloff M, Olive D (1999) Human acute myeloblastic leukemia cells differentiate in vitro into mature dendritic cells and induce the differentiation of cytotoxic T cells against autologous leukemias. Eur J Immunol 29:2567–2578

Chaturvedi P, Hengeveld R, Zechel MA, Lee-Chan E, Singh B (2000) The functional role of class II-associated invariant chain peptide (CLIP) in its ability to variably modulate immune responses. Int Immunol 12:757–765

Chen X, Laur O, Kambayashi T, Li S, Bray RA, Weber DA, Karlsson L, Jensen PE (2002) Regulated expression of human histocompatibility leukocyte antigen (HLA)-DO during antigen-dependent and antigen-independent phases of B cell development. J Exp Med 195:1053–1062

Choudhury A, Gajewski JL, Liang JC, Popat U, Claxton DF, Kliche KO, Andreeff M, Champlin RE (1997) Use of leukemic dendritic cells for the generation of antileukemic cellular cytotoxicity against Philadelphia chromosome-positive chronic myelogenous leukemia. Blood 89:1133–1142

Choudhury BA, Liang JC, Thomas EK, Flores-Romo L, Xie QS, Agusala K, Sutaria S, Sinha I, Champlin RE, Claxton DF (1999) Dendritic cells derived in vitro from acute myelogenous leukemia cells stimulate autologous, antileukemic T-cell responses. Blood 93:780–786

Cignetti A, Bryant E, Allione B, Vitale A, Foa R, Cheever MA (1999) CD34(+) acute myeloid and lymphoid leukemic blasts can be induced to differentiate into dendritic cells. Blood 94:2048–2055

Cignetti A, Vallario A, Roato I, Circosta P, Allione B, Casorzo L, Ghia P, Caligaris-Cappio F (2004) Leukemia-derived immature dendritic cells differentiate into functionally competent mature dendritic cells that efficiently stimulate T cell responses. J Immunol 173:2855–2865

Coulie PG, Karanikas V, Colau D, Lurquin C, Landry C, Marchand M, Dorval T, Brichard V, Boon T (2001) A monoclonal cytolytic T-lymphocyte response observed in a melanoma patient vaccinated with a tumor-specific antigenic peptide encoded by gene MAGE-3. Proc Natl Acad Sci USA 98:10290–10295

Curiel TJ, Wei S, Dong H, Alvarez X, Cheng P, Mottram P, Krzysiek R, Knutson KL, Daniel B, Zimmermann MC, David O, Burow M, Gordon A, Dhurandhar N, Myers L, Berggren R, Hemminki A, Alvarez RD, Emilie D, Curiel DT, Chen L, Zou W (2003) Blockade of B7-H1 improves myeloid dendritic cell-mediated antitumor immunity. Nat Med 9:562–567

Czerniecki BJ, Carter C, Rivoltini L, Koski GK, Kim HI, Weng DE, Roros JG, Hijazi YM, Xu S, Rosenberg SA, Cohen PA (1997) Calcium ionophore-treated peripheral blood monocytes and dendritic cells rapidly display characteristics of activated dendritic cells. J Immunol 159:3823–3837

De Bont ES, Fidler V, Meeuwsen T, Scherpen F, Hahlen K, Kamps WA (2002) Vascular endothelial growth factor secretion is an independent prognostic factor for relapse-free survival in pediatric acute myeloid leukemia patients. Clin Cancer Res 8:2856–2861

De Vries I, Lesterhuis WJ, Scharenborg NM, Engelen LP, Ruiter DJ, Gerritsen MJ, Croockewit S, Britten CM, Torensma R, Adema GJ, Figdor CG, Punt CJ (2003) Maturation of dendritic cells is a prerequisite for inducing immune responses in advanced melanoma patients. Clin Cancer Res 9:5091–5100

Decker WK, Xing D, Li S, Robinson SN, Yang H, Yao X, Segall H, McMannis JD, Komanduri KV, Champlin RE, Shpall EJ (2006) Double loading of dendritic cell MHC class I and MHC class II with an AML antigen repertoire enhances correlates of T-cell immunity in vitro via amplification of T-cell help. Vaccine 24:3203–3216

Delluc S, Tourneur L, Michallet AS, Boix C, Varet B, Fradelizi D, Guillet JG, Buzyn A (2005) Autologous peptides eluted from acute myeloid leukemia cells can be used to generate specific antileukemic CD4 helper and CD8 cytotoxic T lymphocyte responses in vitro. Haematologica 90:1050–1062

Delluc S, Tourneur L, Fradelizi D, Rubio MT, Marchiol-Fournigault C, Chiocchia G, Buzyn A (2006) DC-based vaccine loaded with acid-eluted peptides in acute myeloid leukemia: the importance of choosing the best elution method. Cancer Immunol Immunother 56:1–12

Denzin LK, Sant'Angelo DB, Hammond C, Surman MJ, Cresswell P (1997) Negative regulation by HLA-DO of MHC class II-restricted antigen processing. Science 278:106–109

Dhodapkar MV, Steinman RM, Krasovsky J, Munz C, Bhardwaj N (2001) Antigen-specific inhibition of effector T cell function in humans after injection of immature dendritic cells. J Exp Med 193:233–238

Dissanayake SK, Tuera N, Ostrand-Rosenberg S (2005) Presentation of endogenously synthesized MHC class II-restricted epitopes by MHC class II cancer vaccines is independent of transporter associated with Ag processing and the proteasome. J Immunol 174:1811–1819

Dranoff G, Jaffee E, Lazenby A, Golumbek P, Levitsky H, Brose K, Jackson V, Hamada H, Pardoll D, Mulligan RC (1993) Vaccination with irradiated tumor cells engineered to secrete murine granulocyte-macrophage colony-stimulating factor stimulates potent, specific, and long-lasting anti-tumor immunity. Proc Natl Acad Sci USA 90:3539–3543

Dunn GP, Old LJ, Schreiber RD (2004) The immunobiology of cancer immunosurveillance and immunoediting. Immunity 21:137–148

Dustin ML, Bivona TG, Philips MR (2004) Membranes as messengers in T cell adhesion signaling. Nat Immunol 5:363–372

Egen JG, Allison JP (2002) Cytotoxic T lymphocyte antigen-4 accumulation in the immunological synapse is regulated by TCR signal strength. Immunity 16:23–35

Engels FH, Koski GK, Bedrosian I, Xu S, Luger S, Nowell PC, Cohen PA, Czerniecki BJ (1999) Calcium signaling induces acquisition of dendritic cell characteristics in chronic myelogenous leukemia myeloid progenitor cells. Proc Natl Acad Sci USA 96:10332–10337

Fabre JW (2001) The allogeneic response and tumor immunity. Nat Med 7:649–652

Feller N, van der Pol MA, van SA, Weijers GW, Westra AH, Evertse BW, Ossenkoppele GJ, Schuurhuis GJ (2004) MRD parameters using immunophenotypic detection methods are highly reliable in predicting survival in acute myeloid leukaemia. Leukemia 18:1380–1390

Figdor CG, de V, I, Lesterhuis WJ, Melief CJ (2004) Dendritic cell immunotherapy: mapping the way. Nat Med 10:475–480

Fong L, Brockstedt D, Benike C, Wu L, Engleman EG (2001) Dendritic cells injected via different routes induce immunity in cancer patients. J Immunol 166:4254–4259

Franki SN, Steward KK, Betting DJ, Kafi K, Yamada RE, Timmerman JM (2007) Dendritic cells loaded with apoptotic antibody-coated tumor cells provide protective immunity against B cell lymphoma in vivo. Blood 111:1504–1511

Friedl P, Storim J (2004) Diversity in immune-cell interactions: states and functions of the immunological synapse. Trends Cell Biol 14:557–567

Fujii S, Shimizu K, Fujimoto K, Kiyokawa T, Shimomura T, Kinoshita M, Kawano F (1999) Analysis of a chronic myelogenous leukemia patient vaccinated with leukemic dendritic cells following autologous peripheral blood stem cell transplantation. Jpn J Cancer Res 90:1117–1129

Furumoto K, Soares L, Engleman EG, Merad M (2004) Induction of potent antitumor immunity by in situ targeting of intratumoral DCs. J Clin Invest 113:774–783

Gaiger A, Reese V, Disis ML, Cheever MA (2000) Immunity to WT1 in the animal model and in patients with acute myeloid leukemia. Blood 96:1480–1489

Gaiger A, Carter L, Greinix H, Carter D, McNeill PD, Houghton RL, Cornellison CD, Vedvick TS, Skeiky YA, Cheever MA (2001) WT1-specific serum antibodies in patients with leukemia. Clin Cancer Res 7:761s–765s

Galea-Lauri J (2002) Immunological weapons against acute myeloid leukaemia. Immunology 107:20–27

Galea-Lauri J, Wells JW, Darling D, Harrison P, Farzaneh F (2004) Strategies for antigen choice and priming of dendritic cells influence the polarization and efficacy of antitumor T-cell responses in dendritic cell-based cancer vaccination. Cancer Immunol Immunother 53:963–977

Gao L, Bellantuono I, Elsasser A, Marley SB, Gordon MY, Goldman JM, Stauss HJ (2000) Selective elimination of leukemic CD34(+) progenitor cells by cytotoxic T lymphocytes specific for WT1. Blood 95:2198–2203

Geijtenbeek TB, Krooshoop DJ, Bleijs DA, van Vliet SJ, van Duijnhoven GC, Grabovsky V, Alon R, Figdor CG, van KY (2000a) DC-SIGN-ICAM-2 interaction mediates dendritic cell trafficking. Nat Immunol 1:353–357

Geijtenbeek TB, Torensma R, van Vliet SJ, van Duijnhoven GC, Adema GJ, van KY, Figdor CG (2000b) Identification of DC-SIGN, a novel dendritic cell-specific ICAM-3 receptor that supports primary immune responses. Cell 100:575–585

Glazier KS, Hake SB, Tobin HM, Chadburn A, Schattner EJ, Denzin LK (2002) Germinal center B cells regulate their capability to present antigen by modulation of HLA-DO. J Exp Med 195:1063–1069

Hanks BA, Jiang J, Singh RA, Song W, Barry M, Huls MH, Slawin KM, Spencer DM (2005) Re-engineered CD40 receptor enables potent pharmacological activation of dendritic-cell cancer vaccines in vivo. Nat Med 11:130–137

Harrison BD, Adams JA, Briggs M, Brereton ML, Yin JA (2001) Stimulation of autologous proliferative and cytotoxic T-cell responses by "leukemic dendritic cells" derived from blast cells in acute myeloid leukemia. Blood 97:2764–2771

Hart DN (1997) Dendritic cells: unique leukocyte populations which control the primary immune response. Blood 90:3245–3287

Hawiger D, Inaba K, Dorsett Y, Guo M, Mahnke K, Rivera M, Ravetch JV, Steinman RM, Nussenzweig MC (2001) Dendritic cells induce peripheral T cell unresponsiveness under steady state conditions in vivo. J Exp Med 194:769–779

Hellstrom KE, Hellstrom I (2003) Therapeutic vaccination with tumor cells that engage CD137. J Mol Med 81:71–86

Herr W, Ranieri E, Olson W, Zarour H, Gesualdo L, Storkus WJ (2000) Mature dendritic cells pulsed with freeze-thaw cell lysates define an effective in vitro vaccine designed to elicit EBV-specific CD4(+) and CD8(+) T lymphocyte responses. Blood 96:1857–1864

Hirano N, Takahashi T, Takahashi T, Azuma M, Okumura K, Yazaki Y, Yagita H, Hirai H (1997) Protective and therapeutic immunity against leukemia induced by irradiated B7–1 (CD80)-transduced leukemic cells. Hum Gene Ther 8:1375–1384

Hirano F, Kaneko K, Tamura H, Dong H, Wang S, Ichikawa M, Rietz C, Flies DB, Lau JS, Zhu G, Tamada K, Chen L (2005) Blockade of B7-H1 and PD-1 by monoclonal antibodies potentiates cancer therapeutic immunity. Cancer Res 65:1089–1096

Hirst WJ, Buggins A, Darling D, Gaken J, Farzaneh F, Mufti GJ (1997) Enhanced immune costimulatory activity of primary acute myeloid leukaemia blasts after retrovirus-mediated gene transfer of B7.1. Gene Ther 4:691–699

Holtl L, Ramoner R, Zelle-Rieser C, Gander H, Putz T, Papesh C, Nussbaumer W, Falkensammer C, Bartsch G, Thurnher M (2005) Allogeneic dendritic cell vaccination against metastatic renal cell carcinoma with or without cyclophosphamide. Cancer Immunol Immunother 54:663–670

Hou WS, Van Parijs L (2004) A Bcl-2-dependent molecular timer regulates the lifespan and immunogenicity of dendritic cells. Nat Immunol 5:583–589

Houtenbos I, Westers TM, Ossenkoppele GJ, van de Loosdrecht AA (2003a) Identification of CD14 as a predictor for leukemic dendritic cell differentiation in acute myeloid leukemia. Leukemia 17:1683–1684

Houtenbos I, Westers TM, Stam AG, de Gruijl TD, Scheper RJ, Ossenkoppele GJ, van de Loosdrecht AA (2003b) Serum-free generation of antigen presenting cells from acute myeloid leukaemic blasts for active specific immunisation. Cancer Immunol Immunother 52:455–462

Houtenbos I, Westers TM, de Gruijl TD, Scheper RJ, Ossenkoppele GJ, van de Loosdrecht AA (2004) TNF-alpha receptor 1 expression on acute myeloid leukemic blasts predicts differentiation into leukemic dendritic cells. Leukemia 18:1149–1153

Houtenbos I, Westers TM, Ossenkoppele GJ, van de Loosdrecht AA (2006a) Feasibility of clinical dendritic cell vaccination in acute myeloid leukemia. Immunobiology 211:677–685

Houtenbos I, Westers TM, Ossenkoppele GJ, van de Loosdrecht AA (2006b) Leukaemic dendritic cell vaccination for patients with acute myeloid leukaemia. Br J Haematol 134:445–446

Houtenbos I, Westers TM, Ossenkoppele GJ, van de Loosdrecht AA (2006c) Leukemia-derived dendritic cells: towards clinical vaccination protocols in acute myeloid leukemia. Haematologica 91:348–355

Houtenbos I, Westers TM, Ossenkoppele GJ, van de Loosdrecht AA, Hess CJ, Waisfisz Q (2006d) Flt-3 internal tandem duplication hampers differentiation of AML blasts towards leukemic dendritic cells. Leukemia 20:2219

Houtenbos I, Westers TM, Ossenkoppele GJ, van de Loosdrecht AA, Hess CJ, Waisfisz Q (2006e) Flt-3 internal tandem duplication hampers differentiation of AML blasts towards leukemic dendritic cells. Leukemia 20:2219

Houtenbos I, Westers TM, Dijkhuis A, de Gruijl TD, Ossenkoppele GJ, van de Loosdrecht AA (2007) Leukemia-specific T-cell reactivity induced by leukemic dendritic cells is augmented by 4–1BB targeting. Clin Cancer Res 13:307–315

Hsu FJ, Benike C, Fagnoni F, Liles TM, Czerwinski D, Taidi B, Engleman EG, Levy R (1996) Vaccination of patients with B-cell lymphoma using autologous antigen-pulsed dendritic cells. Nat Med 2:52–58

Hus I, Rolinski J, Tabarkiewicz J, Wojas K, Bojarska-Junak A, Greiner J, Giannopoulos K, Dmoszynska A, Schmitt M (2005) Allogeneic dendritic cells pulsed with tumor lysates or apoptotic bodies as immunotherapy for patients with early-stage B-cell chronic lymphocytic leukemia. Leukemia 19:1621–1627

Ito F, Li Q, Shreiner AB, Okuyama R, Jure-Kunkel MN, Teitz-Tennenbaum S, Chang AE (2004) Anti-CD137 monoclonal antibody administration augments the antitumor efficacy of dendritic cell-based vaccines. Cancer Res 64:8411–8419

Jacobelli J, Andres PG, Boisvert J, Krummel MF (2004) New views of the immunological synapse: variations in assembly and function. Curr Opin Immunol 16:345–352

Jarnjak-Jankovic S, Pettersen RD, Saeboe-Larssen S, Wesenberg F, Gaudernack G (2005) Evaluation of dendritic cells loaded with apoptotic cancer cells or expressing tumour mRNA as potential cancer vaccines against leukemia. BMC Cancer 5:20–30

Jonuleit H, Schmitt E, Schuler G, Knop J, Enk AH (2000) Induction of interleukin 10-producing, nonproliferating CD4(+) T cells with regulatory properties by repetitive stimulation with allogeneic immature human dendritic cells. J Exp Med 192:1213–1222

Kloetzel PM (2004) Generation of major histocompatibility complex class I antigens: functional interplay between proteasomes and TPPII. Nat Immunol 5:661–669

Kolb HJ, Schattenberg A, Goldman JM, Hertenstein B, Jacobsen N, Arcese W, Ljungman P, Ferrant A, Verdonck L, Niederwieser D (1995) Graft-versus-leukemia effect of donor lymphocyte transfusions in marrow grafted patients. European Group for Blood and Marrow Transplantation Working Party Chronic Leukemia. Blood 86:2041–2050

Koski GK, Schwartz GN, Weng DE, Gress RE, Engels FH, Tsokos M, Czerniecki BJ, Cohen PA (1999) Calcium ionophore-treated myeloid cells acquire many dendritic cell characteristics independent of prior differentiation state, transformation status, or sensitivity to biologic agents. Blood 94:1359–1371

Kropshofer H, Vogt AB, Thery C, Armandola EA, Li BC, Moldenhauer G, Amigorena S, Hammerling GJ (1998) A role for HLA-DO as a co-chaperone of HLA-DM in peptide loading of MHC class II molecules. EMBO J 17:2971–2981

Langenkamp A, Messi M, Lanzavecchia A, Sallusto F (2000) Kinetics of dendritic cell activation: impact on priming of TH1, TH2 and nonpolarized T cells. Nat Immunol 1:311–316

Lau R, Wang F, Jeffery G, Marty V, Kuniyoshi J, Bade E, Ryback ME, Weber J (2001) Phase I trial of intravenous peptide-pulsed dendritic cells in patients with metastatic melanoma. J Immunother 24:66–78

Leach DR, Krummel MF, Allison JP (1996) Enhancement of antitumor immunity by CTLA-4 blockade. Science 271:1734–1736

Lee KH, Holdorf AD, Dustin ML, Chan AC, Allen PM, Shaw AS (2002) T cell receptor signaling precedes immunological synapse formation. Science 295:1539–1542

Lee KH, Dinner AR, Tu C, Campi G, Raychaudhuri S, Varma R, Sims TN, Burack WR, Wu H, Wang J, Kanagawa O, Markiewicz M, Allen PM, Dustin ML, Chakraborty AK, Shaw AS (2003) The immunological synapse balances T cell receptor signaling and degradation. Science 302:1218–1222

Levitsky HI, Montgomery J, Ahmadzadeh M, Staveley-O'Carroll K, Guarnieri F, Longo DL, Kwak LW (1996) Immunization with granulocyte-macrophage colony-stimulating factor-transduced, but not B7–1-transduced, lymphoma cells primes idiotype-specific T cells and generates potent systemic antitumor immunity. J Immunol 156:3858–3865

Li L, Giannopoulos K, Reinhardt P, Tabarkiewicz J, Schmitt A, Greiner J, Rolinski J, Hus I, Dmoszynska A, Wiesneth M, Schmitt M (2006) Immunotherapy for patients with acute myeloid leukemia using autologous dendritic cells generated from leukemic blasts. Int J Oncol 28:855–861

Litzow MR, Dietz AB, Bulur PA, Butler GW, Gastineau DA, Hoering A, Fink SR, Letendre L, Padley DJ, Paternoster SF, Tefferi A, Vuk-Pavlovic S (2006) Testing the safety of clinical-grade mature autologous myeloid DC in a phase I clinical immunotherapy trial of CML. Cytotherapy 8:290–298

Lotteau V, Teyton L, Peleraux A, Nilsson T, Karlsson L, Schmid SL, Quaranta V, Peterson PA (1990) Intracellular transport of class II MHC molecules directed by invariant chain. Nature 348:600–605

Lowenberg B, Downing JR, Burnett A (1999) Acute myeloid leukemia. N Engl J Med 341:1051–1062

Mackinnon S, Papadopoulos EB, Carabasi MH, Reich L, Collins NH, Boulad F, Castro-Malaspina H, Childs BH, Gillio AP, Kernan NA (1995) Adoptive immunotherapy evaluating escalating doses of donor leukocytes for relapse of chronic myeloid leukemia after bone marrow transplantation: separation of graft-versus-leukemia responses from graft-versus-host disease. Blood 86:1261–1268

Maldonado RA, Irvine DJ, Schreiber R, Glimcher LH (2004) A role for the immunological synapse in lineage commitment of CD4 lymphocytes. Nature 431:527–532

Masterson AJ, Sombroek CC, de Gruijl TD, Graus YM, van der Vliet HJ, Lougheed SM, van den Eertwegh AJ, Pinedo HM, Scheper RJ (2002) MUTZ-3, a human cell line model for the cytokine-induced differentiation of dendritic cells from CD34+ precursors. Blood 100: 701–703

Menetrier-Caux C, Montmain G, Dieu MC, Bain C, Favrot MC, Caux C, Blay JY (1998) Inhibition of the differentiation of dendritic cells from CD34(+) progenitors by tumor cells: role of interleukin-6 and macrophage colony-stimulating factor. Blood 92:4778–4791

Miga AJ, Masters SR, Durell BG, Gonzalez M, Jenkins MK, Maliszewski C, Kikutani H, Wade WF, Noelle RJ (2001) Dendritic cell longevity and T cell persistence is controlled by CD154-CD40 interactions. Eur J Immunol 31:959–965

Mohty M, Isnardon D, Blaise D, Mozziconacci MJ, Lafage-Pochitaloff M, Briere F, Gastaut JA, Olive D, Gaugler B (2002) Identification of precursors of leukemic dendritic cells differentiated from patients with acute myeloid leukemia. Leukemia 16:2267–2274

Molldrem J, Dermime S, Parker K, Jiang YZ, Mavroudis D, Hensel N, Fukushima P, Barrett AJ (1996) Targeted T-cell therapy for human leukemia: cytotoxic T lymphocytes specific for a peptide derived from proteinase 3 preferentially lyse human myeloid leukemia cells. Blood 88:2450–2457

Monks CR, Freiberg BA, Kupfer H, Sciaky N, Kupfer A (1998) Three-dimensional segregation of supramolecular activation clusters in T cells. Nature 395:82–86

Mullins DW, Sheasley SL, Ream RM, Bullock TN, Fu YX, Engelhard VH (2003) Route of immunization with peptide-pulsed dendritic cells controls the distribution of memory and effector T cells in lymphoid tissues and determines the pattern of regional tumor control. J Exp Med 198:1023–1034

Neefjes JJ, Stollorz V, Peters PJ, Geuze HJ, Ploegh HL (1990) The biosynthetic pathway of MHC class II but not class I molecules intersects the endocytic route. Cell 61:171–183

Nestle FO, Alijagic S, Gilliet M, Sun Y, Grabbe S, Dummer R, Burg G, Schadendorf D (1998) Vaccination of melanoma patients with peptide- or tumor lysate-pulsed dendritic cells. Nat Med 4:328–332

Nestle FO, Farkas A, Conrad C (2005) Dendritic-cell-based therapeutic vaccination against cancer. Curr Opin Immunol 17:163–169

Neves AR, Ensina LF, Anselmo LB, Leite KR, Buzaid AC, Camara-Lopes LH, Barbuto JA (2005) Dendritic cells derived from metastatic cancer patients vaccinated with allogeneic dendritic cell-autologous tumor cell hybrids express more CD86 and induce higher levels of interferon-gamma in mixed lymphocyte reactions. Cancer Immunol Immunother 54:61–66

Obeid M, Tesniere A, Ghiringhelli F, Fimia GM, Apetoh L, Perfettini JL, Castedo M, Mignot G, Panaretakis T, Casares N, Metivier D, Larochette N, van EP, Ciccosanti F, Piacentini M, Zitvogel L, Kroemer G (2007) Calreticulin exposure dictates the immunogenicity of cancer cell death. Nat Med 13:54–61

Oehler L, Berer A, Keil F, Weinlander G, Konig M, Haas OA, Lechner K, Geissler K (2000) Generation of dendritic cells from human chronic myelomonocytic leukemia cells in fetal calf serum-free medium. Leuk Lymphoma 38:577–586

Okada N, Iiyama S, Okada Y, Mizuguchi H, Hayakawa T, Nakagawa S, Mayumi T, Fujita T, Yamamoto A (2005) Immunological properties and vaccine efficacy of murine dendritic cells simultaneously expressing melanoma-associated antigen and interleukin-12. Cancer Gene Ther 12:72–83

Orleans-Lindsay JK, Barber LD, Prentice HG, Lowdell MW (2001) Acute myeloid leukaemia cells secrete a soluble factor that inhibits T and NK cell proliferation but not cytolytic function–implications for the adoptive immunotherapy of leukaemia. Clin Exp Immunol 126:403–411

Orleans-Lindsay JK, Deru A, Craig JI, Prentice HG, Lowdell MW (2003) In vitro co-stimulation with anti-CD28 synergizes with IL-12 in the generation of T cell immune responses to leukaemic cells; a strategy for ex-vivo generation of CTL for immunotherapy. Clin Exp Immunol 133:467–475

Ossenkoppele GJ, Stam AG, Westers TM, de Gruijl TD, Janssen JJ, van de Loosdrecht AA, Scheper RJ (2003) Vaccination of chronic myeloid leukemia patients with autologous in vitro cultured leukemic dendritic cells. Leukemia 17:1424–1426

Panoskaltsis N, Belanger TJ, Liesveld JL, Abboud CN (2002) Optimal cytokine stimulation for the enhanced generation of leukemic dendritic cells in short-term culture. Leuk Res 26:191–201

Panoskaltsis N, Reid CD, Knight SC (2003) Quantification and cytokine production of circulating lymphoid and myeloid cells in acute myelogenous leukaemia. Leukemia 17:716–730

Pistillo MP, Tazzari PL, Palmisano GL, Pierri I, Bolognesi A, Ferlito F, Capanni P, Polito L, Ratta M, Pileri S, Piccioli M, Basso G, Rissotto L, Conte R, Gobbi M, Stirpe F, Ferrara GB (2003) CTLA-4 is not restricted to the lymphoid cell lineage and can function as a target molecule for apoptosis induction of leukemic cells. Blood 101:202–209

Poo WJ, Conrad L, Janeway CA, Jr. (1988) Receptor-directed focusing of lymphokine release by helper T cells. Nature 332:378–380

Powles RL, Crowther D, Bateman CJ, Beard ME, McElwain TJ, Russell J, Lister TA, Whitehouse JM, Wrigley PF, Pike M, Alexander P, Fairley GH (1973) Immunotherapy for acute myelogenous leukaemia. Br J Cancer 28:365–376

Randolph GJ (2001) Dendritic cell migration to lymph nodes: cytokines, chemokines, and lipid mediators. Semin Immunol 13:267–274

Re F, Arpinati M, Testoni N, Ricci P, Terragna C, Preda P, Ruggeri D, Senese B, Chirumbolo G, Martelli V, Urbini B, Baccarani M, Tura S, Rondelli D (2002) Expression of CD86 in acute myelogenous leukemia is a marker of dendritic/monocytic lineage. Exp Hematol 30:126–134

Renkvist N, Castelli C, Robbins PF, Parmiani G (2001) A listing of human tumor antigens recognized by T cells. Cancer Immunol Immunother 50:3–15

Ridgway D (2003) The first 1000 dendritic cell vaccinees. Cancer Invest 21:873–886

Robinson SP, English N, Jaju R, Kearney L, Knight SC, Reid CD (1998) The in-vitro generation of dendritic cells from blast cells in acute leukaemia. Br J Haematol 103:763–771

Roche PA, Cresswell P (1990) Invariant chain association with HLA-DR molecules inhibits immunogenic peptide binding. Nature 345:615–618

Roddie H, Klammer M, Thomas C, Thomson R, Atkinson A, Sproul A, Waterfall M, Samuel K, Yin J, Johnson P, Turner M (2006) Phase I/II study of vaccination with dendritic-like leukaemia cells for the immunotherapy of acute myeloid leukaemia. Br J Haematol 133:152–157

Romagnoli P, Germain RN (1994) The CLIP region of invariant chain plays a critical role in regulating major histocompatibility complex class II folding, transport, and peptide occupancy. J Exp Med 180:1107–1113

Romani N, Gruner S, Brang D, Kampgen E, Lenz A, Trockenbacher B, Konwalinka G, Fritsch PO, Steinman RM, Schuler G (1994) Proliferating dendritic cell progenitors in human blood. J Exp Med 180:83–93

Rosenberg SA, Yang JC, Schwartzentruber DJ, Hwu P, Marincola FM, Topalian SL, Restifo NP, Dudley ME, Schwarz SL, Spiess PJ, Wunderlich JR, Parkhurst MR, Kawakami Y, Seipp CA, Einhorn JH, White DE (1998) Immunologic and therapeutic evaluation of a synthetic peptide vaccine for the treatment of patients with metastatic melanoma. Nat Med 4:321–327

Roskrow MA, Dilloo D, Suzuki N, Zhong W, Rooney CM, Brenner MK (1999) Autoimmune disease induced by dendritic cell immunization against leukemia. Leuk Res 23:549–557

Roucard C, Thomas C, Pasquier MA, Trowsdale J, Sotto JJ, Neefjes J, Van Ham SM (2001) In vivo and in vitro modulation of HLA-DM and HLA-DO is induced by B lymphocyte activation. J Immunol 167:6849–6858

Sallusto F, Lanzavecchia A (1994) Efficient presentation of soluble antigen by cultured human dendritic cells is maintained by granulocyte/macrophage colony-stimulating factor plus interleukin 4 and downregulated by tumor necrosis factor alpha. J Exp Med 179:1109–1118

Santegoets SJ, Masterson AJ, van der Sluis PC, Lougheed SM, Fluitsma DM, van den Eertwegh AJ, Pinedo HM, Scheper RJ, de Gruijl TD (2006a) A CD34(+) human cell line model of myeloid dendritic cell differentiation: evidence for a CD14(+)CD11b(+) Langerhans cell precursor. J Leukoc Biol 80:1337–1344

Santegoets SJ, Schreurs MW, Masterson AJ, Liu YP, Goletz S, Baumeister H, Kueter EW, Lougheed SM, van den Eertwegh AJ, Scheper RJ, Hooijberg E, de Gruijl TD (2006b) In vitro priming of tumor-specific cytotoxic T lymphocytes using allogeneic dendritic cells derived from the human MUTZ-3 cell line. Cancer Immunol Immunother 55:1480–1490

Saudemont A, Buffenoir G, Denys A, Desreumaux P, Jouy N, Hetuin D, Bauters F, Fenaux P, Quesnel B (2002) Gene transfer of CD154 and IL12 cDNA induces an anti-leukemic immunity in a murine model of acute leukemia. Leukemia 16:1637–1644

Saudemont A, Quesnel B (2004) In a model of tumor dormancy, long-term persistent leukemic cells have increased B7-H1 and B7.1 expression and resist CTL-mediated lysis. Blood 104:2124–2133

Sauter B, Albert ML, Francisco L, Larsson M, Somersan S, Bhardwaj N (2000) Consequences of cell death: exposure to necrotic tumor cells, but not primary tissue cells or apoptotic cells, induces the maturation of immunostimulatory dendritic cells. J Exp Med 191:423–434

Scheibenbogen C, Letsch A, Thiel E, Schmittel A, Mailaender V, Baerwolf S, Nagorsen D, Keilholz U (2002) CD8 T-cell responses to Wilms tumor gene product WT1 and proteinase 3 in patients with acute myeloid leukemia. Blood 100:2132–2137

Schnare M, Barton GM, Holt AC, Takeda K, Akira S, Medzhitov R (2001) Toll-like receptors control activation of adaptive immune responses. Nat Immunol 2:947–950

Schui DK, Singh L, Schneider B, Knau A, Hoelzer D, Weidmann E (2002) Inhibiting effects on the induction of cytotoxic T lymphocytes by dendritic cells pulsed with lysates from acute myeloid leukemia blasts. Leuk Res 26:383–389

Schuler (2006) Dendritic cell vaccination of Melanoma: looking back and ahead after 200 patients. Dendritic Cells; 9th International Conference: S04.01

Seya T, Akazawa T, Tsujita T, Matsumoto M (2006) Role of Toll-like receptors in adjuvant-augmented immune therapies. Evid Based Complement Alternat Med 3:31–38

Sloan VS, Cameron P, Porter G, Gammon M, Amaya M, Mellins E, Zaller DM (1995) Mediation by HLA-DM of dissociation of peptides from HLA-DR. Nature 375:802–806

Smits EL, Ponsaerts P, Van de Velde AL, Van Driessche A, Cools N, Lenjou M, Nijs G, Van Bockstaele DR, Berneman ZN, Van Tendeloo V (2007) Proinflammatory response of human leukemic cells to dsRNA transfection linked to activation of dendritic cells. Leukemia 21:1691–1699

Sotomayor EM, Borrello I, Tubb E, Allison JP, Levitsky HI (1999) In vivo blockade of CTLA-4 enhances the priming of responsive T cells but fails to prevent the induction of tumor antigen-specific tolerance. Proc Natl Acad Sci USA 96:11476–11481

Spisek R, Charalambous A, Mazumder A, Vesole DH, Jagannath S, Dhodapkar MV (2007) Bortezomib enhances dendritic cell (DC) mediated induction of immunity to human myeloma via exposure of cell surface heat shock protein 90 on dying tumor cells: therapeutic implications. Blood 109:4839–4845

Stary Bangert C, Altrichter S, Strohal R, Kopp T, Stingle G (2006) Dendritic cells with cytotoxic potential after toll-like receptor 7/8-activation. Dendritic Cells, 9th International Conference: S02.03

Steinman RM, Turley S, Mellman I, Inaba K (2000) The induction of tolerance by dendritic cells that have captured apoptotic cells. J Exp Med 191:411–416

Stumbles PA, Himbeck R, Frelinger JA, Collins EJ, Lake RA, Robinson BW (2004) Cutting edge: tumor-specific CTL are constitutively cross-armed in draining lymph nodes and transiently disseminate to mediate tumor regression following systemic CD40 activation. J Immunol 173:5923–5928

Tamir A, Basagila E, Kagahzian A, Jiao L, Jensen S, Nicholls J, Tate P, Stamp G, Farzaneh F, Harrison P, Stauss H, George AJ, Habib N, Lechler RI, Lombardi G (2007) Induction of tumor-specific T-cell responses by vaccination with tumor lysate-loaded dendritic cells in colorectal cancer patients with carcinoembryonic-antigen positive tumors. Cancer Immunol Immunother 56:2003–2016

Trefzer U, Weingart G, Chen Y, Herberth G, Adrian K, Winter H, Audring H, Guo Y, Sterry W, Walden P (2000) Hybrid cell vaccination for cancer immune therapy: first clinical trial with metastatic melanoma. Int J Cancer 85:618–626

Trefzer U, Herberth G, Wohlan K, Milling A, Thiemann M, Sherev T, Sparbier K, Sterry W, Walden P (2004) Vaccination with hybrids of tumor and dendritic cells induces tumor-specific T-cell and clinical responses in melanoma stage III and IV patients. Int J Cancer 110:730–740

Trefzer U, Herberth G, Wohlan K, Milling A, Thiemann M, Sharav T, Sparbier K, Sterry W, Walden P (2005) Tumour-dendritic hybrid cell vaccination for the treatment of patients with malignant melanoma: immunological effects and clinical results. Vaccine 23:2367–2373

Ullrich HJ, Doring K, Gruneberg U, Jahnig F, Trowsdale J, Van Ham SM (1997) Interaction between HLA-DM and HLA-DR involves regions that undergo conformational changes at lysosomal pH. Proc Natl Acad Sci USA 94:13163–13168

Vakkila J, Lotze MT (2004) Inflammation and necrosis promote tumour growth. Nat Rev Immunol 4:641–648

Valmori D, Dutoit V, Schnuriger V, Quiquerez AL, Pittet MJ, Guillaume P, Rubio-Godoy V, Walker PR, Rimoldi D, Lienard D, Cerottini JC, Romero P, Dietrich PY (2002) Vaccination with a Melan-A peptide selects an oligoclonal T cell population with increased functional avidity and tumor reactivity. J Immunol 168:4231–4240

Van de Loosdrecht AA (2007) The dendritic cell: the piano player in orchestrating the immune response in leukemia. Leuk Lymphoma 48:217–218

Van de Loosdrecht AA, Beelen RH (2006) Emerging immunobiological concepts in macrophage and dendritic cell research and clinical implications. Immunobiology 211:403–406

Van Ham SM, Tjin EP, Lillemeier BF, Gruneberg U, van Meijgaarden KE, Pastoors L, Verwoerd D, Tulp A, Canas B, Rahman D, Ottenhoff TH, Pappin DJ, Trowsdale J, Neefjes J (1997) HLA-DO is a negative modulator of HLA-DM-mediated MHC class II peptide loading. Curr Biol 7:950–957

Van Ham SM, van Lith M, Lillemeier B, Tjin E, Gruneberg U, Rahman D, Pastoors L, van MK, Roucard C, Trowsdale J, Ottenhoff T, Pappin D, Neefjes J (2000) Modulation of the major histocompatibility complex class II-associated peptide repertoire by human histocompatibility leukocyte antigen (HLA)-DO. J Exp Med 191:1127–1136

Van Lith M, Van Ham SM, Griekspoor A, Tjin E, Verwoerd D, Calafat J, Janssen H, Reits E, Pastoors L, Neefjes J (2001) Regulation of MHC class II antigen presentation by sorting of recycling HLA-DM/DO and class II within the multivesicular body. J Immunol 167:884–892

Van Mierlo GJ, den Boer AT, Medema JP, van d, V, Fransen MF, Offringa R, Melief CJ, Toes RE (2002) CD40 stimulation leads to effective therapy of CD40(−) tumors through induction of strong systemic cytotoxic T lymphocyte immunity. Proc Natl Acad Sci USA 99:5561–5566

Vereecque R, Buffenoir G, Preudhomme C, Hetuin D, Bauters F, Fenaux P, Quesnel B (2000) Gene transfer of GM-CSF, CD80 and CD154 cDNA enhances survival in a murine model of acute leukemia with persistence of a minimal residual disease. Gene Ther 7:1312–1316

Waclavicek M, Berer A, Oehler L, Stockl J, Schloegl E, Majdic O, Knapp W (2001) Calcium ionophore: a single reagent for the differentiation of primary human acute myelogenous leukaemia cells towards dendritic cells. Br J Haematol 114:466–473

Watts C (2004) The exogenous pathway for antigen presentation on major histocompatibility complex class II and CD1 molecules. Nat Immunol 5:685–692

Weigel BJ, Panoskaltsis-Mortari A, Diers M, Garcia M, Lees C, Krieg AM, Chen W, Blazar BR (2006) Dendritic cells pulsed or fused with AML cellular antigen provide comparable in vivo antitumor protective responses. Exp Hematol 34:1403–1412

Westers TM, Stam AM, Scheper RM, Regelink JM, Nieuwint AM, Schuurhuis GJ, Van De Loosdrecht AM, Ossenkoppele GM (2003) Rapid generation of antigen-presenting cells from leukaemic blasts in acute myeloid leukaemia. Cancer Immunol Immunother 52:17–27

Westers TM, Houtenbos I, Schuurhuis GJ, Ossenkoppele GJ, van de Loosdrecht AA (2005a) Quantification of T-cell-mediated apoptosis in heterogeneous leukemia populations using four-color multiparameter flow cytometry. Cytometry A 66:71–77

Westers TM, Houtenbos I, Snoijs NC, van de Loosdrecht AA, Ossenkoppele GJ (2005b) Leukemia-derived dendritic cells in acute myeloid leukemia exhibit potent migratory capacity. Leukemia 19:1270–1272

Westers TM, Houtenbos I, van de Loosdrecht AA, Ossenkoppele GJ (2006) Principles of dendritic cell-based immunotherapy in myeloid leukemia. Immunobiology 211:663–676

Westers TM, Ossenkoppele GJ, van de Loosdrecht AA (2007) Dendritic cell-based immunotherapy in acute and chronic myeloid leukaemia. Biomed Pharmacother 61:306–314

Wilcox RA, Tamada K, Flies DB, Zhu G, Chapoval AI, Blazar BR, Kast WM, Chen L (2004) Ligation of CD137 receptor prevents and reverses established anergy of CD8+ cytolytic T lymphocytes in vivo. Blood 103:177–184

Wilson NS, Behrens GM, Lundie RJ, Smith CM, Waithman J, Young L, Forehan SP, Mount A, Steptoe RJ, Shortman KD, de Koning-Ward TF, Belz GT, Carbone FR, Crabb BS, Heath WR, Villadangos JA (2006) Systemic activation of dendritic cells by Toll-like receptor ligands or malaria infection impairs cross-presentation and antiviral immunity. Nat Immunol 7:165–172

Woiciechowsky A, Regn S, Kolb HJ, Roskrow M (2001) Leukemic dendritic cells generated in the presence of FLT3 ligand have the capacity to stimulate an autologous leukemia-specific cytotoxic T cell response from patients with acute myeloid leukemia. Leukemia 15:246–255

Zajac AJ, Murali-Krishna K, Blattman JN, Ahmed R (1998) Therapeutic vaccination against chronic viral infection: the importance of cooperation between CD4+ and CD8+ T cells. Curr Opin Immunol 10:444–449

Zheng R, Friedman AD, Small D (2002) Targeted inhibition of FLT3 overcomes the block to myeloid differentiation in 32Dcl3 cells caused by expression of FLT3/ITD mutations. Blood 100:4154–4161

Index

Printing: Krips bv, Meppel, The Netherlands
Binding: Stürtz, Würzburg, Germany